NJ709 IMP.

Impotence: an integrated approach to clinical practice

For Churchill Livingstone:

Publisher: Georgina Bentliff
Project Editor: Lucy Gardner
Editorial Co-ordination: Editorial Resources Unit
   Copy Editor: Andrew Gardiner
Production Controller: Nancy Henry
Design: Design Resources Unit
Sales Promotion Executive: Douglas McNaughton

Impotence: an integrated approach to clinical practice

Edited by

Alain Gregoire MB BS DRCOG MRCPsych
Consultant Psychiatrist, The Old Manor Hospital, Salisbury, UK

John P. Pryor MS FRCS
Consultant Uroandrologist, King's College and St Peter's Hospitals; Formerly
Dean, Institute of Urology, London University, London, UK

CHURCHILL LIVINGSTONE
EDINBURGH LONDON MADRID MELBOURNE NEW YORK AND TOKYO 1993

CHURCHILL LIVINGSTONE
Medical Division of Longman Group UK Limited

Distributed in the United States of America by Churchill
Livingstone Inc., 650 Avenue of the Americas, New York,
N. Y. 10011, and by associated companies, branches and
representatives throughout the world.

First published 1993

ISBN 0-443-04369-8

British Library Cataloguing in Publication Data
A catalogue record for this book is available from the British
Library.

Library of Congress Cataloging in Publication Data
Impotence : an integrated approach to clinical practice / edited by
    Alain Gregoire, John P. Pryor.
        p.   cm.
    Includes index.
    ISBN 0–443–04369–8 : £45.00
    1. Impotence.   I. Gregoire, Alain, MRCPsych.   II. Pryor, John P.
    [DNLM: 1. Impotence—diagnosis.   2. Impotence—therapy   3. Penis—
physiology. WJ 709 I342]
    RC889.I48   1992
    616.6'92—dc20
    DNLM/DLC
    for Library of Congress   92–13582
                                                        CIP

Produced by Longman Singapore Publishers Pte Ltd
Printed in Singapore

Preface

The simplistic assumption that human disorders have either a physical basis or a psychological one still pervades much of the medical literature. It leads to divisions between professionals which hamper our understanding of many disease processes. There has always been a tendency to explain disorders with no known physical cause as being the result of evil spirits or psychological processes. Psychologists, psychiatrists and social scientists have often been guilty of neglecting the physical and biological aspects of disorders they deal with. Even now, most psychiatric literature reflects a divide between biological and psychological theorists. Similarly, medical and surgical literature still demonstrates little evidence of interest in psychological issues. Fortunately, the modern clinician increasingly recognizes the need to integrate physiological, psychological and pathological aspects of health and disease.

In no field is this integrated approach more important than sexual dysfunction. However, it is only recently that a multifactorial view of erectile dysfunction has been adopted. This book stresses the importance of not conceptualizing physical and psychological issues as distinct and mutually exclusive entities and encourages an eclectic approach to management. Nevertheless, for the sake of clarity, we have observed traditional separations in our chapter headings.

Guided by our belief in the importance of a multidisciplinary approach to impotence, we have placed emphasis in making all chapters accessible to readers from different disciplines and have included cross references wherever appropriate.

The book commences with a critical discussion of the use of the term impotence and the concepts which it embodies. The term is considered by many to have pejorative connotations which are partly the result of the condition it describes. Some clinicians believe that the negative impact of suffering from the disorder can be reduced by changing the term to 'erectile dysfunction'. Others continue to use the term 'impotence' in the belief that the fear and stigma associated with the disorder can only be significantly reduced by the provision of effective treatment services and education.

The remainder of the first section provides a thorough description of current understanding of the many processes involved in normal arousal and erection. This provides the reader with the essential background for the effective assessment and treatment of patients, as well as a basis for understanding future research and developments.

The second section of the book is devoted to the assessment of men with impotence. When assessing problems with such social and psychological impact, a knowledge of key questions and investigations is not enough. Skills in eliciting and interpreting accurate and complete information are essential and demand conscious attention, particularly in the busy clinics with which most clinicians are familiar. Our goal in this section is to provide a logical framework for the confident and skilled application of physical and psychological assessment techniques.

The final section discusses the treatment approaches which are currently available and some potential options which are under development. Although often critical of our knowledge about the outcome of these methods, the authors acknowledge that all have a place in our choice of treatments, even if that place is not entirely clear. The last chapter synthesizes and complements many of the facts and approaches described in earlier chapters by considering the management of the single man.

It is impossible to acknowledge all those who have provided us with the inspiration, ideas and knowledge which have led to the production of this book. However, we would like to express particular thanks to Dr Christopher Bass, Dr Michael Crowe and Professor Giles Brindley and, of course, to all our patients past and present. Finally, we owe a special debt to our wives and families, whose tolerance and whose support of our endeavour has made it all possible.

London   A.G.
1993   J.P.P.

Contributors

John Bancroft MD FRCP FRCP (Edin) FRCPsych
Clinical Consultant, MRC Reproductive Biology
Unit, Royal Edinburgh Hospital, Edinburgh, UK

Martin Cole PhD
Director, Institute for Sex Education and
Research, Birmingham, UK

Ian K. Dickinson MB BS FRCS (Edin)
Consultant in Urology and Andrology, Dartford
and Gravesend Hospitals, Dartford, UK

Alain Gregoire MB BS DRCOG MRCPsych
Consultant Psychiatrist, The Old Manor
Hospital, Salisbury, UK

George O. Klufio MB ChB FRCS FWACS
Consultant Urologist, University of Ghana
Medical School, Accra, Ghana

Michael Murphy MB ChB MRCP MRCPsych
Consultant Psychiatrist, Queen Mary's
University Hospital, Roehampton, London

John P. Pryor MS FRCS
Consultant Uroandrologist, King's College
and St Peter's Hospitals; Formerly Dean,
Institute of Urology, London University,
London, UK

Glenn D. Wilson MA PhD CPsychol FBPS
Senior Lecturer in Psychology, Institute of
Psychiatry, University of London, UK; Adjunct
Professor of Psychology, University of Nevada,
Reno, USA

Contents

Normal erectile function

1. Impotence in perspective

John Bancroft

THE CONCEPT OF IMPOTENCE

Impotence is an emotive word. Recently, I spoke to a 33-year-old man whose wife had left him 18 months earlier. Deeply hurt by this experience, he had since been unable to sustain an erection in his attempts to establish a new sexual relationship. He became depressed and moved from the city to live in the Outer Hebrides, where he was now finding some peace of mind, albeit in relative isolation. 'How are you feeling about yourself now?' I asked. 'I feel impotent,' he replied. This was not a diagnosis but an identity. The pervasiveness of the concept of impotence has a long history.

In the past, and in many parts of the world still today, 'impotence' has been seen as a consequence of witchcraft or evil magic. The witch apparently cast her spell by tying ligatures in threads or strands of leather (Bullough 1976). Until the 19th century, sexual problems were more the province of the church than the medical profession. The *Malleus Maleficarum* of 1486 is often regarded as an early source of comment on sexual psychopathology, both of the times and of its authors. It contained the following interesting comment: 'When the member is in no way stirred and can never perform the action of coitus, this is a sign of frigidity of nature, but, when it is stirred but cannot become erect, it is a sign of witchcraft' (Trethowan 1963). Mystical beliefs still lead to reactions such as Koro (Money & Annecillo 1987) when the penis shrinks, and death is assumed to follow if the penis disappears into the abdominal wall. (The lack of a penis is a defining characteristic of the ghosts of the dead.) Whilst Koro occurs most commonly in South East Asia, it crops up in other parts of the world, although predominantly affecting Asians. The 'Dhat' syndrome, the fixed belief that sperm is leaking from the body through the urine, causing general debility and weakness, stems from the common myth that semen is a vital fluid which should not be wasted. This syndrome is found throughout the Indian continent, affecting both Muslims and Hindus (d'Ardenne 1986).

In European culture, the issue is more one of masculinity, the capacity for a strong erection being symbolic of 'the strong man'. The literal meaning of the word 'impotence' speaks for itself ('want of strength or power; utter inability or weakness; helplessness' *OED*). According to Stekel (1927), 'Impotence impresses its stamp upon a man's whole personality. He loses his feeling of self-regard, his energy, his whole pleasure in productive activity. He has the bitter conviction: You are not a man'. Trethowan (1963), in his review of the demonological literature about impotence, saw a resemblance between the explanations put forward by medieval theologians and more recently by psychoanalysts. I would suggest that this similarity reflects a continuing tendency to interpret 'impotence' as meaning some fundamental disturbance of the individual, resulting from either externally imposed magical forces or internal disturbances of the id. Havelock Ellis (1911) commented, 'the impotent man is made to feel that, while he need not be greatly concerned if he suffers from nervous disturbances of digestion, if he should suffer just as innocently from nervous disturbances of the sexual impulse, it is almost a crime'. But do we, as a modern medical profession, really want to reinforce in any way the idea that the inability to obtain an erection is necessarily a sign of failure as a person and, in particular, as a man?

Until very recently, the medical use of the term 'impotence' has been vague, covering a variety of male sexual problems including premature ejaculation. In an early medical text (Hammond 1887), the term was applied to both men and women, meaning 'an impossibility or difficulty in the accomplishment of the act of copulation', and for men covered 'absence of sexual desire', the inability to ejaculate, as well as erectile failure (although not premature ejaculation). Its legal use infers non-consummation of marriage and has also been applied to the female as well as the male (Johnson 1968). But why, in modern times, is the term being used at all? Its female counterpart, 'frigidity', has more or less disappeared from use in medical writing, because of its unnecessarily pejorative implications. Elliot (1985) investigated this further, perusing the titles in *Psychological Abstracts* between 1940 and 1983. He found that whereas 'frigidity' had virtually disappeared in the last few years of this time span, there had been a *dramatic increase* in the use of 'impotence'. He pointed out that most of the leading authorities in the field of sexology explicitly rejected the term 'frigidity' but continued to use 'impotence'. In 1986 Masters, Johnson and Kolodny, referring to the earlier use of 'frigidity', wrote, 'As this term lacked diagnostic precision and was increasingly used in a negative, disparaging way, portraying women as "cold" or "rejecting", many sexologists abandoned its use'. They continued to use 'impotence' without comment. By interesting contrast, Kaplan (1974) wrote, 'The use of the term impotence is objectionable, not only because it is pejorative, but also because it is inappropriate. In as much as impotence is simply an impairment of penile erection, a more accurate term ... would be "erectile dysfunction". However, the term impotence is widely used; consequently, it has been retained for purposes of this discussion'. Kaplan has continued to retain the term since.

Arentewicz & Schmidt (1983) explicitly stated that they avoided *both* terms, 'impotence' and 'frigidity', first because they are not applied consistently, and secondly because they are judgemental and discriminatory. Those responsible for revising diagnostic systems of classification have rejected both terms. In the first (1952) version of the *Diagnostic and Statistical Manual for Mental Disorders*

(*DSM I*) both 'frigidity' and 'impotence' were used. In the 1968 *DSM II* version only 'impotence' was present. By the 1980 *DSM III* version, both had disappeared. They are also absent from the new *International Classification of Diseases (ICD 10)*. But it is interesting and perhaps surprising that the large majority of professionals have been sensitive to the stigmatizing effects of the pejorative term applied to women, 'frigidity', but not to those of its male counterpart, 'impotence'.

The dramatic increase of use of the term 'impotence' in the psychological literature, reported by Elliot (1985), has been dwarfed by the increase in the surgical literature over the past twenty years. This, of course, reflects an escalation in the number of publications on male sexual dysfunction written by surgeons, mainly urologists, during that time period and suggests a further reason why the term 'impotence' may hold appeal at the present time. The truly dramatic change in this field has been the increase in the amount of surgical treatment, and, more recently, intracavernosal injection treatment, mainly prescribed by urological surgeons. To a very large extent, these new treatment approaches have been obtainable only in the private sector. It has been rediscovered by the surgical profession that many men will part with their money in the search for 'restored potency'. It has become big business, and as such there is a vested interest in reinforcing the more global and stigmatizing concept of 'impotence'. The extent to which the medical profession is colluding with this male propensity for self-denigration, when sexual performance is involved, requires careful consideration. Given the essentially psychosomatic nature of sexual response, we must ask ourselves very seriously whether our approach to assessment, definition and labelling may, in fact, be aggravating the genuine difficulties of our patients. A first step is to consider abandoning the term 'impotence'. Personally, I now have no doubts that this term should be discouraged. It is unlikely to disappear, as it is so deeply rooted in shared concepts of masculinity, but we should not reinforce it. 'Erectile dysfunction' is an appropriate if semantically clumsy term; 'erectile problems' and 'impaired erection' are alternatives which can be used in many contexts.

CHANGING PATTERNS OF HELP FOR ERECTILE PROBLEMS

Medical literature on impotence remained scant until the 20th century. An interesting exception was a book *Sexual Impotence in the Male* by W A Hammond, published in 1883. At that time the principal cause of sexual problems, of most types, was seen to be earlier sexual excess, particularly masturbation, but also other types of sexual activity occurring during childhood and early adulthood. Treatment, according to Hammond, was of two types: *hygienic* and *medical*. In the former category, first and foremost was *rest*; i.e. not only sexual inactivity for at least one year, but also 'rest of mind from lascivious thoughts'. Also advocated were baths, douches, exercise and, of particular importance, a strict rule against sleeping on one's back. As a preventative measure, limitation of sexual activity early in life was strongly encouraged. 'Previous to the twenty first year sexual intercourse should not be practised at all; and between that age and twenty-five, if indulged in, it should certainly not be more frequent than once in ten or twelve days'. If an individual ignored this advice, then he was encouraged to expect early decline of his sexual powers. A large number of devices designed to physically prevent masturbation were patented at the turn of the century (Fig. 1.1).

Of the varieties of medical treatment, Hammond's favourite was *electricity*, and he found little to choose between 'Galvanic', 'Faradic' and 'Statical'.

Every morning I applied statical electricity to the penis and testicles, and to the whole length of the spinal cord, drawing inch sparks from the lower organs, and from three to four inch sparks from the spine. This was continued for about fifteen minutes. Though painful, the effect was all that can be desired: the blood-vessels of the penis became visibly distended, and the whole organ assumed a deeper red color... Twice a week I applied by means of a urethral electrode a galvanic current from eight cells to the membranous and prostatic portions of the urethra, with the object of diminishing the morbid excitability which evidently existed in those parts. (Hammond 1883)

Cauterization of the urethra was apparently also popular, but was strongly criticized by Hammond, who thought it harmful. 'There is nothing that can

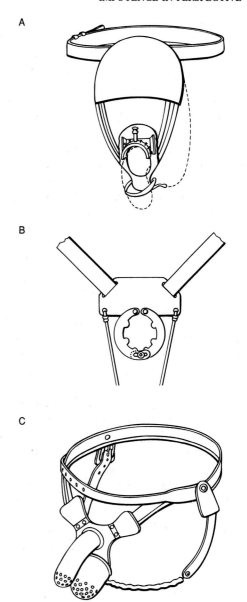

A

B

C

Fig. 1.1 Three examples of antimasturbatory devices patented in the USA at the turn of the century. (From *Some Early Attempts to Modify Penile Erection in Horse and Human: an historical analysis* by P T Mountjoy (1974) The Psychological Record. Reprinted by permission.)

be done by cauterization that cannot be better and more safely effected by electricity'. Other procedures in vogue at the time included massage, percussion, flagellation and urtication (i.e. flagellation with nettles).

During this century we have seen various fashions in the treatment of erectile dysfunction come and go. These have tended to reflect the mind–body dualism that continues to pervade medical thinking: a problem is *either* psychological *or* it is physical. In the earlier part of this century, psychoanalytic opinion, as exemplified by Stekel (1927), saw erectile failure as nearly always traceable to psychological inhibitions and hence potentially responsive to psychotherapy. Needless to say, psychoanalytic psychotherapy was available to very few, and it has always been unclear how often it has been effective with such problems. Before 1970, when Masters & Johnson published their highly influential book, *Human Sexual Inadequacy*, setting in motion the modern approach to directive sex therapy and counselling, a psychological basis for erectile dysfunction was assumed for the large majority of cases — 90 to 95% was the figure often quoted (e.g. Strauss 1950), although its origin was always obscure. Furthermore, with the exception of a few individuals like Hastings (1963), Albert Ellis and the early behaviour therapists, there were very few therapists with coherent therapeutic approaches to the problem (Bancroft 1989a).

Surgical approaches to treatment have surfaced from time to time. Apart from procedures aimed at increasing or stimulating hormonal effects, such as the transplantation of slices of human testis (Lespinasse 1918) or the Steinach procedure of tying the vas, we find ligation of the dorsal vein of the penis advocated in 1902 (Wooten 1902–3). Huhner (1924) was convinced that chronic inflammation and pathological changes in the prostatic urethra were related to sexual 'inefficiency' and he advised local treatment of the verumontanum by irrigation and instillation. Procedures such as cautery and passage of cold sounds had the same aims. Testicular diathermy and galvanic stimulation of perineal musculature were also advocated (Johnson 1968). Lowsley & Bray (1936) devised an operation for shortening the ischiocavernosus muscles and plicating the bulbocavernosus, together with restriction of the dorsal vein. They reported that in 31 out of 51 cases, the 'impotence' was successfully relieved, though they conceded that the long term consequences of the procedure would have to await longer follow-up. This surgical approach bears more than a passing resemblance to the recent procedure of crural plication and dorsal vein ligation (Goldstein & Rothstein 1990).

Attempts to devise pieces of equipment which aid erection or at least vaginal insertion of the non-erect penis, have a long history. Vacuum devices were being tried in the 19th century — Hammond (1883) used the term 'exhausting apparatus' — and there have been various modern versions of this theme in the past few years. Loewenstein's (1947) external penile splint, known as the Coital Training Apparatus, achieved some popularity for a number of years (e.g. Russell 1959). According to Johnson (1968), surgically implanted penile splints go back to 1948 with Loeffler et al (1964) providing an early report in the surgical literature.

In the 1970s the scene started to change dramatically and on two fronts. On the one hand there was the veritable revolution in psychological treatment for sexual dysfunctions, sparked by Masters & Johnson's (1970) book, *Human Sexual Inadequacy*. This was followed soon after by Helen Kaplan's (1974) influential volume *The New Sex Therapy*, in which psychoanalytic principles were married, somewhat awkwardly, to the directive counselling approach of Masters & Johnson. Thus evolved a broad church of sex therapists with backgrounds ranging from hard-line operant behaviour modification to psychoanalysis, and a fair number of eclectic empiricists in between. On the other side of the Atlantic at least, this 'new wave' was accompanied by considerable therapeutic optimism and claims of success. Generally, expectations are by now much more modest.

The other front involved an upsurge of new types of surgically implanted penile splints and increasing interest in the use of vascular surgery for erectile dysfunction (e.g. Michal et al 1974). One important consequence of this surgical revolution was a growing attention to the *investigation* of erectile dysfunction. This was driven by the wish to demonstrate the 'organic' nature of the erectile problem before advocating surgical treatment. The frequency of vascular disease in men with erectile dysfunction was beginning to be recognized when the next crucial development occurred. This was the discovery, by Virag (1982) in Paris, and around the same time, by Brindley

(1983) in London, that the injection of smooth muscle relaxing drugs, such as papaverine, into the corpora cavernosa of the penis could induce an erection. This has been followed by a major escalation of interest in erectile dysfunction amongst urological surgeons, who found themselves empowered, not merely with surgical procedures, but also with a convenient method of inducing erections in their outpatient clinics. The use of such injections for both diagnostic and treatment purposes has increased dramatically over the past four or five years; these developments will be dealt with in the course of this book.

Until very recently, these two new lines of development were taking place largely in isolation from each other. There was remarkably little communication, let alone understanding, between the two professional divisions. In fact, a common message from the surgical field was that sex therapy was ineffective and now unnecessary with the new surgical methods available. Some surgeons made claims of the proportion of cases organically determined, which were no better substantiated than the earlier claims of the 'psychogenic' school (e.g. 'Fact: most impotence — 80 to 90 per cent — is caused by physical, not psychological, problems' Goldstein & Rothstein 1990). Furthermore, from the surgeons' point of view, the problem was now curable! Many sex therapists looked on with considerable suspicion at these surgeons, who, whilst delighted with their pharmaco-mechanical wizardry, appeared unconcerned with the psychological complexities of the human sexual condition. Gradually, and not before time, bridges are being built and interdisciplinary cooperation is following. This volume is an important example. But there is still a considerable amount of crucial ground to be covered by this process. Each of these two contrasting professional fields has an important message to take on board. Let us look at these two messages a little more closely.

Sex therapists have to come to terms with the increasingly demonstrated fact that many men with erectile dysfunction, possibly as many as 50% (Bancroft 1989a), have physical abnormalities which may contribute to their erectile problems. Most commonly, these abnormalities involve the vascular supply of the penis, less commonly its nerve supply. Furthermore, such abnormalities are often not identifiable by means of routine clinical examination. And yet it is important before embarking on sex therapy to have some idea of the extent of possible organic impairment. Such impairment does not necessarily preclude sex therapy, but it does have a bearing on the expectations and goals of both the therapist and the patient. Consequently, sex therapists do need to have working relationships with clinicians who are able to carry out appropriate investigations in such cases. For many otherwise very skilled and capable sex therapists working in non-clinical settings, such as marriage guidance, this can present a problem, which too often is dealt with by denying its existence.

The second message, to the surgeons, is somewhat like a mirror image of the first. In essence, it is that, even when injecting drugs or implanting plastic rods into the penis, it is important to keep in mind that the penis remains, in some sense, in a working relationship with the man attached to it, and in a rather different sense, with the man's sexual partner. The occurrence of an erection is not a guarantee of a sexually satisfactory relationship. Furthermore, the propensity for mind–body dualism has been seduced by the notion that these new developments in investigation and treatment of erectile failure are uncomplicated by psychological mechanisms. Thus investigations using highly sophisticated technology, such as pulse wave Doppler or duplex ultrasound, are seen to be assessing the structural state of the penile blood vessels, whereas intracavernosal injections of smooth muscle relaxants are evoking and evaluating peripheral mechanisms and overriding any influences from the brain. A noteworthy criticism of this rapidly developing and highly technological field is that predominantly it has lacked serious attempts to validate its procedures. At best, validation has involved comparing one uncertain procedure with another. Evidence of abnormality has been too readily taken to indicate organic causation, even though sound evidence of 'normality' is usually lacking. In the private sector, a sophisticated programme of diagnostic investigation adds substantially to the costs of surgery for the desperate patient. The cynical observer might wonder to what extent such investigations are really cost-effective for the patient, or whether they represent an alternative to surgery for boosting professional incomes. (And cost-effectiveness is a crucial issue in seeking to establish these investigative procedures within the National Health Service.)

Fortunately, there have been some working in the field who have sought to apply scientific rigour to the crucial question of validation. Buvat and his colleagues in Lille have provided an example in this respect. From an early stage, this group challenged some of the less well substantiated assumptions. Thus they were able to show that a proportion of men with erectile dysfunction who had demonstrable arterial disease, responded to psychological methods of treatment (Buvat-Herbaut et al 1984). In other words, the existence of organic pathology is not necessarily a sufficient explanation for erectile failure, particularly when vascular pathology is involved, because of the considerable scope for compensatory collateral blood supply. Recently this group has written a valuable and comprehensive review of the recent literature on diagnosis of erectile dysfunction (Buvat et al 1990). They have martialled the evidence that the response to many of the diagnostic procedures, including the most up-to-date ultrasound techniques and the use of intracavernosal injections of drugs, is variable within the same individual. Increasingly it appears that these diagnostic tests are assessing not the prevailing *structural*, but the 'at the time' *functional* status of the erectile mechanisms. Buvat et al (1990) conclude that much of this variance in response during these diagnostic procedures reflects the effect of psychological mechanisms, such as apprehension at the prospect of an intracavernosal injection. It is no longer possible to conclude that an impaired response to papaverine excludes a psychogenic causation. In most respects, any current diagnostic certainty rests on the occurrence of 'normal' responses rather than 'abnormal' ones; a 'normal' NPT is of clear value, a 'normal' response to papaverine excludes certain possibilities. 'Impaired' responses are much more difficult to interpret, and, in addition, with many of the newer procedures, and variables such as 'peak flow velocity' of the penile arterial flow or 'maintenance flow rate'

of dynamic infusion cavernosometry, our knowledge of the normal range is very shaky.

This is not to say that these recent developments are not important and valuable. There is no doubt that as a result of this major investment by surgeons in the investigation of erectile dysfunction, our understanding of the physiology of erection has advanced considerably. Furthermore, we now have at our disposal an impressive array of investigative procedures of considerable potential. But, as far as understanding the aetiology of erectile dysfunction is concerned, the real and important challenge has yet to be taken up.

What are the mechanisms involved in psychological inhibition of erection? The importance of answering this question is not confined to interpreting the variance in these modern diagnostic procedures. It may be the only way that we can substantially improve our psychological, as well as develop alternative, pharmacological methods of treatment. In recent years, Barlow and colleagues, and others (see Cranston-Cuebas & Barlow 1990 for a recent review) have pursued an elegant series of experiments in which psychological variables affecting erectile response have been investigated. By manipulating expectancies and attribution, they have established the foundations of a psychophysiological methodology for pursuing the above question. Most importantly, they have shown that the effects on erectile response of such factors as anxiety, 'feedback' or distraction are not consistent. In particular they have shown that 'functional' men (i.e. without erectile problems) react to these cognitive and affective processes differently to 'dysfunctional' men. But as yet, it is not clear whether these differences precede the dysfunction and thus play an important aetiological role, or whether they are consequences of the dysfunction, and hence no more than an aggravating factor. It is, in any case, questionable whether such factors could account for more than a small proportion of the psychogenic 'erectile failure' that presents in our clinics. Elsewhere I have presented and discussed other psychophysiological approaches which hold some promise for exploring this crucial question (Bancroft et al 1985; Bancroft 1989b, 1990). What is still lacking is a concerted attempt to combine these experimentally rigorous approaches of the psychophysiologist with the physiologically relevant techniques of the surgically oriented diagnostician. It is not only in the clinical but also the research arena that there is a fundamental need for interdisciplinary collaboration in tackling the problem of erectile dysfunction.

How common is erectile dysfunction?

The problem with assessing the frequency of any aspect of sexual behaviour is the sensitivity of the information, and the various factors which might discourage informants from 'telling the truth' or, in fact, being prepared to tell anything (Clement 1990). As a consequence, we have a virtual absence of any proper assessment of a representative sample of the male population. On the face of it, it should be possible to add on questions about erectile function to questionnaires or enquiries involving large representative samples. But 'add on' questions about such matters are highly likely to be suspect in the validity or the response, or, in many cases, simply in the meaning of the question to the respondent. Thus Marsey et al (1984) investigated by questionnaire a large cohort of men in the United States who had undergone vasectomy, and a comparable and equally large control group. Amongst numerous questions about health and many other types of health problem, were one or two questions about erectile function. The incidence of impotence was presented as 17 new cases per 100,000 man years. Not only is this epidemiological statistic difficult to interpret, there is also no indication of what questions were asked. Comhaire et al (1988) reported a further large scale WHO study of 7781 couples consulting for infertility. As presented, the results indicate that 1.3% of the men had 'inadequate coital erection' whereas 5.4% never had an erection during masturbation. Possibly a large proportion of this latter, otherwise surprising figure consists of men who don't masturbate, rather than men who masturbate without an erection, making the figures as presented meaningless. If the questionnaire is answered in such a way, what reliance can be placed on questions about 'adequacy of coital erections'? Valid information about sexual response requires careful as well as sensitive questioning.

The closest we have to a carefully investigated representative sample is that of the original Kinsey survey (Kinsey et al 1948). The representativeness of this sample has been extensively criticized and, in particular, the older age groups were seriously underrepresented (Bancroft 1989a). Within these substantial limitations, the Kinsey survey found that 66 of 4108 males (1.6%) on whom adequate data were available had 'reached more or less permanent erectile impotence'. Such cases were rare in the under 35s, but increased markedly after the age of 55, so that by the age of 70, 27% of their sample came into this category. As far as 'less permanent' erectile failure was concerned, 35% of men reported 'incidental impotence' (i.e. infrequent or justifiable) and 7.1% 'more than incidental' (Gebhard & Johnson 1979).

The 'normal' effects of ageing on erectile response were described by Masters & Johnson (1966). In older men, erections take longer to develop, require more direct tactile stimulation, can be sustained for shorter periods and are more difficult to regain when lost. Spontaneous erections during sleep and on waking become less frequent (Schiavi & Schreiner-Engel 1988). The importance of ageing has been examined in a number of studies (for review see Schiavi 1990). Only one of these can be regarded as representative in its sample: Persson (1980) obtained a systematic and representative sample of 70-year-old individuals born in Sweden in 1901–02. He obtained 85% participation. Forty six per cent of the 166 men reported that they continued to have intercourse. Unfortunately, there was no indication of the proportion who were experiencing erectile difficulty.

Martin (1981) has reported evidence from the Baltimore Longitudinal Study of Ageing, which involved well-educated and generally healthy volunteers attracted to the benefits of periodic medical examination that participation in the study entailed. The proportion of men who had partial or total erectile dysfunction increased from 7% in the 20–30 age group to 57% at ages 70–79. Martin also found a marked relationship between sexual function and activity in later life and that reported when younger. Thus he found that in his least active group (i.e. those with the lowest level of sexual activity in early life) 75% had erectile problems when older; of his moderately active and his most active groups the percentages were 46% and 19% respectively (turning on its head the claim of Hammond (1883) cited above).

In Brecher's (1984) highly unrepresentative but large sample of 2402 older men, 50% reported that they took longer to get an erection, 44% said erection was less rigid when fully erect and 32% were more likely to lose their erection during sexual activity.

Two unrepresentative samples, answering questionnaires published in *Woman* magazine, and selected from 15 000 women and 5000 men who responded, were reported by Sanders (1985, 1987). Noteworthy is the similarity of the figures from the two samples; 7% of the men reported themselves, whereas 8% of the women reported their partners to have erectile problems. In two small, unrepresentative studies, similar figures resulted; Frank et al (1978), in a study of 100 married couples, reported 7% having 'difficulty in getting' and 9% 'difficulty in maintaining' an erection. Nettelbladt & Uddenberg (1979) found that 7% of 58 married men failed to get an erection on at least 50% of occasions.

We have further evidence of a different kind from samples of clinic populations. Best studied in this respect have been male diabetics. Fairburn

et al (1982) reviewed seven prevalence studies and found rates ranging from 35% to 59%. Here again we see a clear relationship with age, the age incidence of erectile dysfunction in diabetic men looking like a grossly amplified version of the age incidence curve reported by Kinsey et al (1948) for men in general (see Fig. 1.2). Other clinic populations have also shown high prevalence rates. Slag et al (1983) surveyed 1180 men attending a medical outpatient clinic and found 34% to have erectile problems. This is obviously a somewhat different type of clinical population to the normal diabetic clinic attender, most of whom will be relatively well, maintained on insulin, whereas the medical outpatient clinic is likely to contain a higher proportion who are currently ill. The association between erectile dysfunction and a variety of medical and surgical conditions is reviewed in Chapter 6.

Amongst men attending sexual problem clinics, erectile dysfunction is by far the most common presenting complaint. In a survey of clinic attenders over a three year period in Edinburgh (Warner et al 1987), 50% of the 533 male presenters had erectile dysfunction as their main complaint. The next most common complaint was 13% with premature ejaculation. Once again

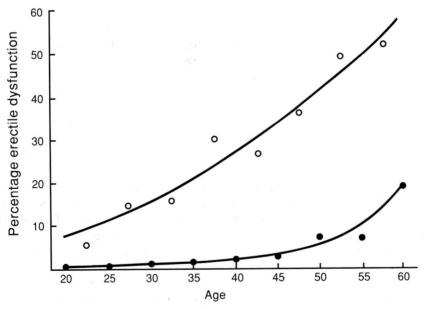

Fig. 1.2 The age incidence of erectile dysfunction in diabetic and non-diabetic men
○ = diabetic men ● = non-diabetic men (Bancroft 1989a)

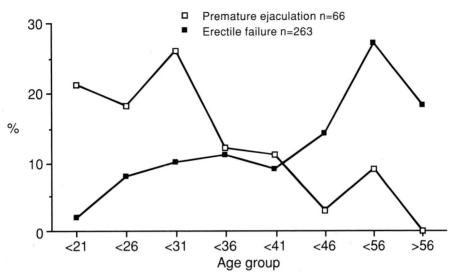

Fig. 1.3 Age distribution of men presenting with erectile failure and premature ejaculation (Warner et al 1987).

there was a clear association between complaints of erectile dysfunction and age (Fig. 1.3), with a peak in the fifties. Of the men with erectile dysfunction, 52% had some concurrent physical disease which may have contributed to their erectile problems: 32% arterial, 21% neurological, 29% urological, 19% diabetes mellitus (Warner et al 1987).

The problems in establishing the extent to which such conditions are contributing to the erectile difficulty will be dealt with at length in this volume. It is, however, common for men to attend such clinics keen, and sometimes determined, to be given a physical explanation for their problem, in spite of the generally much poorer prognosis associated with such aetiology. This is a reflection of the great reluctance that many men have in accepting a psychological explanation for something so central to their identity and self-esteem. It is also often difficult for those who have concurrent physical illness to comprehend the extent to which psychological and physical mechanisms interact — the psychosomatic circle of sex (Bancroft 1989b). Yet this is often crucial to their management. For the professional attempting to help men with concerns about their sexual response, it is important to keep in mind the wide range of diffi-

culty that may be involved, from the man 'turned off' by his partner's response, to the man whose nerve supply to the erectile tissues has been cut during surgery. And in between we will find the complexities of mind–body interaction, still largely mysterious.

SUMMARY

The historical background to the term 'impotence' has been considered and its pejorative meaning emphasized. The use by clinicians of alternative and less stigmatizing terms is strongly encouraged.

The true prevalence of erectile dysfunction remains obscure, though various studies suggest that, overall, it may be in the region of 7 to 8%. It undoubtedly increases with age, reflecting the variety of physical processes that accompany ageing.

The changing fashions of professional help for the man with erectile failure have been briefly reviewed, and serve to remind us of the ephemeral nature of therapeutic enthusiasms. The need for interdisciplinary cooperation in the diagnosis and management of erectile dysfunction is, however, beyond dispute.

REFERENCES

Arentewicz G, Schmidt G 1983 The treatment of sexual disorders. Basic Books, New York

Bancroft J 1989a Human sexuality and its problems, 2nd edn. Churchill Livingstone, London

Bancroft J 1989b Psychosomatic aspects of erectile dysfunction. In: Serio M (ed) Perspectives in andrology. Serono Symposia Publications, Raven Press, New York, vol 53 pp 467–476

Bancroft J 1990 Man and his penis: a relationship under threat? Journal of Psychology & Human Sexuality 2: 7–32

Bancroft J, Bell C, Ewing D J, McCulloch D K, Warner P, Clarke B F 1985 Assessment of erectile function in diabetic and non-diabetic impotence by simultaneous recording of penile diameter and penile arterial pulse. Journal of Psychosomatic Research 29: 315–324

Brecher E M 1984 Love, sex and aging: a Consumer's Union report. Little Brown, Boston

Brindley G S 1983 Cavernosal alpha-blockade: a new technique for investigating and treating erectile impotence. British Journal of Psychiatry 143: 332–337

Bullough V L 1976 Sexual variance in society and history. Wiley-Interscience, New York

Buvat J, Buvat-Herbaut M, Lemaire A, Marcolin G, Quittelier E 1990 Recent developments in the clinical assessment and diagnosis of erectile dysfunction. Annual Review of Sex Research 1: 265–308

Buvat-Herbaut M, Lemaire A, Buvat J 1984 Résultats du traitement non chirurgical d'impuissances érectiles associées à des anomalies sévères d'artères sexuelles. Contraception Fertilité Sexualité 12: 501–506

Clement U 1990 Surveys of heterosexual behavior. Annual Review of Sex Research 1: 45–74

Comhaire F H, Farley T, Rowe P 1988 Sterility and sexuality from the andrologist's standpoint. In: Eicher W, Kockott G (eds) Sexology. Springer-Verlag, Berlin, p 81–102

Cranston-Cuebas M, Barlow D 1990 Cognitive and affective contributions to sexual functioning. Annual Review of Sex Research 1: 119–162

d'Ardenne P 1986 Sexual dysfunction in a transcultural setting: assessment, treatment and research. Sexual & Marital Therapy 1: 23–34

Elliot M L 1985 The use of 'impotence' and 'frigidity': why has 'impotence' survived? Journal of Sex & Marital Therapy 11: 51–56

Ellis H 1911 Studies in the physiology of sex, vol VI. Davis, Philadelphia, p 174

Fairbairn C G, McCulloch D K, Wu F C 1982 The effects of diabetes on male sexual function. Clinics in Endocrinology & Metabolism 11(3): 749–784

Frank E, Anderson C, Rubinstein D 1978 Frequency of sexual dysfunction in 'normal' couples. New England Journal of Medicine 229: 111–115

Gebhard P H, Johnson A B 1979 The Kinsey data. Saunders, Philadelphia

Goldstein I, Rothstein L 1990 The potent male; facts, fiction and future. The Body Press, Los Angeles

Hammond W A 1883 Sexual impotence in the male. Bermingham,

Hammond W A 1887 Sexual impotence in the male and female. Davis, Detroit (*This is the second, enlarged edition of the 1883 volume, which was reprinted in 1974 by Arno Press, New York in the series 'Sex, Marriage and Society'.*)

Hastings D W 1963 Impotence and frigidity. Churchill, London

Huhner M 1924 Impotence in the male: its practical and scientific treatment. Medical Journal & Record 119: 499

Johnson J 1968 Disorder of sexual potency in the male. Pergamon, Oxford

Kaplan H S 1974 The new sex therapy. Brunner Mazel, New York

Kinsey A C, Pomeroy W B, Martin C F 1948 Sexual behavior in the human male. Saunders, Philadelphia

Lespinasse V D 1918 Impotency: its treatment by transplantation of the testicle. Surgical Clinics, Chicago 2: 281

Loeffler R A, Seyegh E S, Lash H 1964 The artificial os penis. Plastic & Reconstructive Surgery 34: 71

Loewenstein J 1947 Treatment of impotence. Hamish Hamilton, London

Lowsley O S, Bray J L 1936 The surgical relief of impotence. Further experience with a new operative procedure. Journal of the American Medical Association 107: 2029–2035

Marsey F J, Bernstein G S, O'Fallon W M et al 1984 Vasectomy and health: results from a large cohort study. Journal of the American Medical Association 252: 1023–1029

Martin C E 1981 Factors affecting sexual functioning in 60-79 year old married males. Archives of Sexual Behavior 10: 399–420

Masters W H, Johnson V E 1966 Human sexual response. Churchill, London

Masters W H, Johnson V E 1970 Human sexual inadequacy. Churchill, London

Masters W H, Johnson V E, Kolodny R C 1986 Sex and human loving. Macmillan, London

Michal V, Kramar R, Bartak V 1974 Femoro-pudendal bypass in the treatment of sexual impotence. Journal of Cardiovascular Surgery 15: 356–359

Money J, Annecillo C 1987 Body-image pathology: Koro, the shrinking-penis syndrome in transcultural sexology. Sexual & Marital Therapy 2: 91–100

Nettelbladt P, Uddenberg N 1979 Sexual dysfunction and sexual satisfaction in 58 married Swedish men. Journal of Psychosomatic Research 23: 141–147

Persson G 1980 Sexuality in a 70-year old urban population. Journal of Psychosomatic Research 24: 335–342

Pietropinto A, Simenauer J 1977 Beyond the male myth. Times Books, New York

Russell G L 1959 Impotence treated by mechanotherapy. Proceedings of the Royal Society of Medicine 52: 872–874

Sanders D 1985 The Woman book of love and sex. Sphere, London

Sanders D 1987 The Woman report on men. Sphere, London

Schiavi R C 1990 Sexuality and ageing in men. Annual Review of Sex Research, 1: 227–249

Schiavi R C, Schreiner-Engel P 1988 Nocturnal penile tumescence in healthy ageing men. Journal of Gerontology 43: 146–150

Slag M F, Morley J E, Elson M K et al 1983 Impotence in medical clinic outpatients. Journal of the American Medical Association 249: 1736–1740

Stekel W 1927 Impotence in male. Boni & Liveright (English translation by Boltz, OH 1955 Liveright, New York)

Strauss B 1950 Impotence from the psychiatric stand point. British Medical Journal 1: 697–704

Trethowan W H 1963 The demopathology of impotence. British Journal of Psychiatry 109: 341–347

Virag R 1982 Intracavernous injection of papaverine for erectile failure. Lancet 2: 938

Warner P, Bancroft J and members of the Edinburgh Human Sexuality Group 1987 A regional service for sexual problems: a 3 year study. Sexual & Marital Therapy 2: 115–126

Wooten J S 1902-3 Ligation of the dorsal vein of the penis as a cure for atonic impotence. Texas Medical Journal 18: 325

2. The psychology of male sexual arousal

Glenn D. Wilson

This chapter is concerned with the psychological processes which determine healthy male sexual arousal, as well as some that might distort or impede it. In this pursuit it is necessary to state at the outset that:

a. Sexual arousal is a function of great evolutionary antiquity and is therefore often best understood within concepts developed by ethologists and sociobiologists.
b. Male sexual arousal is in some respects quite different from female sexual arousal as regards the stimuli and experiences that are optimally exciting (even though the mechanism and experience of orgasm itself may be very similar).
c. Optimal male arousal is not necessarily compatible with the norms of 'respectable' Judeo-Christian society (e.g. life-long, exclusive, monogamous marriage).

Many practising sex therapists, especially those who (like Masters & Johnson) come from a medical background, have sought to keep their advice, and even their theory, within bounds set by the social belief in natural marital compatibility. Unfortunately, this premise cannot be sustained after examination of the scientific facts concerning the biological origins of sexual arousal. Life-long companionship between one man and one woman is an attainable goal, but eternal sexual passion is not very realistic. Failure to recognize this (unfortunate) fact of nature has led to much unnecessary guilt and clinical confusion.

Other writers have sought to bring their conclusions and recommendations into line with a more recent social myth, that of sexual identity — the idea that men and women are just the same 'under the skin'. This, also, is grossly misleading; equality of opportunity is a desirable goal which may be politically organized, but typical men and women will still think and feel differently, especially within the domain of love and sex. This fact, too, is essential to the understanding of normal (and hence also abnormal) sexual functioning.

A central theme of this chapter is that optimal sexual arousal (at least in the human male) depends not just on the stimuli that are currently present in the environment (sights, touch, smells, etc.) but also on internally generated memories, images, desires, etc. (fantasies). Furthermore, fantasies are presumed to add some component to the arousal process that is deficient in the real situation. Therefore, fantasies often tell us more about the underlying nature of sexual desire (the sources of its instinctual power) than everyday sexual behaviour, which of practical necessity must pay more homage to social conventions and reality constraints (see Fig. 2.1).

TRIGGERING OF MALE AROUSAL

One of the striking ways in which male sexuality differs from female sexuality is its active, predatory, target-seeking nature. In connection with the fact that female eggs are more at a premium than male sperm (Trivers 1972), evolution has charged male animals with the responsibility of seeking, pursuing and competing for the favours of females, while the females adopt a relatively passive/receptive, although usually very selective, role. This means it is necessary (evolutionists prefer the term 'advantageous') for males to be equipped with a faster and more sensitive arousal system — one that, in its prime at least, is always 'ready to go'.

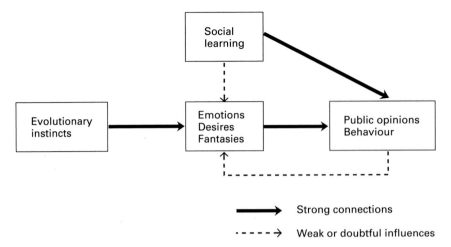

Fig. 2.1 A model for causation of amatory and sexual behaviour.

Among the more obvious manifestations of this easily activated male 'starter motor' are the higher rates of masturbation among young men (compared with young women) and their greater interest in looking at nudes, pornography, etc. Softcore men's magazines sell millions of copies annually, whereas direct female reflections of that formula have never appealed much to women. (Even *Playgirl* could not survive commercially without its male purchasers, whereas romantic novels are sold in their millions.) Male fantasies also have a 'pornographic' quality about them, dwelling much more on group sex scenarios and anonymous visual details such as breast size, pubic hair and the colour of underwear, than on the identities and feelings of the individuals involved (Wilson 1987; Table 2.1).

Table 2.1 Main elements of anonymously reported sexual fantasies (percentages). (Columns add to more than 100 because categories are not mutually exclusive).

	Men(%) (n = 291)	Women(%) (n = 409)
Group sex	31	15
Voyeuristic/fetishistic	18	7
Steady partner incorporated	14	21
Identified people (other than partner)	8	8
Setting romantic/exotic	4	15
Rape/force	4	13
Sadomasochism	7	7
No fantasies	5	12
Everything	3	0
No answer	21	19

(From Wilson 1987)

Sexual deviations (paraphilias) are an almost entirely male phenomenon, and these appear as overly-rigid exaggerations of typical male sexuality. The targets of paraphilia are usually impersonal, often visual/fetishistic and sadomasochistic in character and require a frequent 'turnover' of fresh exemplars to offset habituation. These points will be returned to later in the chapter. (For a fuller discussion of male–female differences in sexual arousability and their sociobiological origins, see Symons 1979; Wilson 1981a, 1989).

ORIGINS OF MALE SEX TARGETS

A striking thing about the 'blueprints' for male sexual arousal is how early in life they seem to be established. This, together with their rigidity, is one of the main reasons for supposing that they may constitute a form of imprinting (Wilson 1987).

There is increasing evidence that a rough outline of the biologically appropriate sexual target (reproductive age females) is stored innately somewhere between the limbic region and temporal cortex of the male brain (Flor-Henry 1987; Kolarsky et al 1967). In Jungian terminology, this would correspond to an 'archetype' or 'racial memory', but since aspects of it may go back in evolution as far as the reptilian era (Eibl-Eibesfeldt 1990), it is probably better understood in terms of the ethological concept of the *innate releasing mechanism* (IRM). It seems that all animals from sticklebacks to human beings have neural cells (or circuits) that are preset to respond to stimulus configurations that have powerful survival significance. Examples might be the colour red, the sound of a baby crying, or the shape of a human face. The primary IRM for male sexual arousal appears to be a visual configuration consisting of paired, pink, fleshy hemispheres separated by a mysterious dark cleavage (Wickler 1967; Morris 1971) (see Fig. 2.2), although certain tactile and olfactory (pheromonal) stimuli may also operate as innate releasers.

While these IRMs set up general guidelines as to what will be found erotically exciting, it seems that these may be further specified or modified by early childhood *imprinting*. Just as ducklings are primed to follow the first moving object that resembles their mother in certain visual aspects, and as adult drakes to mate with this same imprint, so human males attach their sexual responses to certain stimuli that they find in the environment that are the best available approximation to the innate blueprint (Bateson 1981). Usually this is a female (especially her breasts and genitals) but the process can go wrong, which may be one of the origins of fetishism, sadomasochism, paedophilia and various other 'paraphilias'.

The early childhood origins of sex targets is confirmed by many different observations:

a. People choose partners that are reminiscent of their opposite-sex parent in certain respects (Wilson & Barrett 1987).
b. Deviant sex targets are associated with minor temporal lobe damage occurring within the first three years of life (Kolarsky et al 1967).

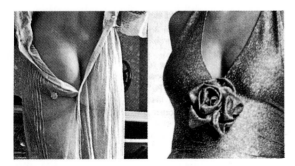

Fig. 2.2 The similarity between breasts and buttocks, illustrating the innate releaser of sexual arousal for the human male (paired, pink, fleshy hemispheres). Breasts may be regarded as a near-universal fetish, or as a 'genital echo' in Desmond Morris's terminology.

c. Most fetishists recall being excited by their fetish object from a very young age (Gosselin & Wilson 1980).
d. Many deviations include infantile components (nappies, dummies, comforters, knicker-wetting, discipline, etc.), suggesting that they date from critical experiences or periods in childhood.

The imprinting theory of sexual targets explains why fetish objects usually bear a close similarity to females and their genitals. The colours pink, red and black are favoured, as are flesh-like textures such as leather, rubber and silk. Intimate female garments are also common fetish objects because they are closely associated with women (and perhaps absorb their pheromones). Since parents are usually exercising a disciplinarian role at the same time as a boy is imprinting sex targets, it is not surprising that sadomasochistic elements such as belts, whips, punishment and humiliation are often taken into the blueprint for arousal. The fact that high-heeled shoes are a much more common fetish object than women's hats may be due to their leather composition, but possibly also to the fact that shoes are more salient in the sightline of a crawling infant.

Among the fetishisms observed clinically by Chalkey & Powell (1983) was one focused on plucked chickens. While at first this might appear ridiculous, it does come close to the innate releasing mechanism (IRM) description of paired, pink, fleshy hemispheres, and is even about the right size!

This sensory connection between fetishisms and the presumed IRMs for sexual arousal is one reason for preferring the imprinting model over 'conditioning theory', which suggests that we are sexually excited by stimuli that have appeared in simple conjunction with an innately active stimulus (like Pavlov's dogs learning to salivate at the sound of a bell). While there have been experimental demonstrations of conditioned sexual arousal (Rachman & Hodgson 1968; McConaghy 1970), the conditioning model does not explain why naturally occurring fetish objects nearly always have a close association with females. No lawn-mower fetishisms have appeared in the clinic, but many men are excited by rubber and leather. Nor does conditioning theory explain why fetishists are nearly always men, why the 'unconditioned stimulus' (actual women) ceases to be exciting after the conditioned response has become established, or why the conditioned response (the fetishism) is so resistant to extinction. Conditioned responses usually disappear after a while if they are not reinforced by the unconditioned stimulus.

In these and several other respects conditioning fails to explain the origins of male sexual arousal. A model which assumes innate releasing mechanisms modified by early childhood imprinting is, however, quite effective in explaining the known facts. Male targets (whether normal or fetishistic) are established early in life, are extremely inflexible, are closely related to IRMs and are more likely to occur in the absence of the IRM rather than its presence.

This description of fetishism may seem like a diversion in relation to the stated aim of describing 'healthy' male arousal, but the main point being made is that the ideal fantasies/desires/targets of normal men have visual/fetishistic qualities about them, and there is a continuum bridging clinical fetishism and normal male sexuality. Men are turned on by partners that conform to certain sensory configurations (e.g. long black hair, large pink breasts, shaved pubic hair, etc.). Their sexual arousal is typically keyed to aspects of women such as these (albeit idiosyncratic — differing from one male to the next) rather than being tied exclusively to the identity of a particular woman with whom they have fallen in love. Men are thus capable of responding to (and indeed may desire) a variety of different partners in the course of their lifetime, all of them being within a certain range of the ideal blueprint or 'prototype'.

This may sound chauvinistic, and may be deplored by wives, moralists and feminists, but it remains an inescapable fact concerning the process of sexual arousal in the average male (not just of 'our society' but of all societies at all times in history). Also unfortunate, but equally inescapable, is the preference of most men for youthful partners, which also seems to be biologically programmed because of the higher fertility of young women; the reciprocal is much less true because males remain reproductive longer than females, and their primary commodity (power, or the capacity to provide and protect) often increases with age.

RESPONSE TO EROTICA

Consistent with what has been said above, men differ from women in their reactions to pornography in predictable ways.

1. Men are more interested in seeking out and viewing explicit representations of sex than are women. Women usually decline opportunities to look at pornography unless they feel particularly safe (usually in the company of a man they love).
2. Men are more attracted to anonymous, mechanical, anatomical, lustful and group sex representations than women, especially scenes in which the woman is young and being exploited, raped, humiliated or otherwise treated as a sex object. Loving, romantic, relationship-oriented scenes are of greater interest to women.
3. Visual pornography seems to be more attractive to men; women are usually more interested in auditory or written material (especially when details of the people concerned and their relationships are described). This appears to reflect a generally more visual/spatial orientation in men, compared with a preference for the verbal/semantic mode in women (Gillan & Frith 1979).

Laboratory studies have shown little difference between men and women in either self-reported arousal or physiological responses to a wide variety of erotic stimuli (for a review see Rosen & Beck 1988). There is no doubt that women do become aroused by depictions of explicit sexual activity once persuaded to view it, and that romantic storylines are not a prerequisite to arousal. The outstanding sex difference is that of interest in pornography, willingness to view it, and attitudes towards it (Symons 1979). (In fact, selective volunteering renders many of the laboratory studies difficult to interpret; female subjects are more self-selected and therefore likely to be less representative of women in general than male samples are of men in general.) What is clear is that the majority of women would rather read romantic novels than look at pornographic pictures and they express disgust concerning certain types of pornography (e.g. depictions of coercive sex leading to orgasm) even though these have the capacity to arouse them if actually viewed.

Again, feminists and social learning theorists are inclined to attribute these sex differences to upbringing and the media and to suppose that they will disappear with greater social equality between men and women or as a result of deliberate campaigns. However, these differences are exactly what would be predicted on the basis of ethological theory and are therefore deeply rooted in our biology. Thus changes brought about by social pressures and ideals, however desirable to modern human society, are likely to be fragile and sometimes superficial.

It should be noted that within male samples there are considerable individual differences in the extent to which erotic pictures are arousing (Schmidt et al 1969). While the vast majority of men are excited to some extent (as indexed by self-ratings, penile plethysmograph readings and increase in masturbation rates following exposure), this effect is less strong in men who are conservative or non-permissive (as measured by church affiliation, political preference and attitudes to pre-marital sex). The usual interpretation of this is that negative attitudes towards hedonistic sex introduce cognitive factors that interfere with, or inhibit, the sexual arousal process. However, the work of Eysenck (1976) on the genetic relationship between permissiveness and libido suggests another interpretation. Permissiveness and libido are so highly correlated that it may not be possible to separate them; both are apparently reflecting the same genetic and hormonal factors, as though the permissive attitudes have developed as a rationalization for the kinds of behaviour that a high libido would dictate. In other words, while individual differences linking permissiveness to arousability are undeniable, their origin may also be biochemical rather than (or as well as) learned within the family, religion or other context.

In a study confirming a link between male hormones and libido, Wilson (1984) found that within a sample of opera singers, basses and baritones reported higher libido and more backstage affairs than tenors. The most likely interpretation of this is that the hormonal factors determining depth of voice (whether prenatal or pubertal) are at the same time responsible for setting levels of libido/permissiveness. Whenever differences between typical men and women are discussed it is necessary to remember that there are considerable individual differences within each sex and that these also may be due to biological factors.

In passing, it is worth noting that a frequently used diagnostic description, 'inhibited sexual desire' (Kaplan 1979), which even appears in the DSM-III, carries within it an unjustifiable theoretical presumption — that some hypothetical inhibitory force is blocking the manifestation of 'normal' libido. Another possibility that should be considered is that the libido is naturally (i.e. physiologically rather than pathologically) low or non-existent. There is, to date, no satisfactory evidence that the majority of men (or women) diagnosed as suffering from ISD are victims of excessive 'inhibitory forces', whether psychodynamic, conditioned or anything else. They may simply be people with libido that is towards the low end of a wide normal distribution. These two different types of sexual unresponsiveness are illustrated in Figure 2.3. Perhaps a parallel diagnostic presumption would be to describe homosexuals as inhibited (or perverted) heterosexuals; such a description, which has been common in the past, is understandably offensive to homosexuals and most scientists today contest its validity (Ellis and Ames 1987).

LEARNING AND COGNITIVE FACTORS

Although the importance of instinctual and early imprinting processes in male sexual arousal has been stressed above, there is no doubt that later learning and cognitive factors, such as beliefs and expectations about the role of men and women, are influential.

For example, previously experienced sexual behaviours often form the basis of present sexual fantasy. Sue (1979) found that 43% of male and 41% of female college students had fantasized about a former lover during intercourse with a current lover. Also, Griffitt (1975) has produced

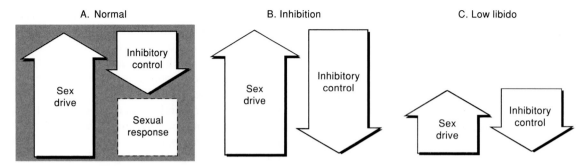

Fig. 2.3 Two models of 'inhibited sexual desire' based on the relative strengths of positive drive (libido) and inhibitory forces (guilt, fear, anxiety, etc.). Different treatments would be required for these different types of sexual dysfunction. (From Wilson & Nias 1976)

evidence that prior experience of a sexual act is linked with heightened arousal to imagery depicting that act. In the latter case, of course, the direction of cause and effect is questionable, but it is nevertheless reasonable to suppose that sexual experiences can modify our future responsiveness to reminiscent situations and partners.

It has often been speculated by clinicians that traumatic or unsatisfactory relations with parents and caretakers in childhood, and unfortunate encounters with female partners during the formative (especially pubescent) years, may be responsible for inadequate functioning or even distortions of sex targets in later life (Stoller 1976). Thus the psychoanalysts attribute homosexuality to 'castration anxiety' which might arise in early childhood as a result of exposure to an over-dominant mother and become exaggerated by 'castrating' experiences with threatening women in adulthood. Although scientific evidence to support such ideas has been elusive, there are laboratory studies which show that 'self-talk' (as suggested by an experimenter) can alter sexual responsiveness to erotica (Dekker & Everaerd 1989). If the things that experimenters tell us to concentrate on can alter our sexual arousal, then it is likely that the things we tell ourselves (based on past experience) will be at least equally influential.

An interesting experimental demonstration of the effects of ego-deflation was reported by La Torre (1980). Male students were asked to choose females they would like to date out of a selection of photographs. They were then repeatedly given feedback either to the effect that they had been rejected by these women (failure) or that those

potential partners were keen to meet them (success). These decisions on the part of the women were supposedly based on reciprocally viewing photographs and hearing biographical descriptions of the male students. Subsequent testing using a variety of visual stimuli ranging from images of complete women to impersonal approximations, such as parts of the body, shoes and underwear, revealed the beginnings of a fetishistic tendency in the 'unsuccessful' males who believed that women found them unattractive. The rejected men were becoming more responsive to the 'partial' women pictures than to the complete women.

Such a finding is consistent with the work of Gosselin & Wilson (1980) showing that most types of deviant men are shy and introverted, as well as the clinical picture of fetishists as being sexually inexperienced and frequently suffering from socially stigmatizing conditions such as psoriasis, dermatitis or epilepsy (Chalkley & Powell 1983).

It was noted earlier that conditioning can influence responsiveness to erotic stimuli. This applies not only to the classical (Pavlovian) conditioning paradigm described above, but also to operant conditioning, which is concerned not with the juxtaposition of stimuli, but with the relationship between some behaviour and its consequences (rewarding or punishing). This is especially true when biofeedback of sexual arousal is provided by penis plethysmograph or some such device (see Dekker & Everaerd 1989, for a review of such studies). There are several studies showing that erections may be voluntarily facilitated or inhibited, presumably by self-manipulation of internal imagery, and that biofeedback (allowing subjects to monitor their sexual arousal) can assist in the gaining of voluntary control.

Perhaps the most interesting study using the conditioning paradigm is that of Kantorowitz (1978). Eight men were asked to masturbate to orgasm in each of eight sessions while different erotic slides were paired with the plateau, resolution and refractory phases of the sexual response cycle as described by Masters & Johnson 1966 (see Fig. 2.4). Slides presented in the preorgasmic (plateau) phase showed gains in arousability (i.e., they were subsequently more exciting) while those seen after orgasm (the refractory phase) showed a loss of erotic stimulation value.

In human terms, this effect might help to explain why men are more excited by women with whom they have not yet had sex. It might also suggest that the man who turns away from his partner immediately after sex may even be doing her a favour (as well as himself) by avoiding a conditioned loss of interest in her physical appearance. Of course, the same effect might apply to women as regards their attraction to men, but the study does not seem to have been replicated across gender.

In passing, we might note that Kantorowitz also observed personality differences in the ease with which positive and negative conditioning occurred. Extroverts were more strongly conditioned in the preorgasmic (positive) phase while introverts were more prone to the deconditioning effect after orgasm. This is consistent with the fact that introverts generally encounter more sexual difficulties of an inhibitory nature (e.g., impotence and diminished desire — see Wilson 1981b).

HABITUATION AND NOVELTY

One of the striking effects observed in laboratory studies of erotic arousal is the tendency for repeated exposure to the same erotic stimulus to evoke progressively less arousal (O'Donohue & Geer 1985). This is commonly referred to as *habituation*, and it implies that novelty is a major requirement of sexual arousal. In this sense, sexual arousal to erotic stimuli is more than a knee-jerk reflex — an image that begins as highly exciting soon loses its capacity to arouse.

This novelty need extends to sex partners as well. Laboratory animals tire of the same partner but rates of intercourse are quickly restored if a fresh partner is supplied (Michael & Zumpe 1978). This is referred to as the 'Coolidge Effect' after the well-known story about the visit of President and Mrs Coolidge to a Government farm, in which Mrs Coolidge is greatly impressed by the rooster's prowess before being told that his performance figure of 'dozens of times a day' was with a different hen each time (Bermant 1976). Farm animals, such as bulls and rams, have a notorious preference for novel females (Fig. 2.5) and the 'Don Juan syndrome' is well-recognized in the human male.

Although women also find the idea of novel partners exciting (see, for example, Fisher & Byrne 1978) men typically place more emphasis

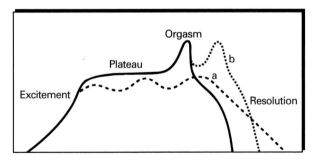

Fig. 2.4 Diagrammatic representation of human sexual response cycles. The solid line is the typical male pattern, which is also quite common in females. The dotted lines show two fairly common female variants: failure of orgasm (**a**) and multiple orgasm (**b**). (From Wilson & Nias 1976)

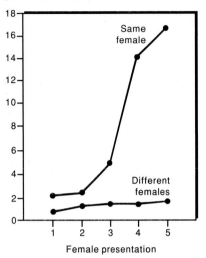

Fig. 2.5 A demonstration of the Coolidge Effect in sheep. Rams introduced to the same female time after time show progressively retarded ejaculation. This does not happen if a fresh female is supplied on each occasion. (Modified from Beamer, Bermant & Clegg 1969)

on partner novelty. This, too, is just what would be predicted on the basis of evolutionary theory. Males can benefit genetically from multiple partners because they have the capacity to impregnate many females in parallel. Females have greater interest in retaining the continued help of the male they have chosen to impregnate them. Once again, the difference between men and women is not absolute, but about twice as many men as women express a desire for more different partners to idealize their sex lives (Wilson 1989; Table 2.2).

There is a possibility that habituation explains the incest avoidance behaviour of advanced mammals, since studies of captive primates, as

Table 2.2 Male/female differences in what constitutes an ideal sex life.

		%Males		%Females	
	Age	<30	>30	<30	>30
Not getting enough sex at the moment		55	56	41	41
If not enough, ideal would be:					
More sex with spouse or steady partner		37	38	62	63
More exciting variations with partner		34	38	24	26
More different partners		38	37	20	18

(From Wilson 1989)

well as humans in the Israeli kibbutzim, indicate that individuals avoid sexual contact with others with whom they have been raised in close proximity, regardless of whether they are genetically related. In other words, incest avoidance behaviour occurs not because of genetic recognition or fear of punishment (although the latter may also be involved) but primarily as a result of the process of 'familiarity breeds contempt'. Close family members reared apart often experience powerful sexual attraction, whereas those who have spent most of their lives together are sexually disinterested. This being the case, the sexual indifference that frequently develops between married couples may be construed as a special case of incest avoidance. Alternatively, both may be attributed to the habituation of sexual drive with continuous exposure.

Marriage guidance counsellors see many couples whose sex life has virtually ceased and they often try to interpret this in terms of psychological conflict between the couple, with interpersonal bitterness actively impeding the sexual relationship. While there may be some truth in this position, and indeed it may be the only positive way to proceed with therapy, the real source of the problem may well be simply a loss of sexual passion due to over-familiarity. Similarly, sex therapists see many men suffering from 'impotence' that, whether recognized or not by the patient, is specific to their wife or long-term partner. Though it may be unethical or unacceptable to test the hypothesis by promoting affairs, their potential functioning with novel, young women may be totally unimpaired. Again, it may be clinically convenient to work on the assumption that 'unconscious hostilities' within the relationship, or some such positive inhibition, are responsible, but simple habituation may be a much more significant factor.

While the importance of novelty to sexual arousal is well documented scientifically, and generally fairly widely appreciated by lay people if not always the clinical professionals, it remains something of a theoretical challenge. Novelty effects on what psychologists call the *orienting response* (a constellation of physiological indicators of alertness and anxiety which seem to reflect the animal's attempt to assess the survival threat of new stimuli) are reasonably understandable in terms of a 'comparator' in the hippocampus which progressively reclassifies a familiar stimulus as non-threatening (Gray 1982). But it is rather more difficult to conceive of the brain processes that are required to mediate sexual habituation (though exist they must).

The problem is that we have, on the one hand, a positive blueprint or 'prototype' for arousal set by innate releasing mechanisms and imprinting-type processes in early childhood, and on the other, a program for ensuring that any one exemplar of the prototype progressively loses its power to excite. The masochist, for example, can never be satisfied with one particular picture of a woman with boots and whip; he needs a continuing supply of slight variations on that theme. For the fetishist, no one pair of shoes will do; constantly changing details within the same basic framework are required. And for the majority of 'normal' men, no one nude picture (or particular partner) can offer life-long optimal stimulation; some degree of wanderlust seems inevitable. Changing clothes, sexual positions, venues for intercourse, diminished lighting, etc., all assist in the novelty search, but are in a sense substitutes for the 'real thing', which in evolutionary terms is nothing less than a change of partner. The evolutionary significance of such a pattern is clear (the 'reproductive imperative' once again prompting relative promiscuity in males in order to maximize gene distribution) but its physiological mechanism remains mysterious.

The interesting theoretical question arises: what if a particular partner and the activities which she enjoyed happened to correspond precisely to the optimal blueprint we have been discussing? Would this be true love? Would the novelty mechanism cease to function? Presumably such an event would be statistically very unlikely, but might be approached closely every so often. Indeed, monogamous, swan-like attachments in human couples do sometimes occur and might be explained in these terms. This would presume that the constant need for novelty occurs only because each concrete exemplar departs from the blueprint in some respect so as to generate instability.

It seems more likely, however, that novelty per

se has excitement value and that something akin to the orienting response or even the 'fight/flight' emergency system is responsible. There is some evidence that threat can contribute to sexual arousal (hence masochism, wartime romances and the extra spice that illegitimacy often seems to bestow on a relationship). Indeed, novelty is psychophysiologically very much akin to threat; novel stimuli are treated as dangerous by the 'behavioural inhibition system' of the brain until proved otherwise (Gray 1982). Thus novel partners may 'turn us on' partly because they frighten us to some extent.

SYMPATHETIC EXCITATION AND SEXUAL AROUSAL

Zillmann (1986) notes that sexual arousal shares with the extreme emotions of anger and fear an element of sympathetic dominance of the autonomic nervous system, and is thus closely related to the emergency/survival system. He maintains that this assessment is valid even though there are some parasympathetic components to sexual capacity (notably vasocongestion of the genitals). Hence Zillmann refers to the 'fight-flight-coition trichotomy' as a group of comparable hypersympathetic states.

The association among these three emotions is confirmed at several levels. Brain research reveals interconnections in the limbic system such that excitation of amygdaloid structures (thought to control fight and flight) often spill over into septal structures (believed to control sexual behaviour), and vice versa. There are also endocrine links, in that the adrenal cortex secretes androgens that simultaneously potentiate sexual and aggressive behaviours in both men and women. At the behavioural level, erotica produces sympathetic excitation that is virtually indistinguishable from fear and anger in terms of its physiological manifestations. For a more detailed discussion of the central and peripheral psychophysiological associations between sexual and autonomic arousal see Chapter 3.

From these commonalities among fear, anger and sexual arousal, Zillmann proposes that arousal from a prior emotion will facilitate a subsequent emotion in the same group by a process of excitation transfer. There is indeed anecdotal and experimental evidence that fear and anger may promote sexual arousal and activity. For example, male rats subjected to electric shock in the presence of an oestrous female are more likely to copulate than unshocked rats (Caggiula & Eibergen 1969). Similarly, studies with human subjects show that prearousal by fear or anxiety induction can increase sexual responsiveness (e.g. Hoon, Wincze & Hoon 1977; Wolchik et al 1980; Barlow et al 1983) and romantic attraction (Dienstbier 1979). There are, however, gender differences in this respect. Generally speaking, women are more likely to be excited by fear of their mate and men are more likely to be inhibited (Medicus & Hopf 1990) (see Table 2.3).

Research such as this suggests that the attempt to treat sexual dysfunction by relaxation techniques such as desensitization or antianxiety drugs (whether in men or women) may be mistaken in its basic premise that relaxation facilitates sexual arousal. This might explain the repeated clinical failure of such an approach, especially with female patients (Riley & Riley 1986). It is also consistent with the finding that alcohol has a depressing effect upon sexual potency even though it may be socially liberating (Rosen & Beck 1988).

However, it is likely that there are certain types of anxiety that are dysfunctional, at least for certain men. Beck et al (1984) found that although heightened anxiety increased the sexual responsiveness of sexually functional men, the reverse was true with dysfunctional men. For a group of men with sexual difficulties, anxiety seemed to exert an inhibitory influence on penile response. It is also possible that the level of anxiety is critical. Very high levels of anxiety may be more universally inhibitory to sexual arousal.

It is perhaps slightly disturbing that the scientific evidence appears to suggest some possible benefits of antisocial activities such as infidelity

Table 2.3 Effects of fear and aggression on male and female sexual behaviour in many animal species, including humans.

	Fear (of mate)	Aggression (towards mate)
Males	Neutral to inhibit	Neutral to facilitate
Females	Neutral to facilitate	Neutral to inhibit

(Modified from Medicus & Hopf 1990)

and sadomasochism, even rape, identifying them as potential facilitators of sexual excitement in normal men. At this point, the value of sexual satisfaction has to be weighed against other values that we might call moral or civilized. Certainly, extreme forms of coercive sex, such as rape, or dangerous practices, such as self-strangulation, must be deplored even if their motivation may be better understood in the light of the above theory.

Performance demands

A particular form of anxiety or destructive self-talk that is frequently cited by clinicians as a cause of men's sex problems is that of performance stress — a feeling that stud-like prowess is called for and that failure to measure up would be intensely humiliating. This is said to set up a vicious spiral whereby the fear of failure increases the likelihood of actual failure, which in turn increases the failure anxiety on future occasions (Masters & Johnson 1970; Kaplan 1979).

Intuitively, this seems plausible enough and a number of laboratory studies have set out to verify such an effect. Farkas et al (1979) attempted to create differential demand for erection in 32 functional men by telling them that the video they were going to watch either would or would not be sexually arousing. Neither tumescence nor self-reported arousal were affected by these instructions. Lange et al (1981) used a more direct approach, instructing 24 functional men either to become sexually aroused (performance demand condition) or to focus on internal pleasurable sensations (sensate focus) while watching erotic videos. Again, no effect was observed except for a slight tendency toward greater arousal in the demand condition. Heiman & Rowland (1983) replicated this study but added a group of dysfunctional men, in whom the reverse (a decrease in penile response) was found.

Perhaps the most interesting study in this area is that of Barlow et al (1983) who induced performance demand by threatening electric shock if insufficient erectile arousal was not achieved while viewing erotic films. This yielded greater tumescence in a group of normal men than did a nonshock control condition. However, a non-contingent threat of shock produced the same increase in tumescence (c.f. discussion of excitation transfer).

Such findings suggest that performance demand is not an inhibitory factor in its own right, though it may become so after an experience of failure in the manner suggested by Masters & Johnson and other sex therapists. In other words, performance demand is inhibitory to actual performance only when it is accompanied by an expectation of failure. It is also likely that individual differences are important; as suggested earlier, neurotic introverts are probably more prone to inhibitory effects.

A similar conclusion concerning the selective effect of performance demand was provided by Beck et al (1983), who studied the effects of varied levels of perceived partner arousal on the extent to which men were sexually aroused by erotic videos. When the stimulus partner was perceived as highly aroused, dysfunctional men showed *lower* tumescence, while functional men showed *increased* responsiveness. Post-experimental interviews confirmed that, in real life, functional men were more 'turned on' by an aroused partner, while dysfunctional men felt this increased the pressure on them to perform. Thus it appears that performance demand is detrimental to the sexual performance only of men who have already had sexual difficulties; functional men are either unaffected or prompted to greater achievement.

DOMINANCE AND SELF-ESTEEM

This discussion leads naturally to an important prerequisite of male sexual functioning, which is a sense of power, competence and self-esteem, whether related to the female partner or the environment in general. The natural order in most mammals appears to be one of intense inter-male competition, with the dominant males gaining reproductive privileges and submissive (unsuccessful) males being relegated to the sexual wilderness. In most primates, including humans, the top 20% of males enjoy 80% of the copulations (Wilson 1989). To a large extent this is mediated by female choice (Henry Kissinger is among those to observe that 'power is the ultimate aphrodisiac') but males who triumph in competition,

sports events or battle are apparently prepared to capitalize sexually upon their conquest by changes in brain chemistry that are linked with changes in sex hormones (Rose et al 1975).

At the opposite end of triumph is depression, which may occur as a result of repeated experiences of failure and helplessness. A rapid fall in social status (equivalent to loss of position in an animal dominance hierarchy) is often observed to be a precursor of depressive illness and loss of libido is a well-documented symptom of depression. This withdrawal from competition might function to protect a defeated male from total annihilation, so that he lives to fight another day.

Thus for effective sexual functioning a man requires a sense of social potency; he needs to feel 'on top' and 'good about himself'. In contrast, submission is more likely to facilitate the sexual responsiveness of a woman; females seldom show courtship behaviour toward males over whom they are dominant (Eibl-Eibesfeldt 1990). Treatment programmes for male impotence might therefore usefully include elements of assertiveness training and focus on rebuilding feelings of worth, competence and efficacy in much the same way as do modern behavioural treatments for depression.

SUMMARY

Male sexual arousal typically displays the following characteristics:

1. Images of an ideal 'target' are generated as a result of innate guidelines and early childhood imprinting processes. Whether normal or deviant, these are difficult to alter and may be called up as fantasies to assist in arousal during adult intercourse. Visual elements predominate (especially including aspects such as pink, round, black, hairy) but pheromones and other sensory qualities are also involved.
2. Conditioning, learning and cognitive factors such as expectations of success/failure and feelings of self-esteem have some capacity to enhance or inhibit sexual functioning from early childhood through to adult life. One of the most important of these is the feeling of social dominance, competence or ego-security. Some measure of perceived 'adequacy', and

perhaps even dominance over the partner, is essential to male arousal.

3. Novelty and youthfulness in the partner are major factors determining the ease with which sexual arousal occurs. Romantic love is seldom a prerequisite for male arousal and over-familiarity with a particular partner commonly leads to habituation (progressive loss of sexual excitement). This almost inevitably leads to strains within long-term marriage.

4. Threat or anxiety are not necessarily antithetical to male sexual arousal, and may even enhance arousal in normal men by a process of excitement transfer. This may explain the special attraction of illicit sex as well as the popularity of sadomasochistic images and behaviours such as pain, bondage and humiliation. However, performance anxiety, combined with an expectation of likely failure, constitutes a special type of anxiety that is inhibitory in men with a history of dysfunction, and there are important individual differences in the effects of anxiety upon arousal.

Some treatment programmes in the past have been unrealistic in ignoring the above characteristics of 'normal' male functioning in favour of social myths, such as gender identity and natural monogamy, and medical myths, such as the universal destructiveness of anxiety and the pathology of 'deviant' sources of arousal. Open-minded therapists have much to learn from pornographers and the streetwise and may usefully develop techniques for reconciling fantasies with reality as far as this is practical. At the same time, those who recommend radical changes in lifestyle, such as divorce, 'swinging' or surrogate partners, have to be aware of the enormous ethical responsibility they assume.

REFERENCES

Barlow D H, Sakheim D K, Beck J G 1983 Anxiety increases sexual arousal. Journal of Abnormal Psychology 92: 49–54

Bateson P 1981 Control of sensitivity to the environment during development. In: Immelmann K, Barlow G W, Petrinovitch L, Main M (eds) Behavioural development. Cambridge University Press, Cambridge, Mass.

Beamer W, Bermant G, Clegg M 1969 Copulatory behaviour of the ram. Ovis Aires II: Factors affecting copulatory satiation. Animal Behaviour 17: 706–711

Beck J G, Barlow, D H, Sakheim D K 1983 The effects of attentional focus and partner arousal on sexual responding in functional and dysfunctional men. Behaviour Research and Therapy 21: 1–8

Beck J G, Barlow D H, Sakheim D K, Abrahamson D J 1984 Sexual responding during anxiety: clinical and non-clinical patterns. Paper presented at annual meeting of the Association for Advancement of Behaviour Therapy, Philadelphia

Bermant G 1976 Sexual behaviour: hard times with the Coolidge Effect. In: Siegel M H, Zeigler H P (eds) Psychological research: the inside story. Harper & Row, New York

Caggiula A R, Eibergen R 1969 Copulation of virgin male rats evoked by painful peripheral stimuli. Journal of Comparative and Physiological Psychology 69: 414–419

Chalkley A J, Powell G E 1983 The clinical description of forty-eight cases of sexual fetishism. British Journal of Psychiatry 142: 292–295

Dekker J, Everaerd W 1989 Psychological determinants of sexual arousal: a review. Behaviour Research and Therapy 27: 353–364

Dienstbier R A 1979 Emotion-attribution theory: establishing roots and exploring future perspectives. In:

Howe H E, Dienstbier R A (eds) Nebraska Symposium on Motivation 26: 227–306 University of Nebraska Press, Lincoln

Eibl-Eibesfeldt I 1990 Dominance, submisson and love: sexual pathologies from the prespective of ethology. In: Feierman J R (ed) Pedophilia: biosocial dimensions. Springer-Verlag, New York

Ellis L, Ames M A 1987 Neurohormonal functioning and sexual orientation: a theory of homosexuality-heterosexuality. Psychological Bulletin 101: 223–258

Eysenck H J 1976 Sex and personality. Open Books, London

Farkas G M, Sine L F, Evans I M 1979 The effects of distraction, performance demand, stimulus explicitness and personality on objective and subjective measures of male sexual arousal. Behaviour Research and Therapy 17: 25–32

Fisher W A, Byrne D 1978 Sex differences in response to erotica: love versus lust. Journal of Personality and Social Psychology 36: 117–125

Flor-Henry P 1987 Cerebral aspects of sexual deviation. In: Wilson G D (ed) Variant sexuality: research and theory. Johns Hopkins University Press, Baltimore

Gillan P, Frith C 1979 Male-female differences in response to erotica. In: Cook M, Wilson G D (eds) Love and attraction: an international conference. Pergamon Press, Oxford

Gosselin C C, Wilson G D 1980 Sexual variations: fetishism transvestism and sadomasochism. Faber & Faber, London

Gray J A 1982 The neuropsychology of anxiety: an enquiry into the functions of the septo-hippocampal system. Oxford University Press, New York

Griffitt W 1975 Sexual experience and sexual responsiveness: sex differences. Archives of Sexual Behaviour 4: 529–540

Heiman J R, Rowland D L 1983 Affective and physiological sexual response patterns: the effects of instructions on sexually functional and dysfunctional men. Journal of Psychosomatic Research 27: 105–116

Hoon P W, Wincze J P, Hoon E 1977 A test of reciprocal inhibition theory: are anxiety and arousal in women mutually inhibitory? Journal of Abnormal Psychology 86: 65–74

Kantorowitz D A 1978 An experimental investigation of preorgasmic reconditioning and postorgasmic deconditioning. Journal of Applied Behavioural Analysis 11: 23–34

Kaplan H S 1979 Disorders of sexual desire. Brunner/Mazel, New York

Kolarsky A, Freund K, Machet J, Polak O 1967 Male sexual deviation: association with early temporal lobe damage. Archives of General Psychiatry 17: 735–743

Lange J D, Wincze J P. Zwick W, Feldman S, Hughes K 1981 Effect of demand for performance, self-monitoring of arousal and increased sympathetic nervous system activity on male erectile response. Archives of Sexual Behaviour 10: 443–464

La Torre R A 1980 Devaluation of the human love object: heterosexual rejection as a possible antecedent to fetishism. Journal of Abnormal Psychology 89: 295–298

McConaghy N 1970 Penile response conditioning and its relationship to aversion therapy in homosexuals. Behaviour Therapy 1: 213–221

Masters W H, Johnson V E 1966 Human sexual response. Little Brown, Boston

Masters W H, Johnson V E 1970 Human sexual inadequacy. Little Brown, Boston

Medicus G, Hopf S 1990 The psychology of male/female differences in sexual behaviour. In: Feierman J R (ed) Pedophilia: biosocial dimensions. Springer-Verlag, New York

Michael R P, Zumpe D 1978 Potency in male rhesus monkeys: effects of continuously receptive females. Science 200: 451–453

Morris D 1971 Intimate behaviour. Jonathan Cape, London

O'Donohue W T, Geer J H 1985 The habituation of sexual arousal. Archives of Sexual Behaviour 14: 233–246

Rachman S, Hodgson R J 1968 Experimentally induced 'sexual fetishism': a replication and development. Psychological Record 16: 293–296

Riley A J, Riley E J 1986 The effect of single dose diazepam on female sexual response induced by masturbation. Sexual and Marital Therapy 1: 49–53

Rose R M, Bernstein I S, Gordon T P 1975 Consequences of social conflict on plasma testosterone levels in rhesus monkeys. Psychosomatic Medicine 37: 50–61

Rosen R C, Beck J G 1988 Patterns of sexual arousal: psycho-physiological processes and clinical applications. Guilford Press, New York

Schmidt G, Sigusch V Meyberg U 1969 Psychosexual stimulation in men: emotional reactions, changes of sex behaviour and measures of conservative attitudes. Journal of Sex Research 5: 199–217

Stoller R J 1976 Perversion — the erotic form of hatred. Delta Books, New York

Sue D 1979 Erotic fantasies of college students during coitus. Journal of Sex Research 15: 299–305

Symons D 1979 The evolution of human sexuality. Oxford University Press, New York

Trivers R L 1972 Parental investment and sexual selection. In: Campbell B (ed) Sexual selection and the descent of man. Aldine, Chicago

Wickler W 1967 Sociosexual signals and their intra-specific imitation among primates. In: Morris D (ed) Primate ethology. Weidenfeld & Nicolson, London

Wilson G D 1981a Love and instinct. Temple Smith, London

Wilson G D 1981b Personality and sex. In: Lynn R (ed) Dimensions of personality. Pergamon Press, Oxford

Wilson G D 1984 The personality of opera singers. Personality and Individual Differences 5: 195–201

Wilson G D 1987 Variant sexuality: Research and theory. Johns Hopkins University Press, Baltimore

Wilson G D 1989 The great sex divide. Peter Owen, London

Wilson G D, Nias D K B 1976 Love's mysteries: the psychology of sexual attraction. Open Books, London

Wilson G D Barrett P T 1987 Parental characteristics and partner choice: some evidence for Oedipal imprinting. Journal of Biosocial Science 19: 157–161

Wolchik S A, Beggs V E, Wincze J P, Sakheim D K, Barlow D H, Mavissakalian Z 1980 The effect of emotional arousal on subsequent sexual arousal in men. Journal of Abnormal Psychology 89: 595–598

Zillmann D 1986 Coition as emotion. In: Byrne D, Kelley K (eds) Alternative approaches to the study of sexual behaviour. Lawrence Erlbaum Associates, Hillsdale, N J

3. The neuroanatomy and neurophysiology of erection

Michael Murphy

In 1863 Eckhard induced penile erection in the dog by electrically stimulating the pelvic nerves (nervi erigentes). Thirteen years later Nikolsky discovered that the anticholinergic drug, atropine, prevented this effect, suggesting that erection resulted from activation of sacral parasympathetic pathways. In contrast, electrical stimulation of sympathetic pathways was found to cause penile shrinkage, suggesting that the sympathetic system's role was in subsidence (detumescence) of erection (Semans & Langworthy 1938). This suggestion was further supported by the recent discovery that alpha-adrenoceptor blocking drugs (drugs that block some of the effects of the sympathetic nervous system on tissue) induce erection (Brindley 1983).

Taken together, these findings fit into the familiar picture of autonomic control of visceral function, with parasympathetic cholinergic effects being opposed by sympathetic noradrenergic effects. However, this picture has been modified by new and sometimes conflicting findings; the control of erection is more complex. For example, stimulation of sympathetic pathways sometimes appears to cause erection, as well as shrinkage of the penis. In addition, discoveries of new neurotransmitters and neuromodulators acting in autonomic pathways have led to new concepts of autonomic function. For example, it has been shown that small peptides are frequently released from presynaptic fibres along with 'conventional' neurotransmitters, facilitating or inhibiting the action of the latter. In the case of the parasympathetic supply to the penis, one such peptide, vasoactive intestinal polypeptide (VIP), may be more important for erection than acetylcholine (Gu et al 1983; Steers et al 1984; Andersson et al 1984).

It is widely accepted that the vascular events leading to erection are under neural control. However, some of these events are not directly mediated by neuroeffector junctions (the sites at which nerve fibres make chemical contact with muscle fibres, causing them to contract or relax), but involve the release of chemical messengers from non-neural tissue, such as the endothelium (the layer of cells that lines the blood vessels and erectile tissue). However, in the case of the one endothelium-derived relaxing factor (EDRF) identified so far, nitric oxide, its release is still dependent on nerve signals. In this case these are transmitted via parasympathetic fibres.

From a neurophysiological point of view, three peripheral mechanisms are involved in erection: a parasympathetic 'vascular mechanism', a sympathetic 'inhibitory mechanism' and a somatomotor 'muscular mechanism' (Junemann et al 1989a). Each of these is discussed in detail below. The main function of the autonomic nervous system (parasympathetic and sympathetic divisions) is to regulate the tone of the smooth muscle in the arterioles and trabeculae of the penis. This in turn determines the volume of blood in the erectile tissue. Thus, with parasympathetically mediated relaxation of smooth muscle there is dilatation of arterioles and relaxation of the trabecular smooth muscle leading to expansion of the corporal space. The somatomotor 'muscular mechanism' involves activation of striated muscle, the bulbocavernosus and ischiocavernosus muscles, via the pudendal nerve. This is part of the 'voluntary' nervous system, rather than the autonomic nervous system, although it is usually activated reflexly, rather than by will.

In view of recent changes in our understanding

of the autonomic nervous system (ANS) and the importance of these changes to our understanding of erection, the anatomy and physiology of the ANS in general is reviewed at the beginning of this chapter. This is followed by a description of the peripheral nerve supply of the penis, and a discussion of the functional significance of each type of fibre. The neurotransmitters involved in these pathways are briefly discussed (they are discussed more fully in Ch. 5). The subsequent section deals with the central nervous system. We have little information on how the brain influences erection, and what we know is based largely on animal models. Nevertheless, observations made on patients with spinal cord injuries have taught us about the contribution of spinal reflexes and supraspinal influences. Finally, the role of gonadal steroids is discussed. The brain is rich in receptors for these hormones, and they are found in their highest concentration in the medial preoptic area (MPOA), anterior hypothalamic area (AHA) and the hippocampus. Thus, as well as the brain controlling the genitals, the genitals influence the brain through the hormones they produce.

THE AUTONOMIC NERVOUS SYSTEM — GENERAL CONSIDERATIONS

This major subdivision of the nervous system is concerned with the regulation of involuntary visceral activity. It is involved in numerous biological functions, including the control and coordination of digestion, respiration and circulation of the blood. Its control of erection is mainly exerted through its regulatory effect on the tone of the smooth muscle in erectile tissue. Its component parts are situated in the brain, spinal cord and peripheral nervous system. The autonomic nervous system (ANS) also has receptors in the organs and the walls of blood vessels it controls, which relay local information via peripheral nerve fibres (afferent fibres) to the central components of the system. The fibres transmitting information from the brain to the target organ (efferent fibres) have a distinct anatomical organization (c.f. the somatic or voluntary nervous system) consisting of preganglionic and postganglionic neurones. The preganglionic neurone has its cell body in the central nervous system (in the case of the nerve supply to the penis that means the spinal cord) and its axons terminate on postganglionic nerve cells. The postganglionic cells are outside the central nervous system and are grouped together to form autonomic ganglia. Their axons terminate on effector organs, e.g. smooth muscle, which they can either excite or inhibit.

The ANS has two divisions, sympathetic and parasympathetic. This distinction is based on four differences:

1. They originate in different parts of the CNS: the cell bodies of sympathetic preganglionic neurones are in the thoracic and upper lumbar spinal cord (T1–12), while those of the parasympathetic division are in the brain stem and sacral spinal cord (S2–S4). Both types of spinal preganglionic cell are located in the intermediolateral cell column of the cord.
2. Their peripheral ganglia have a different anatomical relationship with the effector organ: sympathetic ganglia are some distance from the effector in the paravertebral chain or prevertebral ganglia, while parasympathetic ganglia are in close proximity to the effector organ (parasympathetic postganglionic cells are often loosely aggregated in smaller groups in the wall of the effector organ).
3. The transmitter released at the effector organ is different: at sympathetic postganglionic neuroeffector junctions this is generally noradrenaline (thus adrenergic), at parasympathetic postganglionic junctions it is usually acetylcholine (thus cholinergic). There are, however, important exceptions to this, e.g. some postganglionic sympathetic fibres are cholinergic, as in the case of the sympathetic pathway for erection (there is some controversy about whether these fibres belong to the sympathetic system — see below). Furthermore, there is increasing evidence of the existence of nonadrenergic, noncholinergic autonomic neurotransmission involving peptides, gamma-aminobutyric acid (GABA) and other substances. Erection is again a case in point: the postganglionic fibres of the parasympathetic erectile pathway involve a nonadrenergic noncholinergic mechanism (Ottsen et al 1984). In some sites these neurotransmitters, or substances that modulate neurotransmission

(neuromodulators), may be released along with the 'classical' neurotransmitter — cotransmission (Lundberg 1981). This may occur in the control of erection when VIP and acetylcholine are coreleased.

4. Sympathetic and parasympathetic divisions usually have opposing effects on the same effector organ. For example, activation of the sympathetic system increases heart rate, while parasympathetic activity slows heart rate. Sympathetic responses tend to be generalized and more sustained, as in the 'fight or flight' response seen in stressful situations. In contrast, parasympathetic responses tend to be localized and brief and are often involved in conservation of bodily energy.

In addition to the peripheral and spinal structures described above, the preganglionic cells of both divisions are subject to facilitatory and inhibitory influences from autonomic centres in the brain stem (via the reticulospinal pathways), hypothalamus and other parts of the brain (see below).

These traditional principles of autonomic organization provide the basic framework for understanding the peripheral control of erection. However, it should be clear from the above discussion that they do not always hold true for erection, having frequently been contradicted by clinical and experimental data. It is worth noting at this stage that although growth of the basic neurosciences has added to our understanding of erection, it has frequently been empirical clinical discoveries which have preceded and instigated work in the neuroscience of erection.

PERIPHERAL NERVE PATHWAYS

Three groups of peripheral nerve fibre play a role in erection. These are classified anatomically as parasympathetic, sympathetic and somatic (sensorimotor). Peripheral nerves supplying the penis (see Fig. 3.1) may contain combinations of these fibres, but particular nerves are predominantly made up of either autonomic or somatic fibres. Thus the pelvic nerves are mainly parasympa-

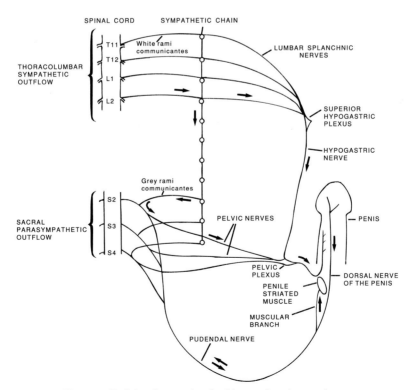

Fig. 3.1 Peripheral nerves involved in erection. Arrows denote direction of neural conduction.

thetic, but receive some sympathetic fibres; the hypogastric nerves contain most of the sympathetic supply to the penis and the pudendal nerve provides the somatic fibres, but contains some autonomic fibres as well.

PARASYMPATHETIC PATHWAYS — ANATOMY

The spinal nuclei for preganglionic neurones involved in this pathway are in the intermediolateral grey matter of the spinal cord at the S2 to S4 level. From these nuclei, axons travel anteriorly and join the axons from the spinal centres involved in bladder and rectal control to form the sacral visceral efferent fibres which emerge in the anterior roots of S2 to S4 (Lue et al 1984). Electrical stimulation of the sacral roots, S2, S3 or S4, may cause erection in men (Habib 1967). In most men S3 is the main source of erectogenic fibres, with a smaller supply coming from either S2 or S4. Only two roots are effective in any one man (Brindley et al 1982).

The preganglionic fibres from the sacral roots cross the medial surface of the levator ani muscles in the pelvic nerves (pelvic splanchnic nerves, nervi erigentes) (Walsh & Donker 1982). These nerves also receive sympathetic fibres from the sacral sympathetic chain ganglia, via the grey rami (Pick & Sheehan 1946). The number of distinct pelvic nerves varies from 3 to 6 between subjects. The pelvic nerves are then joined by fibres from the inferior hypogastric nerves (sympathetic) to form the pelvic plexus (sometimes called the inferior hypogastric plexus) in the pelvic fascia on the lateral side of the rectum, seminal vesicles, prostate and posterior bladder.

Damage to the pelvic plexus is a main cause of erectile dysfunction after pelvic surgery. Because of this, the pelvic plexus and its efferent fibres to the corpora cavernosa (the cavernous nerves) have been the subject of several recent detailed human anatomical studies. Walsh & Donker (1982) traced the autonomic innervation of the corpora cavernosa in stillborn neonates and fetuses. They demonstrated that the important branches of the pelvic plexus were situated between the rectum and urethra, and that they penetrated the urogenital diaphragm near or in the muscular wall of

the urethra. They concluded that impotence following radical retropubic prostatectomy could result from damage to these fibres at two points: during division of the lateral pedicle or during apical dissection when the urethra is transected.

The course of the cavernous nerves from the pelvic plexus to the penis has been further studied in serial sections of the pelvis removed en bloc from cadavers (Lue et al 1984; Lepor et al 1985). They have been traced from ganglia in the pelvic fascia across the posterolateral aspect of the seminal vesicle and prostate to the apex of the gland. Here they are close to the membranous urethra, which they accompany through the urogenital diaphragm. They are then located on the lateral aspect of the membranous urethra, ascending to the 1 and 11 o'clock positions in the proximal bulbous urethra. Some fibres then supply the corpus spongiosum while others enter the penile crura with branches of the pudendal artery and cavernous veins. They innervate both the helicine arteries that supply the corporal space and the trabecular smooth muscle. In addition to being damaged during radical prostatectomy and radical cystectomy, damage to the pelvic plexus and cavernous nerves may occur with abdominoperineal resection of the rectum, transurethral resection of the prostate, external sphincterotomy, internal urethrotomy and prostatic abscess (Lue et al 1984). Rupture of the membranous urethra with pelvic fracture may be followed by neurogenic impotence, but this may also be the result of surgery at a time when anatomical landmarks are obscured by oedema and haemorrhage.

Radical prostatectomy is the most effective treatment for localized prostatic adenocarcinoma, but it has been eschewed in favour of less effective treatments because of the complication of impotence (Lepor et al 1985). However, the precise localization of the microscopic cavernosal nerves and their relations to other structures in the adult male pelvis has led to modifications of surgical technique which spare these nerves and preserve potency (Walsh et al 1983; Brendler et al 1990; Bigg et al 1990).

Parasympathetic supply — neurophysiology

In the pelvic plexus, preganglionic fibres make

synaptic contacts with the postganglionic neurones that innervate the penis. As in other autonomic ganglia, transmission through these small pelvic ganglia is inhibited by drugs that block nicotinic acetylcholine receptors. Parasympathetic postganglionic transmission, however, is not prevented, as it is at other sites in the autonomic nervous system, by muscarinic receptor blockade (atropine). This is presumably because VIP, and not acetylcholine, is the important neurotransmitter (see above).

The effect of parasympathetic neural activity is to increase blood flow through both the corpora cavernosa (cavernosal space) and the corpus spongiosum and glans (spongiosal space). The exact neurotransmitter mechanisms controlling blood flow through each of these spaces may be different: while sacral nerve root stimulation increases blood flow through both spaces, intracavernosal injection of an alpha-blocker causes an increase in cavernosal blood flow without a corresponding increase in spongiosal flow (Brindley 1985). This observation might, however, be due to the technique of injecting the drug into the corpus cavernosum, rather than reflecting a difference in the number of alpha-adrenoceptors in the two structures.

Once the arterial vessels supplying the erectile tissue have dilated during the development of erection they remain so for the duration of the erection (Brindley 1985). Earlier theories that explained the regulation of blood flow into the penis in terms of arteriovenous shunting and the contraction and relaxation of intravascular valves (polsters) have received little support from recent anatomical studies (Aboseif & Lue 1988).

In addition to arterial dilatation, occlusion of the veins draining the penis must occur before erection can be maintained (see Ch. 4). While there is general agreement that dilatation of penile arteries and relaxation of trabecular smooth muscle of the sinusoids are neurally-mediated, there is disagreement about the mechanism of venous occlusion. It is possible that the obstruction to venous outflow during erection is an entirely mechanical effect of raised intracavernosal pressure. It has been shown that venous compression occurs within the corpora cavernosa during full erection, when veins are compressed between the distended sinusoidal walls and the noncompliant tunica albuginea (Lue & Tanagho 1987). On the other hand, it has been argued that outflow resistance is not apparent in an erection artificially maintained by saline infusion, despite high intracavernosal pressure, unless there is also sexual stimulation. This suggests that outflow resistance is under the control of the central nervous system (Brindley 1985).

While the sacral parasympathetic nerves form the efferent pathway for reflex erection, psychogenic erections can still occur after extensive damage to these nerves, demonstrating that another pathway must be involved. This second erectile pathway is formed by fibres from the lower thoracic and upper lumbar roots and belongs to the sympathetic system.

The sympathetic pathways — anatomy

The sympathetic preganglionic fibres to the penis arise from cells in the intermediolateral grey cell column of the upper lumbar and lower thoracic segments of the cord. There is some variation, amongst individuals, in the segmental origin of fibres supplying the penis, but mostly they are from T11 to 12 (see Fig. 3.1).

The organization of the sympathetic outflow to the penis is principally the same as that to other viscera. Preganglionic fibres leave the cord in the ventral roots of the corresponding spinal nerve and then pass via the white rami communicantes to the paravertebral sympathetic chain. Having entered the sympathetic chain, preganglionic fibres behave differently. Some descend to ganglia at a lower lumbar or sacral level and synapse with ganglion cells that project via the pudendal and pelvic nerves to the penis. Others pass through the corresponding chain ganglia without making synaptic contact and travel in lumbar splanchnic nerves to synapse in the ganglia of the superior hypogastric plexus. This plexus lies in front of the bifurcation of the aorta in extraperitoneal connective tissue. Complete lesions of the hypogastric plexus occur during para-aortic lymph node dissection for carcinoma of the testes, but normal erections usually persist (Brindley 1985).

The superior hypogastric plexus divides inferiorly into left and right hypogastric nerves which descend to the two pelvic (inferior hypo-gastric) plexuses. As well as postganglionic fibres, these nerves also contain preganglionic fibres that synapse on cells in the pelvic plexuses. A smaller number of sympathetic postganglionic fibres also reach the pelvic plexuses via the pelvic nerves. As described above, parasympathetic fibres also relay in the pelvic plexus. It has been suggested that penile postganglionic neurones in the plexus might receive excitatory inputs from both para-sympathetic and sympathetic pathways, as occurs in the pelvic ganglia of the cat (de Groat et al 1979). Both sympathetic and parasympathetic fibres travel from the pelvic plexus to the penis in the cavernous nerves, the anatomy of which are discussed above.

The sympathetic pathways — neurophysiology

The sympathetic pathways to the penis are thought by some neurophysiologists to contain both erectile and anti-erectile fibres. This is con-sistent with the observation that stimulation of the superior hypogastric plexus can cause either erec-tion or penile shrinkage (Brindley 1985). Others believe that the erectile effect of hypogastric stimulation may not be the result of sympathetic excitation, but rather result from stimulation of parasympathetic fibres which join the hypogastric plexus from the sacral outflow (Junemann et al 1989b). If the sympathetic pathways to the penis are extensively damaged, normal erection usually still occurs (Brindley 1985). Thus, the parasym-pathetic pathway is sufficient for normal erectile function. Seminal emission is lost in sympathetic lesions, but orgasm still occurs.

Junemann et al (1989b) have studied the neuro-physiological role of the sympathetic nervous system by examining the effects of hypogastric (sympatheic) nerve stimulation and cavernous (parasympathetic) nerve stimulation, alone and in combination. Stimulation of the cavernous nerves alone induced full erection. When this was com-bined with stimulation of the hypogastric nerves, however, erection was blocked. Similarly, when erection was established by cavernous nerve stimu-lation, additional hypogastric nerve stimulation caused rapid detumescence (within 15 seconds),

suggesting a direct sympathetic effect on erec-tile tissue. When sympathetic stimulation was stopped and parasympathetic maintained, erec-tion rapidly returned. This is strong evidence that the sympathetic system inhibits erection and causes detumescence.

Somatic nerve pathways and their functional significance

Penile sensory fibres belong to spinal segments S2, S3 and S4 and travel from the penis in the dorsal nerve of the penis which joins the pudendal nerve. The pudendal nerve also supplies the motor innervation of the ischiocavernosus, bulbocav-ernosus (penile muscles) and other pelvic mus-cles. These muscles are thought to play a role in achieving rigidity of the erect penis (see below).

The pudendal nerve leaves the pelvis through the lower part of the greater sciatic foramen and enters the gluteal region close to the ischial spine, on the medial side of the internal pudendal ves-sels. It then travels through the lesser sciatic foramen into the pudendal canal with the internal pudendal artery. After giving off the inferior rectal nerve, it divides into the perineal nerve and the dorsal nerve of the penis. The perineal nerve has muscular branches that supply the perineal mus-cles, sphincter urethrae and part of the external sphincter, and a branch which supplies the corpus spongiosum.

The dorsal nerve of the penis runs along the ramus of the ischium and along the inferior ramus of the pubis with the pudendal artery on the deep surface of the urogenital diaphragm. It gives a branch to the corpus cavernosum and then travels with the dorsal artery of the penis and ends in the glans. This nerve is vulnerable to trauma in pelvic fracture.

Functional significance

The dorsal nerve of the penis transmits sensory information from the glans, prepuce, frenulum and skin of the shaft, as well as from the corpora. Its fibres thus form the afferent pathway for reflex erection (discussed below). Sensory fibres are of the A-delta or C-type, and most end in free nerve endings, rather than in corpuscles (Halata & Munger 1986).

The motor neurone cells of the pudendal nerve form a ventrolateral group in the anterior grey column of the cord known as 'the nucleus of Onufrowicz' or Onuf's nucleus. The axons of these motor neurones supply striated muscles of the penis (bulbocavernosus and ischiocavernosus) and perineum. The nucleus has not received much attention in man. However, there is a comparable structure in the rat, the spinal nucleus of the bulbocavernosus (SNB), which has attracted interest. The SNB of the male rat contains the motor neurones innervating the penile striated muscles (bulbocavernosus and ischiocavernosus). In females it is much smaller or undetectable; in other words the SNB shows sexual dimorphism (Breedlove & Arnold 1980). The development of this nucleus depends on exposure to the hormone testosterone or its androgenic metabolites in early life, and it will develop in female animals after a single injection of testosterone in the neonatal period (Breedlove et al 1982). In the adult rat, the motor neurones of the SNB accumulate androgens. Androgens facilitate penile reflexes (involved in copulation), which in turn involve contraction of the bulbocavernosus muscle (Hart 1967, 1979; Hart & Melese-D'Hospital 1983). It seems likely, therefore, that the hormone-sensitive SNB is a site at which androgens influence copulatory behaviour in male rats.

In man, the functional significance of this somatomotor system in erection is unclear. Contractions of the penile muscles clearly play a role in the so-called 'rigid erection phase' (Aboseif & Lue 1988). This term refers to one of six haemodynamic phases seen during the development and loss of an erection. These six phases are as follows:

1. flaccid phase;
2. latent (filling) phase, with increased blood flow but no change in intracavernous pressure;
3. tumescent phase, when intracavernous pressure rises;
4. full erection phase, when intracavernous pressure is just below systolic blood pressure;
5. rigid erection (skeletal) phase, when there is a further rise in intracavernous pressure with skeletal muscle contraction;
6. detumescent phase.

Full erection results from activation of the autonomic mechanisms described above. Electrical stimulation of the cavernous nerves causes full erection, without complete rigidity (Junemann et al 1989b). Rigid erection is the result of somatic efferent impulses in the pudendal nerve causing contraction of the ischiocavernosus muscles which compress the proximal ends of the corpora cavernosa, causing the intracavernosal pressure to rise above that of the systolic blood pressure, giving greater rigidity to the penis. These periods of increased rigidity are brief and are readily observed as small rhythmic movements of the penis. It has been suggested that rigid erection occurs during sexual activity when tactile stimulation of the penis triggers the 'bulbocavernosus reflex' (Aboseif & Lue 1988). This is a spinal reflex, and is more accurately called the glandipudendal reflex since its receptive field is the glans, and the responding muscles, including the bulbocavernosus and the ischiocavernosus, are supplied by the pudendal nerve (Brindley & Gillan 1982).

While such a reflex response might facilitate penetration, it is not essential for potency. On the other hand, absence of the glandipudendal reflex has been found in association with anorgasmia in men and women (Brindley & Gillan 1982). The reflex is sometimes useful in the neurological assessment of patients with impotence, when its absence suggests a lower motor neurone lesion involving sacral segments 2, 3 and 4. It is assessed by palpating the perineum or anus for contraction and compressing the glans. However, it is clinically detectable in only 70% of normal men and thus its presence is more useful in excluding lower motor neurone lesions than its absence is for a positive diagnosis.

In some men contraction of the penile muscles occurs prior to the rigid erection phase. Around 25% of men tested in a laboratory showed rhythmic contractions from the onset of tumescence. Most were aware of these and able to inhibit them. Similarly, many men voluntarily contract these muscles to create a pump action and facilitate erection, although it is not known whether this has its intended effect (Bancroft 1989). These contractions are also seen with sleep-related erections. In an electromyographic study of bulbocavernosus and ischiocavernosus muscle activity during sleep, bursts of activity in the muscles slightly preceded and accompanied penile pulsations, after which there was usually a slight increase in penile circumference. This led Karacan et al (1983) to suggest that muscle contractions sporadically pump blood into the penis to assist in the initiation and maintenance of erection.

In animals, the dorsal nerve of the penis contains autonomic efferents in addition to somatic fibres. It has been suggested that this may also be true of man (de Groat & Steers 1988). Such autonomic efferents may modulate the sensitivity of cutaneous sensory receptors (Johnson et al 1986). This hypothesis might help to explain why idazoxan, an alpha$_2$-adrenoceptor antagonist, enhances penile sensation and the erectile response to tactile stimuli (see Ch. 5).

NEUROCHEMICAL CONTROL OF PENILE TUMESCENCE

Cholinergic mechanisms

Since Nikolsky demonstrated that atropine prevented electrically stimulated erection in the dog, numerous experiments on the effects of acetylcholine and atropine have been published. The results of these are at odds with one another. Some investigators have found that atropine partially inhibits erection from nerve stimulation in dogs and rabbits (Sjorstrand & Klinge 1979; Andersson et al 1984), but others have found no effect (Dorr & Brody 1967; Henderson & Roepke 1933). In a study of normal male volunteers, atropine had no effect on erection induced by erotic films or mechanical vibration (Wagner & Brindley 1980). Furthermore, intracavernosal injection of atropine does not inhibit erection (Brindley 1986).

Studies of acetylcholine's effect in vivo on a variety of species have also been contradictory. Injection of acetylcholine intravenously or into the aorta and penile artery has no erectile effect, but a partial response to intracavernosal acetylcholine has been reported (Andersson et al 1987). In man, intracavernosal neostigmine (a cholinergic agent) also has no effect (Brindley 1986). These findings suggest that many textbooks and clinical reports have overemphasized the significance of muscarinic transmission in the physiology of erection, and that anticholinergic drug effects have been wrongly implicated in cases of impotence.

Despite the above findings, it is evident from studies using a variety of techniques that cholinergic neurotransmission occurs in the human corpus cavernosum (Polak et al 1981; Gu et al 1983; Lincoln et al 1987; Dail & Hamill 1989). A recent hypothesis is that cholinergic nerves, rather than having a direct effect on the corpus cavernosum, modulate other neuroeffector systems (Saenz de Tejada et al 1988). Muscarinic receptors on noradrenergic nerve terminals have been identified in other autonomic pathways (Burnstock 1986; Hedlund et al 1984). Their activation inhibits the release of noradrenaline. There is evidence of this type of interaction in the penis: atropine enhances adrenergically induced sinusoidal muscle contraction in vitro (Saenz de Tejada et al 1988). In addition to inhibiting adrenergic control of smooth muscle tone, cholinergic modulation of peptidergically mediated relaxation of sinusoidal muscle may also occur (Fig. 5.1).

There is also evidence of the converse: alpha$_2$-adrenoceptors have been identified on cholinergic nerve terminals (Steers et al 1984; Hedlund & Andersson 1985).

A further mechanism through which cholinergic transmission facilitates erection involves the release of a factor from arterial and cavernosal endothelium; this is discussed below.

Adrenergic mechanisms

The simple technique of injecting drugs into the corpus cavernosum has demonstrated the importance of adrenergic mechanisms in erection. Injection of the alpha-blockers, phenoxybenzamine and phentolamine, causes erection; while the alpha-agonist, metaraminol, causes shrinkage of both the erect and flaccid penis (Brindley 1983a, 1983b, 1984a, 1986). Neither a beta-blocker (propranolol) nor a selective alpha$_2$-antagonist (idazoxan) have effects when given by this route (Brindley 1986). These findings suggest that the tone of the trabecular smooth muscle in the flaccid penis is maintained by continuous alpha$_1$-adrenoceptor stimulation.

Beta-adrenoceptors that mediate smooth muscle relaxation are present in the corpus cavernosum, but they appear to be of little physiological significance (Hedlund & Andersson 1985). However, beta-blockers, especially propranolol, can induce impotence. The mechanism is not known (see Ch. 5).

The alpha$_2$-adrenoreceptor antagonist, yohimbine, is reported to be effective in the treatment of impotence, but the sites and mechanism of its action are unknown (see Ch. 9). Idazoxan, a more potent and selective alpha$_2$-adrenoreceptor antagonist, has no effect on penile tumescence per se, but enhances penile sensation and responsiveness to tactile stimuli in normal men (see Ch. 5, p. 60).

Peptidergic mechanisms

Stimulation of autonomic nerves causes relaxation of human corpus cavernosal muscle in spite of cholinergic and adrenergic blockade. This suggests that non-adrenergic, non-cholinergic neurotransmission is important in erection (Hedlund & Andersson 1985; Saenz de Tejada et al 1988). The chemical identity of this neurotransmitter is not clearly established. The nerves innervating the erectile tissue of the penis contain several regulatory peptides. The most favoured candidate for the role of principle neurotransmitter in erection at present is vasoactive intestinal polypeptide (VIP).

VIP is a 28 amino acid peptide with a potent vasodilatory action (Said 1981). VIP-immunoreactive fibres innervate arterial, arteriolar and nonvascular smooth muscle in penile erectile tissue (Polak et al 1981; Gu et al 1983). Gu et al (1984) have compared erectile tissue obtained during surgery for impotence with tissue from men with normal erectile function, undergoing gender reassignment operations. They found that almost all the impotent men had fewer VIP nerves than controls, regardless of the cause of impotence, suggesting that loss may be secondary to other causes. The lack of VIP nerves was most obvious where impotence was severe or of long duration. This neuronal depletion was, however, not specific to VIP fibres and may have been part of a more generalized loss of neural elements in the penis. Nevertheless, most of the fibres related to blood vessels contain VIP immunoreactivity.

VIP fibres follow the same anatomical course as cholinergic fibres and ultrastructural examination

of human penile tissue shows that VIP containing vesicles are colocalized with other vesicles that probably contain acetylcholine (Polak et al 1981; Steers et al 1984; Gu et al 1983). In the rat, VIP has been identified in pelvic ganglion cell bodies that have cholinergic projections to the penis (Dail et al 1986).

VIP is found in sympathetic as well as parasympathetic postganglionic fibres at various sites in the autonomic nervous system where there is again evidence that it is a cotransmitter with acetylcholine (Lundberg 1981; Burnstock 1986). Although the above observations are consistent with VIP having a neurotransmitter function, it is not a proven neurotransmitter.

Elevated concentrations of VIP have been found in penile venous blood during erection in men (Virag et al 1982); VIP relaxes adrenergically contracted cavernosal smooth muscle in vitro (Steers et al 1984; Hedlund 1985; Adaikan et al 1986) and has caused slight tumescence in vivo (Ottsen et al 1984).

Several other peptides have been identified in cavernous nerve fibres; substance P and neuropeptide Y (NPY) may prove to have physiological roles (Gu et al 1983; Adrian et al 1984; Wespes et al 1989). Like VIP, substance P has an inhibitory effect on cavernosal muscle, but is found in smaller concentrations and is localized mainly in nerves around the corpuscular receptors beneath the epithelium of the glans penis, rather than in relation to vascular or trabecular smooth muscle (Gu et al 1983). NPY has both direct and indirect vasoconstrictor actions and is found in high concentrations in the penis (Adrian et al 1985). It will no doubt be the focus of future research.

Indirect chemical mechanisms

The vasodilatory effect of acetylcholine has been shown to require the presence of the vascular endothelium, indicating that the relaxation of arterial smooth muscle may not be mediated by muscarinic neuromuscular junctions, but rather by endothelium-derived relaxing factor(s) (EDRF) (Furchgott & Zawadski 1980). Acetylcholine also relaxes contracted strips of human cavernosal smooth muscle in vitro, and there is evidence that this, too, depends on an intact endothelium (Saenz de Tejada et al 1988). Research on the chemical identity of this factor suggests that it is nitric oxide, a vasodilator with an action on intracellular 3', 5'-cyclic guanosine monophosphate, similar to the vasodilatory and erectogenic drug, sodium nitroprusside (Palmer et al 1987). A study of cavernosal tissue from diabetic men with impotence has suggested that impairment of this endothelium-mediated mechanism may partly account for the high prevalence of impotence in this population (Saenz de Tejada et al 1989). There is also a possibility that there is more than one EDRF (Vanhoutte 1987).

Prostaglandins relax cavernosal muscle in vitro (Hedlund & Andersson 1985) and induce erection with intracavernosal injection; these findings are discussed in Chapter 5. Prostacyclin is synthesized under muscarinic control in human cavernosal tissue, suggesting a physiological role for prostaglandins in erection (Jeremy et al 1986).

CENTRAL MECHANISMS

We do not have as clear a picture of the central pathways and mechanisms of erection as we have of the peripheral system. The information we have about central neural control in man comes from observations made in paraplegic subjects and patients who have impaired erection after neurosurgery. Other than this, we have to rely on findings from animal experiments to understand the central organization of the mammalian male sexual response, keeping in mind the likelihood of differences between species.

One difference between studying peripheral nerve mechanisms and brain mechanisms is the difficulty, in the latter, of isolating simple responses, like erection, from the more complex behaviours into which these responses are normally integrated. For example, electrical stimulation at particular sites in the brain of a primate elicits erection, but usually along with other behaviours, such as bearing of fangs. This complex response is typical of the animal's dominance behaviour, rather than sexual behaviour. Thus, the brain structure or pathway identified by this technique may not be relevant to erections that occur in sexual behaviour. Research on the central control of sexual responses, therefore, has to be sensitive to the context in which experimentally induced responses occur. This applies regardless of the technique used, whether it involves neuroanatomical lesions or localized manipulation of monoamine and peptide neurotransmitters.

Reflex and psychogenic erections

A distinction has been made between reflex and psychogenic erections on the basis of the pathways and mechanisms involved. During normal sexual activity, reflex and psychogenic mechanisms interact, but studies of paraplegic patients with lesions at various levels have suggested that the two mechanisms can operate independently (Talbot 1949; Bors & Comarr 1960; Chapelle et al 1980). The validity of the distinction between the two types of erection has been challenged recently (Krane 1986; Wein et al 1986).

Entirely reflex erection can be observed in men with complete spinal cord lesions above the sacral segments. In such men there is obviously no sensation and erection depends on a sacral cord mechanism in isolation from the rest of the central nervous system. In normal men, the receptive field for this reflex is probably the penis only; the erectile inducing effect of tactile stimulation at other sites is likely to be a learnt or 'psychogenic' effect. The receptors for the reflex are concentrated in the glans, frenulum and the corpora cavernosa (Brindley 1985). The afferent pathway is in the dorsal nerve of the penis and the pudendal nerve. Afferent impulses activate spinal interneurons, which in turn activate the parasympathetic preganglionic neurones (S2 and S3).

Erection in response to sexual thoughts only, without tactile stimulation, occurs in most normal men and is called psychogenic. Although this response is psychogenic in the first instance, it seems likely that once an erection is developing, receptors in the penis are stimulated by the tumescence and the reflex mechanism is also activated.

If the sacral cord is damaged, reflex erections disappear, but psychogenic erections still occur. Psychogenic erections occur in men with complete lesions of the cord as high as T12, suggesting that they are mediated by the sympathetic pathway in these men. Psychogenic erections in paraplegic men are usually short-lived, only partial and lack the rigidity needed for coitus; they involve swelling of the corpora cavernosa, but not the corpus spongiosum (Chapelle et al 1980). Reflex erections are characterized by greater rigidity and involve the corpus spongiosum.

Spinal mechanisms and pathways

In addition to the reflex mechanisms controlling erection, the neural systems underlying ejaculation and other elements of sexual behaviour are also integrated at the level of the spinal cord (Beach 1967; Hart 1969). Hart (1967) transected the spinal cords of dogs and found that mechanical stimulation of the penis caused erection, ejaculation, pelvic thrusting, lordosis and leg kicking — characteristics of canine coital behaviour. In addition, he demonstrated that the refractory period (the time after ejaculation for which the animal was sexually unresponsive) had been shortened by the transection. This suggests that the descending influences from the brain inhibit the spinal reflexes after copulation; transection of the cord above the level of these spinal mechanisms freed them from normal inhibitory supraspinal control.

Recent experiments with rats suggest that the brain exerts both excitatory and inhibitory influences on the spinal mechanisms that regulate erections (Sachs & Bitran 1990). Sachs and Bitran examined the effects of spinal block with local anaesthesia on rats that had copulated to sexual satiety. They found that thoracic spinal block did not reverse the complete abolition of reflex erections, establishing that copulation has direct inhibitory effects on the spinal cord's intrinsic system (this was in addition to results suggesting that copulation also acted via the brain to inhibit spinal centres). Their results also suggested that the two variables studied, erection latency (the time taken to induce erection) and production (the number and intensity of erections), were regulated by separate neural systems. For example, they found that, in the sexually rested rat, the net influence of the brain was to inhibit the latency system and excite the production system.

The spinal pathways transmitting information between the brain and spinal mechanisms have still not been clearly identified. A few observations made after spinal neurosurgery have yielded some information. Bilateral anterolateral cordotomy at the upper thoracic level for pain relief is followed by variable effects on sexual function. Most patients become impotent, while others retain erections and ejaculation but loose erotic sensations and orgasm. As touch and two-point discrimination are not affected by this procedure, it seems likely that the erotic quality of genital stimulation depends on ascending fibres that run with the spinothalamic pathways for pain and temperature. This is supported by studies on monkeys in which the anterolateral spinothalamic tracts were electrically stimulated. This induced manipulation of the genitals, erection and ejaculation (de Groat & Steers 1988). The relevant fibres could be traced to the caudal thalamic intralaminar nuclei, which may be the receiving area for erotic genital sensation. Electrical stimulation of these nuclei in humans has been reported to cause erotic feelings and orgasm.

It is difficult to judge from available data whether anterolateral cordotomy also interrupts descending pathways for psychogenic erection. There is evidence from animal experiments of an efferent hypothalamospinal pathway for erection running in the dorsal funiculus of the cord (Swanson 1977; Swanson & Sawchenko 1983).

Cerebral mechanisms

In the early 1960s, MacLean and colleagues set out to establish the cerebral representation of penile erection using a combination of neurophysiological and neuroanatomical methods. Using the squirrel monkey, they explored midline cortical and subcortical structures with electrical stimulation and identified sites at which erection was consistently produced. Positive loci (points in the brain where stimulation elicited erection) were found in the medial frontal lobe, the most strongly positive being in precallosal cingulate gyrus and subcallosal region, and caudal part of the gyrus rectus (the most medial convolution on the ventral surface of the frontal lobe) (Dua & MacLean 1964). Positive loci then followed a course, starting anteriorly (rostrally) from the gyrus rectus into the medial portion of the septum and then into the medial preoptic area (MPOA), a region rostral to and contiguous with the anterior hypothalamic area (see Fig. 3.2).

The medial preoptic area

The MPOA has subsequently been shown in numerous experiments to be a critically important component of the neural circuitry underlying the expression of male copulatory behaviour in mammals. Destruction of the nerve cell bodies of the MPOA by a neurotoxin which spares axons passing through the region seriously disrupts the male animal's ability to copulate (Hansen 1982). The effect of such a lesion is specific to copulatory behaviour (consummatory behaviour) and does not affect sexual appetitive behaviour (sexual motivation).

The neurones of the MPOA also possess receptors for sex steroids, and the integrity of the area is critical for steroid effects on sexual behaviour (Hansen 1982). Beta-endorphin also influences male sexual behaviour by an effect on the MPOA-anterior hypothalamus continuum. As with neurotoxic lesions in this area, beta-endorphin inhibits copulation specifically: sexual motivation and non-sexual consummatory behaviours, such as feeding, remain unaltered (Hughes et al 1987). Beta-endorphin does not have this effect when injected into other brain structures.

Changes in neuronal activity in the MPOA of the male monkey have been shown to coincide with the commencement of sexual behaviour and penile erection (Oomura et al 1988). Other changes in electrical activity are seen at ejaculation, which coincides with the onset of the refractory period. Similarly, changes in the MPOA of female monkeys have been related to the commencement of sexual behaviour. The MPOA is not the only site of altered activity during copulation: increased neuronal activity in the dorsomedial hypothalamic nucleus (DMH) in the male monkey and in the ventromedial hypothalamic nucleus (VMH) in the female monkey have also been recorded (Oomura et al 1988).

Caudal to the MPOA, MacLean found that positive loci followed two separate courses, suggesting two efferent systems for erection. Laterally, positive loci extended into the lateral hypothalamus (LH) where they joined the course of the medial forebrain bundle (MFB) to the ventral tegmentum of the midbrain. It is worth noting that lesions of the MFB disrupt copulatory behaviour in male, but not in female rats (Hitt et al 1970). Also, involvement of the LH in erection is interesting in light of self-stimulation studies showing that animals derive more reward or pleasure from electrical stimulation of this region than any other in the brain. However, many ascending and descending fibres travel through the LH, so the two findings may not be functionally related.

The paraventricular nucleus of the hypothalamus

Another group of positive loci were traced by MacLean and Ploog (1964) into the anteromedial hypothalamus, where they ran into the paraventricular nucleus (PVN) of the hypothalamus. Evidence gathered since MacLean's experiments suggests that the PVN has an important role in integrating autonomic, neuroendocrine and behavioural responses to the environment, including sexual responses. To understand how erection may be integrated with other components of the sexual response at the hypothalamic level, it is necessary to examine the PVN in more detail.

The PVN has two main subdivisions: the magnocellular division, whose axons project to the neurohypophysis (posterior pituitary gland), and the parvocellular division, which has projections to various sites within the central nervous system (brain and spinal cord). The magnocellular division is part of the neuroendocrine system responsible for the secretion of oxytocin, a peptide hormone with well defined physiological roles in lactation and parturition. Recent studies in men have found that oxytocin is released into the circulation during sexual activity (Murphy et al 1987). This implies activation of the magnocellular division of the PVN during coitus. The function of this hormone in sexual activity is unknown; it reaches maximum plasma levels at the time of ejaculation and then rapidly disappears from the circulation. Oxytocin in the circulation may therefore play a role in ejaculation or the refractory period, rather than erection.

However, oxytocin is also synthesized in the parvocellular division of the PVN and is contained in fibres that project from the PVN to the autonomic centres in the spinal cord. These have been anatomically demonstrated by immunohistochemical methods (Swanson 1977; Swanson & Sawchenko 1983) and follow a pathway that overlaps the erectile pathway suggested by MacLean's electrophysiological studies. The oxytocinergic fibres leave the paraventricular nucleus and descend initially through the medial forebrain bundle and continue caudally through the ventral tegmental region, the ventrolateral reticular formation and enter the dorsolateral funiculus of the cord. These fibres run the entire length of the cord supplying oxytocinergic innervation to preganglionic autonomic neurones, both sympathetic and parasympathetic, at all levels. They are unlikely to be involved exclusively in sexual function, and probably have a role in other visceral functions, such as feeding.

It has also been hypothesized, on anatomical evidence, that oxytocinergic fibres from the PVN modulate the processing of nociceptive (pain perception) and thermal information in the spinal cord (Swanson & Sawchenko 1983). As was mentioned above, erotic sensation travels a similar course to pain and temperature and may thus also be modulated by this descending oxytocinergic influence. This could be another aspect of the PVN's role in integrating the neural inputs and outputs underlying the sexual response.

Several of the points made above are speculative, and are made in an effort to pull together different pieces of experimental animal work and construct a model that might have heuristic value in humans. There are, of course, many gaps in our basic data on humans. For example, the release of oxytocin into the circulation during sexual activity in man cannot be taken to imply that there is concurrent central oxytocinergic activity. However, there is evidence in animals that oxytocin release into the blood with coitus is associated with central release (Stoneham et al 1987).

Other evidence that oxytocin plays a role in erection comes from pharmacological studies. Microinjection of oxytocin into the PVN has been shown to elicit erection in the rat (Melis et al 1986), an effect not seen when nearby structures were injected. This effect is thought to be mediated by oxytocin receptors located on cell bodies of oxytocinergic neurones and suggests that there is a positive feedback effect of oxytocin on its own neurones (Swanson & Sawchenko 1983). Dopamine receptor agonists, such as apomorphine, given systemically also induce erection in man and rats via an effect on the brain, probably by acting on the PVN which contains dopaminergic neurones of the incerto-hypothalamic system (Melis et al 1987). There is evidence that these dopaminergic neurones induce erection by activating oxytocinergic neurones (Argiolas et al 1987).

The role of the hippocampus

The hippocampus appears to act in concert with the PVN in erection. MacLean noted that the areas discussed above (septum, MPOA and anterior hypothalamus), as well as positive loci in the anterior and midline thalamus, coincided with the anatomical distribution of hippocampal projections (via the fornix). He also found electroencephalographic evidence of an interaction between the hippocampus and these medial structures during experimentally induced erection. Thus, erection was frequently associated with after-discharges in the hippocampus even though electrical stimulation had been applied in a medial structure, such as the hypothalamus. During this hippocampal activity the erections became throbbing in character and reached their maximal size, often waxing and waning in size for 10 minutes following the after-discharge. When certain diencephalic sites were stimulated, e.g. anterior thalamus, erection followed the termination of stimulation, rather than occurring with it. These rebound erections were concurrent with hippocampal discharges and are evidence of the intimate anatomical and functional organization of the inhibitory and excitatory mechanisms involved.

Other evidence of the link between hippocampus and the PVN in erection is the finding that bilateral microinjection of oxytocin into a specific region in the hippocampus (CA1 field) also causes erection in rats (Melis et al 1986). Specific oxytocin receptors as well as fibres containing oxytocin, almost certainly originating from the PVN, have been identified in the hippocampus (Raggenbass et al 1989). As in the spinal cord, however, oxytocinergic innervation of the hippocampus is involved in functions other than sexual behaviour.

Other sites in the limbic forebrain where electrical stimulation induced erection were identified by MacLean and Ploog (1962). These were thought to belong to two separate neuroanatomical systems: one comprising the mammillary bodies, mammillothalamic tract, anterior thalamic nuclei and cingulate gyrus, the second involving the medial dorsal nucleus of the thalamus and anatomically related structures. There has been little further exploration of these structures in the context of the male sexual response by neuroscientists.

Midbrain and hindbrain

Mapping of midbrain and pontine structures involved in erection suggest that the effector pathway travels from the ventral tegmentum through the substantia nigra. MacLean et al (1962) speculated that three forebrain systems might contribute to the integration of the visceral response of erection (tumescence) with the somatic aspects of sexual behaviour at this level. The three systems are the limbic, extrapyramidal and neocortical outflows (MacLean et al 1963).

Observations in man

Direct study of the human brain is restricted to observations made during neurosurgery. Even then, exploration is restricted by ethical considerations. However, some reports are worth noting. For example, the difference between electrical stimulation of the neocortex and electrical stimulation of the phylogenetically older medial temporal structures. In the case of the neocortex, Penfield & Jasper (1954) observed that stimulation of most parts of the human neocortex has not elicited any responses of a sexual nature. Stimulation of the genital receiving area of the parietal cortex causes contralateral affectively neutral genital sensations, i.e. they do not have an erotic quality. In contrast, stimulation of the amygdala, a limbic structure, can elicit erotic feelings identical to those experienced during intercourse (Gloor 1986). Analogous observations have been made in contrasting the experiences of epileptic patients with parietal lobe foci and those with mediobasal temporal foci (Toone 1986).

There has been a report of impotence in patients following surgery that involved damage to diencephalic brain structures bilaterally (Meyers 1962). The aim of the operation was to alleviate myoclonus by cutting the ansa lenticularis, a bundle of fibres from the globus pallidus to the thalamus. The total impotence that followed is unlikely to have been caused by damage to this structure, but rather from damage caused in gaining access to it. This can be substantiated by the observation that alternative stereotactic procedures for lesioning the ansa do not leave patients impotent. The surgical approach responsible for the impotence involved penetrating the wall of the third ventricle and making a cut through the anterior hypothalamus. This lesion involved 'the dorsomedial hypothalamic nucleus, the adjacent fornix and perifornical gray matter, the posterior septal region and the posterior-inferior aspect of the anterior commissure' (Meyers 1962). Damage to the fornix and perfornical area would include damaging the PVN outflow to the medial forebrain bundle (Everitt BJ — personal communication). As described above, this is a descending pathway for erection in the monkey, and it might therefore be the site of the lesion responsible for impotence in Meyers' cases. Postoperative assessment of these cases supported the idea that the impotence was due to the neural lesion and not secondary to endocrine changes.

These clinical observations suggest that, as in other mammals, the mediobasal temporal lobe and the anterior diencephalon are important CNS structures in the sexual response of man.

Neuroendocrine aspects of erectile function

In animal studies, many elements of mammalian sexual behaviour have been shown to depend on androgens. In man, however, the relationship between sexual behaviour and plasma hormone levels is not a simple correlation. In men with normal gonadal function there is no correlation between circulating testosterone levels and measures of sexual interest, activity or erectile function.

In animals, some elements of sexual behaviour persist for weeks or months after castration, depending on the species. In man, erections may continue for years (Heim 1981). In all mammals,

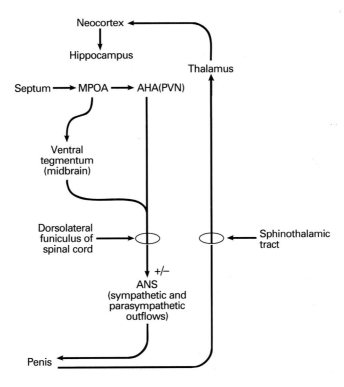

Fig. 3.2 Diagram showing central nervous system structures and pathways likely to be involved in erection. MPOA: medial preoptic area; AHA: anterior hypothalamic area; PVN: paraventricular nucleus of the hypothalamus; MFB: medial forebrain bundle; ANS: autonomic nervous system.

sexual behaviour continues after testosterone and its metabolites have disappeared from the circulation. Likewise, there is a delay before testosterone replacement gradually restores male sexual behaviour after chronic androgen deficiency.

Information about the role of androgens in man comes mainly from studies of hypogonadism and castration. These demonstrate that lack of androgens leads to reduced sexual interest and activity. Effects on erectile funtion are more complex (Kwan et al 1983). For example, one study of hypogonadal men found that erections in response to erotic films were unaffected by androgen withdrawal and replacement (Bancroft & Wu 1983). In contrast, androgens did make a difference to whether or not these men developed erections with sexual fantasy: there were fewer fantasy-induced erections after androgen withdrawal and an increase in fantasy-induced erections with androgen replacement. These findings suggest that

androgens have more effect on the brain systems involved in the cognitive and affective aspects of the sexual response, than they do on the neural mechanisms controlling the vascular mechanism of erection.

However, sleep erections are impaired by androgen withdrawal (Cunningham et al 1982). Furthermore, administering testosterone to normal men increases the rigidity of sleep erections, without affecting their frequency (Carani et al 1990). This suggests that testosterone acts on the motor neurones that supply the striated muscles of the penis, the contraction of which give the erect penis its rigidity (see p. 35).

Testosterone's effects on the expression of male sexual behaviour are mediated at many sites. These include sites in the forebrain, especially the medial preoptic area and anterior hypothalamus, and the spinal cord. Some of the neural effects of testosterone are not the result of testosterone per se, but rather of its metabolites, oestradiol and dihydrotestosterone (DHT). For example, there is evidence that the nerve cells of the MPOA aromatize testosterone to oestradiol, which then stimulates the cellular processes leading to activation of male copulatory behavior (Watson et al 1989). Thus, testosterone acts both as hormone and prohormone and its specific effects depend on the enzyme activity of target tissue. This also means that testosterone, as well as acting through the androgen receptor, acts in tissues with a high aromatase level as an oestrogen via the oestrogen receptor. Furthermore, the other main metabolite of testosterone, DHT, also binds to the oestrogen receptor and thereby can act as an inhibitor of oestrogen action (see Mooradian et al 1987 for review). Different metabolites of testosterone probably affect different components of sexual behaviour through actions at different sites (Michael et al 1987).

Gonadal steroid receptors in the brain are localized to specific well defined areas, and their distribution is similar in all vertebrates. Androgen and oestrogen receptors are often localized in the same regions. As well as the MPOA–anterior hypothalamic region, other sites of high steroid receptor density relevant to sexual behaviour are the medial and cortical amygdaloid nuclei (mainly oestrogen receptors) and the hippocampus (mainly androgen receptors). They are also found in other hypothalamic nuclei concerned with the regulation of gonadotrophin release.

The steroid hormone's interaction with its receptor is an unusual one. The hormone diffuses into brain cells where it binds to the receptor protein, either in the cytoplasm or in the nucleus. This steroid–receptor complex becomes attached to the genome and is able to alter gene expression and thus protein synthesis. The protein end-product of this depends on the cell: it might be a pre-hormone, such as the precursor for prolactin, or a receptor protein, such as a progesterone receptor. This mechanism of action involves delay between receptor activation and response and may account, in part, for the slow clinical action of testosterone replacement therapy or antiandrogenic drugs. But testosterone also has rapid electrophysiological effects, and these are probably mediated by different receptors on the cell membrane. Testoster-

one's rapid facilitatory effect on penile reflexes in the rat is probably mediated by this second type of neuronal receptor, since inhibition of protein synthesis does not reduce it (Meisel et al 1986). Also, a rapid effect of testosterone on bulbocavernosus muscle activity has been demonstrated electrophysiologically (Sachs & Leipheimer 1988). This might help to explain testosterone's effect on the rigidity of sleep erections (see above), since contraction of the bulbocavernosus increases intracavernosal pressure in the erect penis and thus adds to its rigidity.

Prolactin, a hormone secreted by the anterior pituitary gland, under the control of the hypothalamus, may also play a role in regulating erection. This is suggested by clinical observations in men with pathologically elevated levels of prolactin (hyperprolactinaemia). This is usually due to a prolactin secreting pituitary tumour and impotence is almost always present. Erectile function recovers rapidly in most of these men when their hyperprolactinaemia is treated.

However, hyperprolactinaemia impairs gonadal function and is associated with reduced libido, making it difficult to ascertain what the mechanism for erectile dysfunction is. Animal experiments indicate that hyperprolactinaemia affects erectile function independently of libido and gonadal function, and that it acts at a supraspinal level (Doherty et al 1986). It has been suggested, on pharmacological evidence, that the impotence in hyperprolactinaemia results from an effect of prolactin on the central dopaminergic control of erection (Buvat et al 1985, see Ch. 5, p. 64).

SUMMARY

The peripheral nerves supplying the penis are:

1. the pelvic nerves (mainly parasympathetic)
2. the hypogastric nerves (mainly sympathetic), and
3. the pudendal nerve (mainly somatic).

1. and 2. join to form the pelvic plexus and give rise to the cavernous nerves which supply the erectile tissues; 3. supplies the striated muscles of the penis and receives the sensory fibres of the dorsal nerve of the penis.

Three peripheral neurphysiological mechanisms

are involved in erection: a parasympathetic 'vascular mechanism', a sympathetic 'inhibitory mechanism' and a somatic 'muscular mechanism'. The main function of the autonomic nervous sytem (parasympathetic and sympathetic divisions) is to regulate the tone of the smooth muscle in the arterioles and trabeculae of the penis. The somatic mechanism contributes to the rigidity of the erect penis.

Animal experiments on the role of cerebral areas and pathways indicate the importance of the diencephalon, and in particular the medial preoptic area and adjacent anterior hypothalamic area. The hippocampus probably interacts with the diencephalon in the expression of erection.

The medial forebrain bundle is a major pathway by which erectogenic impulses descend from the forebrain to the ventral tegmentum of the midbrain and thence caudally. A second hypothalamospinal pathway, in which the neuropeptide oxytocin may have particular functional significance, may also be important.

REFERENCES

Aboseif M D, Lue T F 1988 Hemodynamics of penile erection. Urologic Clinics of North America 15(1): 1–8

Adaikan P G, Kottegoda S R, Ratnam S S 1986 Is vasoactive intestinal polypeptide the principle transmitter involved in human penile erection? Journal of Urology 135: 638–640

Adrian T E, Gu J, Allen J M, Takemoto K, Polak J M, Bloom S R 1984 Neuropeptide Y in the human genital tract. Life Sciences 35: 2643–2648

Andersson P O, Bloom S R, Mellander S 1984 Haemodynamics of pelvic nerve induced penile erection in the dog: possible mediation by vasoactive intestinal polypeptide. Journal of Physiology 350: 209–224

Argiolis A, Melis M R, Gessa G L 1986 Oxytocin: an extremely potent inducer of penile erection and yawning in male rats. European Journal of Pharmacology 130: 264–373

Argiolas A, Melis M R, Mauri A, Gessa G L 1987 Paraventricular nucleus lesion prevents yawning and penile erection induced by apomorphine and oxytocin, but not by ACTH, in rats. Brain Research 421(1–2): 349–352

Bailey D J, Dolan A L, Phoroah P D P, Herbert J 1984 Role of gonadal and adrenal steroids in the impairment of the male rat's sexual behaviour by hyperprolactinaemia. Neuroendocrinology 39: 555–562

Bancroft J 1989 Human sexuality and its problems. 2nd edition. Churchill Livingstone, Edinburgh

Bancroft J, O'Carroll R, McNeilly A, Shaw R W 1984 The effects of bromocriptine on the sexual behaviour of hyperprolactinaemic men: a controlled case study. Clinical Endocrinology 21: 131–137

Bancroft J, Wu F C W 1983 Changes in erectile responsiveness during androgen replacement therapy. Archives of Sexual Behaviour 12: 59

Bigg S W, Kavoussi L R, Catalona W J 1990 Role of nerve-sparing radical prostatectomy for clinical stage B2 prostate cancer. Journal of Urology 144(6): 1420–1424

Blanco R, Saenz de Tejada I, Goldstein I, Krane R J, Wotiz H H, Cohen R A 1988 Cholinergic neurotransmission in human corpus cavernosum II. Acetylcholine synthesis

Bors E, Comarr A E 1960 Neurological disturbances in sexual function with special reference to 529 patients with spinal cord injury. Urology Survey 10: 191–222

Breedlove S M, Arnold A 1980 Hormone accumulation in a sexually dimorphic motor nucleus of the rat spinal cord. Science 210: 564–566

Breedlove S M, Jacobson C D, Gorski R, Arnold A P 1982 Masculinization of the female rat spinal cord following a single neonatal injection of testosterone propoinate but not estradiol benzoate. Brain Research 237: 173–181

Brendler C B, Steinberg G D, Marshall F F, Mostwin J L, Walsh P C 1990 Local recurrence and survival following nerve-sparing radical cystoprostatectomy 144(5): 1137–40

Brindley G S 1983 Cavernosal alpha-blockade: a new technique for investigating and treating erectile impotence. British Journal of Psychiatry 143: 332–337

Brindley G S 1985 Pathophysiology of erection and ejaculation. In: Whitfield H N, Hendry W F (eds) Textbook of genito-urinary surgery. Churchill Livingstone, Edinburgh

Brindley G S 1986 Pilot experiments on the actions of drugs injected into the human corpus cavernosum penis. British Journal of Pharmacology 87: 495–500

Brindley G S, Gillan P W 1982 Men and women who do not have orgasms. British Journal of Psychiatry 140: 351–356

Brindley G S, Polkey C E, Rubston D N 1982 Sacral anterior root stimulators for bladder control in paraplegia. Paraplegia 20: 365–381

Burnstock G 1986 The changing face of autonomic neurotransmission. Acta Physiologica Scandinavica 126: 67–91

Buvat J, Lemaire A, Buvat-Herbaut M, Fourlinnie J, Racedot A, Fossati P 1985 Hyperprolactinaemia and sexual function in men. Hormone Research 22: 196–203

Carani C, Scuteri A, Marrama P, Bancroft J 1990 The effects of testosterone administration and visual erotic stimuli on nocturnal penile tumescence in normal men. Hormones and Behaviour 24(3): 435–41

Carter J N, Tyson J E, Tolis G, Van Vliet S, Faiman C, Friesen H G 1987 Prolactin secreting tumors and hypogonadism in 22 men. New England Journal of Medicine 299: 847–852

Chapelle P A, Durand J, Lacert P 1980 Penile erection following complete spinal cord injury in man. British Journal of Urology 52: 216–219

Cunningham G R, Karacan I, Ware J C, Lantz C D, Thornby J I 1982 The relationship between serum testosterone and prolactin levels and nocturnal penile tumescence (NPT) in impotent men. Journal of Andrology 3: 241–247

Dail W G, Hamill R W 1989 Parasympathetic nerves in penile erectile tissue of the rat contain choline acetyltransferase. Brain Research 487(1): 165–170

Dail W G, Moll M A, Weber K 1983 Localization of vasoactive intestinal polypeptide in penile erectile tissue and in the major pelvic ganglion of the rat. Neuroscience 10: 1379–1386

Dail W G, Manzanares K, Moll M A, Minorsky N 1985 The hypogastric nerve innervates a population of penile neurones in the pelvic plexus. Neuroscience 16: 1041–1046

Dail W G, Minorsky N, Moll M A, Manzanares K 1986 The hypogastric nerve pathway to penile erectile tissue: histochemical evidence supporting a vasodilator role. Journal of the Autonomic Nervous System 15: 341–349

de Groat W C, Booth A M, Krier J 1979 Interaction between sacral parasympathetic inputs to pelvic ganglia. In: Brooks C M, Koizumi K, Sato A (eds) Integrative function of the autonomic nervous system. University of Tokyo Press, Tokyo

de Groat W C, Steers W D 1988 Neuroanatomy and neurophysiology of penile erection. In: Tanagho E A, Lue T F, McLure R D (eds) Contemporary management of impotence and infertility. Williams and Wilkins, Baltimore

Doherty P C, Bartke A, Smith M S 1985 Hyperprolactinemia and male sexual behaviour: effects of steroid replacement with estrogen plus dihydrotestosterone. Physiology and Behaviour

Doherty P C, Baum M J, Todd B R 1986 Effects of chronic hyperprolactinaemia on sexual arousal and erectile function in male rats. Neuroendocrinology 42: 368–375

Dorr L D, Brody M J 1967 Hemodynamic mechanisms of erection in the canine penis. American Journal of Physiology 213: 1526–1531

Dua S, MacLean P D 1964 Localization for penile erection in medial frontal lobe. American Journal of Physiology 207: 1425–1434

Eckhard C 1863 Untersuchungen uber die erection des penis beim hunde. Beitrage zur Anatomie und Physiologie 3: 123–150

Ellis W J, Grayhack J T 1963 Sexual function in ageing males after orchidectomy and estrogen therapy. Journal of Urology 89: 895

Furchgott R F 1984 The role of endothelium in the responses of vascular smooth muscle to drugs. Annual Review of Pharmacology and Toxicology 24: 175–197

Gloor P 1986 Role of the human limbic system in perception, memory, and affect: lessons from temporal lobe epilepsy. In: Doane B K, Livingston K E (eds) The limbic system: functional organization and clinical disorders. Raven Press, New York

Gu J, Polak J M, Probert L et al 1983 Peptidergic innervation of human male genital tract. Journal of Urology 130: 386–391

Gu J, Lazarides M, Pryor J P et al 1984 Decrease of vasoactive intestinal polypeptide in the penises from impotent men. Lancet ii: 315–318

Habib H N 1967 Experience and recent contribution in sacral nerve stimulation for voiding in both human and animals. British Journal of Urology 39: 73–83

Halata Z, Munger B 1986 The neuroanatomical basis for the protopathic sensibility of the human penis. Brain Research 271: 205–230

Hansen S, Kohler C, Goldstein M, Steinbusch H V M 1982 Effects of ibotenic acid-induced neuronal degeneration in the medial preoptic area and the lateral hypothalamic area on sexual behaviour in the male rat. Brain Research 239: 213–232

Hart B L 1967 Testosterone regulation of sexual reflexes in spinal male rats. Science 155: 1283–1284

Hart B L 1979 Activation of sexual reflexes by

dihydrotestosterone but not estrogen. Physiology and Behaviour 23: 107–109

Hart B L, Melese-D'Hospital P Y 1983 Penile mechanisms and the role of the striated penile muscle in penile reflexes. Physiology and Behaviour 31: 807–813

Hedlund H, Andersson K E 1985 Effects of some peptides on isolated human penile tissue and cavernous artery. Acta Physiologica Scandinavica 124: 413–419

Heim N 1981 Sexual behaviour of castrated sex offenders. Archives of Sexual Behaviour 10: 11

Henderson V E, Roepke M H 1933 On the mechanism of erection. American Journal of Physiology 106: 441–448

Hitt J C, Hendricks S E, Ginsberg S J, Lewis J H 1970 Disruption of male but not female sexual behavior in rats by medial forebrain bundle lesions. Journal of Comparative Physiology and Psychology 73: 377–384

Hughes A M, Everitt B J, Herbert J 1987 Selective effects of beta-endorphin infused into the hypothalamus, preoptic area and the bed nucleus of the stria terminalis on the sexual and ingestive behaviour of male rats. Neuroscience 23: 1063–1073

Hyndman O R, Wolkin J, 1943 Anterior cordotomy. Further observation on physiologic results and optimum manner of performance. Archives of Neurology and Psychiatry 50: 129–148

Johnson R D, Kitchell R L, Gilanpour H 1986 Rapidly and slowly adapting mechanoreceptors in the glans penis of the cat. Physiology and Behaviour 37: 69–78

Junemann K P, Persson-Junemann C, Tanagho E A, Alken P 1989a Neurophysiology of penile erection. Urology Research 17(4): 213–217

Junemann K P, Persson-Junemann C, Lue T F, Tanagho E A, Alken P 1989b Neurophysiological aspects of penile erection: the role of the sympathetic nervous system. British Journal of Urology 64(1): 84–92

Kalra P S, Simpkins J W, Luttge W G, Kalra S P 1983 Effects on male sexual behavior and preoptic dopamine neurons of hyperprolactinemia induced by MtTW15 pituitary tumors. Endocrinology 113: 2065–2071

Karacan I, Aslan C, Hirshkowitz M 1983 Erectile mechanisms in man. Science 220: 1080–1081

Krane R J 1986 Sexual function and dysfunction. In: Walsh P C, Gittes R F, Perlmutter A D et al (eds) Campbell's Urology, 700–735. W B Saunders, Philadelphia

Kwan M, Greenleaf W, Mann J et al 1983 The nature of androgen action on male sexuality: a combined laboratory/ self-report study on hypogonadal men. Journal of Clinical Endocrinology and Metabolism 57: 557

Lal S, Ackman D, Thavundayil J X, Kiely M, Etienne P 1984 Effect of apomorphine, a dopamine receptor agonist, on penile tumescence in normal subjects. Progress in Neuro-Psychopharmacology and Biological Psychiatry 8: 695–699

Lepor H, Gregerman M, Crosby R, Mostofi F R, Walsh P C 1985 Precise localization of the autonomic nerves from the pelvic plexus to the corpora cavernosa: a detailed anatomical study of the adult male pelvis. Journal of Urology 133: 207–212

Lue T F, Tanagho E A 1987 Physiology of erection and pharmocological management of impotence. Journal of Urology 137: 829–836

Lue T F, Zeineh S J, Schmidt R A, Tanagho E A 1984 Neuroanatomy of penile erection: its relevance to iatrogenic impotence. Journal of Urology 131: 273–280

Lundberg J M 1981 Evidence of coexistence of vasoactive intestinal polypeptide (VIP) and acetylcholine in neurons of cat exocrine glands. Morphological, biochemical and functional studies. Acta Physiologica Scandinavica [suppl] 496: 1–57

Lundberg J M, Hedlund B, Bartfai T 1982 Vasoactive intestinal polypeptide enchances muscarinic ligand binding in cat submandibular salivary gland. Nature 295: 147–149

McEwen B S 1981 Neural gonadal steroid actions. Science 211: 1303–1311

MacLean P D, Ploog D W 1962 Cerebral representation of penile erection. Journal of Neurophysiology 25: 29–55

MacLean P D, Denniston R H, Dua S 1963 Further studies on cerebral representation of penile erection: caudal thalamus, midbrain, and pons. Journal of Neurophysiology 26: 273–293

Mas M, Zahradnik M A, Martino V, Davidson J M 1985 Stimulation of spinal serotonergic receptors facilitates seminal emission and suppresses penile erectile reflexes. Brain Research 342: 128–134

Meisel R L, Leipheimer R E, Sachs B D 1986 Anisomycin does not disrupt the activation of penile reflexes by testosterone in rats. Physiology and Behaviour 37(6): 951–956

Melis M R, Ariolis A, Gessa G L 1986 Oxytocin-induced penile erection and yawning: sites of action in the brain. Brain Research 398: 259–265

Melis M R, Ariolis A, Gessa G L 1987 Apomorphine-induced penile erection and yawning: sites of action in the brain. Brain Research 415: 98–104

Meyers R 1962 Three cases of myoclonus alleviated by bilateral ansotomy, with a note on postoperative alibido and impotence. Journal of Neurosurgery 17: 71–81

Michael R P, Bonsall R W, Zumpe D 1987 Testosterone and its metabolites in male cynomolgus monkeys (Macaca fascicularis): behavior and biochemistry. Physiology and Behaviour 40(4): 527–537

Mooradian A D, Morley J E, Korenman S G 1987 Biological actions of androgens . Endocrinology Reviews 8(1): 1–28

Murphy M R, Seckle J R, Burton S, Checkley S A Lightman S L 1987 Changes in oxytocin and vasopressin secretion during sexual activity in men. Journal of Clinical Endocrinology and Metabolism 65: 738–741

Murray F T, Cameron D, Ketchum C 1984 Return of gonadal function in men with prolactin-secreting pituitary tumors. Journal of Clinical Endocrinology and Metabolism 59: 79–85

Nagulesparen M, Ane V, Jenkins J C 1978 Bromocriptine treatment of males with pituitary tumors, hyperprolactinemia and hypogonadism. Clinical Endocrinology 9: 73–80

Nikolsky W 1879 Einbeitrag zur physiologie der nervi erigentes. Archiv für Anatomit und Physiologie Jahrgang 209: 221

Onuf (Onufrowicz) B 1900 On the arrangement and function of the cell groups of the sacral region of the spinal cord in man. Archives of Neurology and Psychopathology 3: 387–11

Oomura Y, Aou S, Koyama Y, Fujita I, Yoshimatsu H 1988 Central control of sexual behavior. Brain Research Bulletin 20(6): 863–870

Ottsen B, Wagner G, Virag R, Fahrenkrug J 1984 Penile erection: possible role for vasoactive intestinal polypeptide as a neurotransmitter. British Medical Journal 288: 9–11

Padma-Nathan H, 1988 Neurologic Evaluation of Erectile Dysfunction. Urologic Clinics of North America, 15(1): 77–80

Palmer R M J, Ferrige A G, Moncada S 1987 Nitric oxide release accounts for the biological activity of endothelium-derived relaxing factor. Nature 327: 524–526

Penfield W, Jasper H 1954 Epilepsy and the functional anatomy of the human brain. Little, Brown, Boston

Perryman R L, Thorner M O 1981 The effects of hyperprolactinemia on sexual and reproductive function in men. Journal of Andrology 5: 233

Pick J, Sheehan D 1946 Sympathetic rami in man. Journal of Anatomy 80: 12–20

Polak J M, Gu J, Mina S, Bloom S R 1981 Vipergic nerves in the penis. Lancet ii: 217–219

Raggenbass M, Tribollet E, Dubois-Dauphin M, Dreifuss J J 1989 A correlation between oxytocin neuronal sensitivity and receptor binding: an electrophysiological and autoradiographical study comparing rat and guniea-pig hippocampus. Procedings of the National Acadamy of Science 86: 750–754

Sachs B D, Bitran D 1990 Spinal block reveals roles for brain and spinal cord in the mediation of reflexive penile erections in rats. Brain Research 528(1): 99–108

Sachs B D, Leipheimer R E 1988 Rapid effect of testosterone on striated muscle activity in rats. Neuroendocrinology 48(5): 453–458

Siad S I 1981 VIP overview. In: Bloom S R, Polak J M (eds) Gut hormones, 2nd edn. Churchill Livingstone, Edinburgh p. 379–384

Saenz de Tejada I, Blanco R, Goldstein I et al 1988 Cholinergic neurotransmission in human corpus cavernosum I. Responses of isolated tissue. American Journal of Physiology 254: H459–H467

Saenz de Tejada I, Goldstein I, Krane R J 1988 Local control of penile erection: nerves, smooth muscle, and endothelium. Urologic Clinics of North America 15(1): 9–16

Saenz de Tejada I, Goldstein I, Azadzoi K, Krane R J, Cohen R A 1989 Impaired neurogenic and endothelium-mediated relaxation of penile smooth muscle from diabetic men with impotence. New England Journal of Medicine 320(16): 1025–1030

Semans J H, Langworthy O R 1938 Observation on the neurophysiology of sexual function in the male cat. Journal of Urology 40: 836–846

Schroder H D, 1981 Onuf's nucleus X: a morphological study of a human spinal nucleus. Anatomy and Embryology 162: 443–453

Schwartz M F, Banman J E, Masters W H 1982 Hyperprolactinemia and sexual disorders in men. Biological Psychiatry 17: 861–876

Sjostrand N O, Klinge E 1979 Principal mechanisms controlling penile retraction and protrusion in rabbits. Acta Physiologica Scandavica 106: 199–214

Steers W D, McConnell J, Benson G 1984 Anatomical localization and some pharmacological effects of vasoactive intestinal polypeptide in human and monkey corpus cavernosum. Journal of Urology 132: 1048–1053

Stoneham M D, Everitt B J, Hansen S, Lightman S L, Todd K 1985 Oxytocin and sexual behaviour in the male rat and rabbit. Journal of Endocrinology 107: 97–106

Swanson L W 1977 Immunohistochemical evidence for a neurophysin containing autonomic pathway arising in the paraventricular nucleus of the hypothalamus. Brain Research 128: 346–353

Swanson L W, Sawchenko P E 1983 Hypothalamic integration: organization of the paraventricular and supraoptic nuclei. Annual Review of Neuroscience 6: 269–324

Talbot H S 1949 A report on sexual function in paraplegics. Journal of Urology 61: 265–270

Toone B 1986 Sexual disorders in epilepsy. In: Tedley T A, Meldrum B S (eds) Recent advances in epilepsy 3. Churchill Livingstone, Edinburgh p. 233–261

Virag R, Ottesen J, Fahrenkrug J, Levy C, Wagner G 1982 Vasoactive intestinal polypeptide release during penile erection in man. Lancet ii: 1166

Wagner G, Brindley G S 1980 The effect of atropine and beta blockers in human penile erection: a combined pilot study. In: Zorgniotti A W, Ross G (eds) Vasculogenic impotence. Charles C Thomas, Springfield, Illinois, p. 77

Walsh P C, Donker P 1982 Impotence following radical prostatectomy: insight into etiology and prevention. Journal of Urology 128: 492–497

Walsh P C, Lepor H and Eggleston J C 1983 Radical prostatectomy with preservation of sexual function: anatomical and pathological considerations. Prostate 4: 473

Walsh P C, Mostwin J L 1985 Radical prostatectomy and cystoprostatecomy with preservation of potency: results utilizing a new nerve-sparing technique. British Journal of Urology

Watson J T, Adkins-Regan E 1989 Testosterone implanted in the preoptic area of male Japanese quail must be aromatized to activate copulation. Hormones and Behaviour 23(3): 432–47

Weber R F A, Ooms M P, Vreeburg J T M 1982 Effects of a prolactin-secreting tumor on copulatory behaviour in male rats. Journal of Endocrinology 903: 223–229

Wein A J, Van Arsdalen K N, Hanno P M et al 1986 Physiology of male sexual function. In: Rajfer J (ed) Urologic Endocrinology. W B Saunders, Philadelphia pp. 249–274

4. Haemodynamic aspects of erection

John P. Pryor   George O. Klufio

Erection requires the inflow of a sufficient amount of blood into the penis to raise the intracorporeal pressure to the level of mean arterial pressure. Relaxation of the cavernous smooth muscle and obstruction to venous outflow contribute to the attainment of this pressure by trapping the blood within the corpora. The whole of this process is under neural control. This is the basis of erection but it is first necessary to consider the anatomy of the penis.

ANATOMICAL CONSIDERATIONS

Structure of the penis

The penis is comprised of three corpora (Figs 4.1 & 4.2) and it is the paired corpora cavernosa that become rigid during erection. The adjacent corpus spongiosum is expanded at its distal end to become the glans penis and the urethra runs through the central part of it.

The crura of the penis (the proximal parts of the corpora cavernosa) are attached to the pubic arch and are fixed, whereas the pendulous part of the penis enlarges during erection. The corpora cavernosa are attached to the symphysis pubis and the linea alba of the anterior abdominal wall by suspensory ligaments. The fundiform part of the suspensory ligament prevents retraction of the penis and the remainder of the suspensory ligament at the base of the penis provides stability at the time of erection.

The corpora cavernosa (Fig. 4.3) comprise a dense outer layer of fibrous tissue which is relatively inelastic, and an inner vascular sponge. Fibrous septa extend into the erectile tissue from the investing tunica albuginea. The crura of the corpora cavernosa, which are covered by the ischiocavernosus muscle in the perineum, converge and are adherent to each other in the penis. The septum between the two corpora is perforated and the two function as a single unit. The corpora cavernosa consist of large vascular spaces lined by endothelium covering the underlying smooth

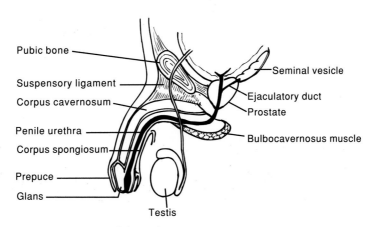

Fig. 4.1 Anatomy of the penis.

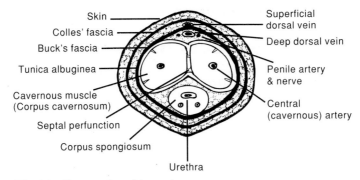

Skin — Superficial dorsal vein
Colles' fascia — Deep dorsal vein
Buck's fascia —
Tunica albuginea — Penile artery & nerve
Cavernous muscle (Corpus cavernosum) — Central (cavernous) artery
Septal perfunction —
Corpus spongiosum —
Urethra

Fig. 4.2 Cross section of the penis.

muscle. The whole has a rich and complex inner-vation and blood supply.

Histological examination of the penis has been periodically reviewed (Conti & Virag 1989) and more recently the fine structure has been exam-ined by electron microscopy (Persson et al 1989; Jevitch et al 1990; Meuleman et al 1990). These studies have shown that the proportion of fibrous tissue within the corpora cavernosa increases with age (Ruzbarksy & Michal 1977). The increase in fibrous tissue reduces penile extensibility and this correlates with a decrease in erectile capacity (Bondil et al 1990).

Arterial supply

The arterial supply to the penis is derived from the two internal pudendal arteries, which are branches of the anterior division of the internal iliac arteries. Each internal pudendal artery reaches the perineum by passing along the lateral wall of the ischiorectal fossa and emerging through Alcock's canal to become the penile artery. The penile artery has a branch to the bulb of the ure-thra and one to the corpus spongiosum. The main penile artery divides into the dorsal artery of the penis, which also supplies the glans penis, and a deeper cavernous branch (Fig. 4.4) which supplies the corpus cavernosum. On entering the corpus, the artery divides into numerous fine branches which are enclosed and supported within the cav-ernous tissue. Some of these branches open di-rectly into the cavernous spaces whilst others are spiral shaped, helicine arteries and in addition to

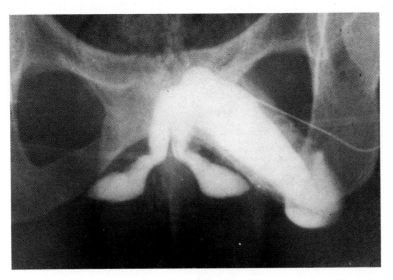

Fig. 4.3 Cavernosogram to show the relationship of the crura to the pubic arch. There has been some filling of the glans penis (corpus spongiosum).

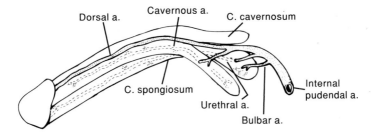

Fig. 4.4 Blood supply of the penis.

opening into the sinusoidal spaces, give off capillary branches to nourish the cavernous muscle. The detailed anatomy of the cavernous artery wall has been the subject of much discussion (Conti 1952; Wagner et al 1982), particularly with regard to the presence or absence of polsters. The arterial supply to the penis is subject to some individual variation but the cavernous arteries are the only ones essential for an erection (Lue et al 1985).

Venous drainage

Small venules originate within the corpora and unite into larger venules that subsequently form the subtunical plexus between the sinusoidal walls and the tunica albuginea. In the distal and middle part of the corpora, these venules drain into emissary veins that pierce the tunica albuginea to form the circumflex veins. These circumflex veins drain into the deep dorsal vein of the penis and this also receives tributaries from the glans penis. The deep dorsal vein empties into the preprostatic plexus of veins and thence into the internal iliac veins.

The proximal corpora are drained by the cavernous and crural veins. These empty into the preprostatic plexus and the internal pudendal vein.

The bulbar vein, which drains the bulb of the corpus spongiosum, empties into the internal pudendal vein. The skin of the penis and prepuce drain into the superficial dorsal vein which, in the majority of people, empties into the saphenous veins. The venous drainage of the penis is shown in Figure 4.5.

MECHANISM OF ERECTION

Our understanding of the mechanism of erection has been revised in the past decade and undoubtedly will be modified further. Observations made by Uhrenholdt & Wagner (1980), Shirai & Ishii (1981) and Newman & Northrup (1981) reflect the increase in interest in the paraphysiology of erectile dysfunction, and Lue's animal work has greatly clarified our views (Lue et al 1984; Lue 1986). The neurological and biochemical changes associated with erection are discussed in Chapter 3; this chapter is concerned with the vascular events taking place within the penis.

Flaccidity

The small, soft penis of the resting state is associated with a low inflow of blood. This is sufficient

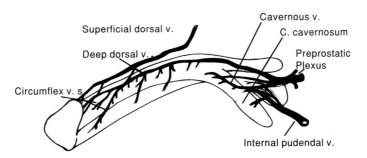

Fig. 4.5 Venous drainage of the penis.

to nourish the cavernous muscle and is too small to be measured by standard doppler ultrasound techniques. Sympathetic nervous activity causes constriction of the arteries and maintains contraction of the cavernous smooth muscle (Wagner et al 1989). The low resting flow through the cavernous tissue would appear to be the result of the peripheral resistance rather than the polster mechanism (Aboseif & Lue 1988). Shunt mechanisms (Wagner et al 1982) may exist but their role is uncertain. It should be emphasized that the muscle of the corpus cavernosum is actively contracting during flaccidity and *relaxes* during erection.

Erection

During erection, the penis enlarges and becomes hard. The vascular changes may be divided into different phases and Lue (1986) described five of these.

1. **Latent Phase**. The start of an erection is preceded by relaxation of arterial and cavernous smooth muscle. This leads to a drop in vascular resistance, resulting in rapid inflow of blood into the cavernous spaces. For a short period there is no increase, or even a slight fall, in the intracorporeal pressure. This period of isometric filling of the sinusoidal spaces is associated with the highest flow rate of the whole erectile process and may be more than double the resting value. During this phase there is only slight elongation and fullness of the penis.

2. **Tumescence Phase**. As the inflow of blood continues, it becomes associated with increasing intracavernous pressure. When the intracavernous pressure rises above diastolic pressure, flow occurs only during systole. This phase is characterized by rapid expansion and elongation of the penis to its full size. The duration of this phase is age dependent and is influenced by the strength of stimulation.

3. **Full Erection Phase**. The continued inflow of blood, and distension of the sinusoidal spaces, compresses the subtunical plexus against the non-compliant tunica albuginea. This impedes the outflow of blood through the emissary veins (Wespes & Schulman 1990)

and the intracavernous pressure rises further. A stage of full erection is reached when the intracorporeal pressure equals mean systolic pressure. The pressure remains steady during this phase, indicating that the rate of arterial inflow is lower than during the tumescence phase and equals the venous outflow.

4. **Rigid Erection Phase**. Penile rigidity is achieved by contraction of the ischiocavernosus muscles and this raises the intracavernous pressure to well above systolic blood pressure (Lavoisier et al 1986; Wespes et al 1990). There is no flow in the cavernosus artery at this stage and, at the same time, there is further obstruction of the venous channels and flow in them also approaches zero. Consequently, for a short period of a few minutes, the corpora cavernosa become functionally dead spaces with hardly any inflow or outflow. This phase occurs naturally during sexual intercourse or masturbation and its duration is limited by muscle fatigue which obviates the risk of tissue ischaemia.

5. **Detumescence Phase**. This commences with the relaxation of the ischiocavernosus muscles, but detumescence is also an active process due to the contraction of the cavernosal smooth muscle under sympathetic nervous stimulation. This contraction expels blood from the sinusoidal spaces and it is accompanied by arterial vasoconstriction to reduce the inflow to the resting level. The penis becomes smaller and shorter and eventually flaccid.

The changes described above all take place in the corpora cavernosa, but similar changes take place in the corpus spongiosum, including the glans penis. However, the pressure rise is not so great as there is no limiting investing layer of tunica albuginea. Furthermore, the venous outflow into the deep dorsal vein is unimpeded. There is a valvular mechanism in these veins (Fitzpatrick & Cooper 1975; Fitzpatrick 1982) and it may be that these are regulated by non-adrenergic mechanisms — possibly neuropeptide Y (NPY) (Crowe et al 1991). There is some compression of the deep dorsal vein between the overlying stretched skin and the expanded corpora during full erection. This raises the pressure in the glans and increases

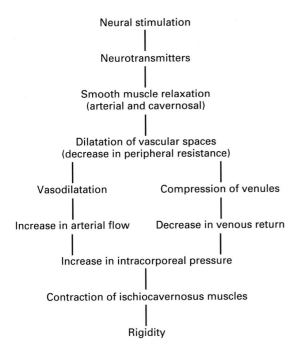

Neural stimulation

|

Neurotransmitters

|

Smooth muscle relaxation
(arterial and cavernosal)

|

Dilatation of vascular spaces
(decrease in peripheral resistance)

Vasodilatation   Compression of venules

Increase in arterial flow   Decrease in venous return

Increase in intracorporeal pressure

|

Contraction of ischiocavernosus muscles

|

Rigidity

Fig. 4.6 Mechanisms of erection.

its engorgement and firmness. There is a further increase in venous resistance with contraction of the ischiocavernosus and bulbocavernosus muscles during the rigid phase of erection.

SUMMARY

Erection is essentially a vascular phenomenon which is under neural control. It is summarized in Figure 4.6. It involves increased arterial inflow into the corpora cavernosa with relaxation of a fully compliant cavernous smooth muscle. Concurrently there is obstruction to venous outflow, which is largely passive in nature. These factors, combined with the non-distensible tunica albuginea, cause a rise in intracavernous pressure to the level of mean arterial pressure and the penis becomes erect. Contraction of the pelvic floor muscles, particularly at the time of orgasm, may raise the intracorporeal pressure to levels above systolic pressure, thereby producing increased penile rigidity.

REFERENCES

Aboseif M D, Lue T F, 1988 Hemodynamics of penile erection. Urologic Clinics of North America 15(1): 1–8

Bondil P, Louis J F, Dauves J P, Costa P, Lopez C, Navratil H 1990 Clinical measurement of penile extensibility: preliminary results. International Journal of Impotence Research 2: 193–201

Conti G 1952 L'érection du pénis humain et ses bases morphologico vasculaires. Acta Anat 14: 217–262

Conti G, Virag R 1989 Human penile erection and organic impotence: normal histology and histopathology. Urology International 44: 303–308

Crowe R, Burnstock G, Dickinson I K, Pryor J P 1991 The human penis: an unusual penetration of NPY-immunoreactive nerves within the medial muscle coat of the deep dorsal vein. Journal of Urology 145: 1292–1296

Fitzpatrick T J 1982 The penile intercommunicating venous valvular system. Journal of Urology 127: 1099–1100

Fitzpatrick T J, Cooper J F 1975 A cavernosogram study on the valvular competence of the human deep dorsal vein. Journal of Urology 113: 497–499

Jevitch M J, Khawand N Y, Vidic B 1990 Clinical significance of ultrastructural findings in the corpora cavernosa of normal and impotent men. Journal of Urology 143: 289–293

Lavoisier P, Courtois F, Barres D 1986 Correlation between intracavernous pressure and ischiocavernosus muscle in man. Journal of Urology 136: 936–939

Lue T F 1986 Mechanism of penile erection in the monkey. Seminars in Urology 4: 217–224

Lue T F, Takamura T, Umraiya M, Schmidt R A 1984 Haemodynamics of canine corpora cavernosa during erection. Urology 24: 347–352

Lue T F, Hricak H, Maeick K N, Tanogho E A 1985 Vasculogenic impotence evaluated by high resolution ultrasonography and pulsed doppler spectrum analysis. Radiology 153: 777–781

Meuleman E J H, ten Cate N L, de Wilde P C M, Voogs C P, Debruyne F M J 1990 The use of penile biopsies in the detection of end organ disease: a histomorphometric study of the human cavernous body. International Journal of Impotence Research 2: 161–166

Newman H F, Northrup J D 1981 Mechanism of human penile erection: an overview. Urology 17: 399–408

Persson L, Diederichs W W, Lue T F, Yen T S B, Fishman I J, McLin P H, Tanagho E A 1989 Correlation of altered penile ultrastructure with clinical arterial evaluation. Journal of Urology 142: 1462–1468

Ruzbarksy V, Michal V 1977 Morphological changes in the arterial bed of the penis with ageing. Relationship to the pathogenesis of impotence. Investigative Urology 15: 194–199

Shirai M, Ishii N 1981 Haemodynamics of erection in man. Archives of Andrology 6: 27–32

Uhrenholdt A, Wagner G 1980 Blood flow measurement by the clearance method in human corpus cavernosus in the flaccid and erect states. In: Zorgniotti A W, Rossi G (eds) Vasculogenic impotence. Charles C Thomas, Springfield: 41–46

Wagner G, Bro-Rasmussen F, Willis E A, Nielsen M H 1982 New theory on the mechanism of erection involving hitherto undescribed vessels. Lancet ii: 416–418

Wagner G, Gerstenberg T, Levin R J 1989 Electroactivity of

the corpus cavernosus during flaccidity and erection of the human penis. Journal of Urology 142: 723–724

Wespes E, Schulman C C 1990 Study of human penile venous system and hypothesis on its behaviour during erection. Urology 36: 68–72

Wespes E, Nogueira M C, Herbaut A G, Caufriez M, Schulmann C C 1990 Role of the bulbocavernosus muscles on the mechanism of human erection. European Urology 18: 45–48

5. The pharmacology of erection and erectile dysfunction

Michael Murphy

This chapter is about drugs that affect erection and the neurotransmitter mechanisms involved. The subject is complex, and data are often conflicting or inconsistent. Thus, many aspects of the pharmacology of erection remain unclear. Despite this, our understanding of the subject is rapidly increasing. This is because of developments in the basic sciences, and the discovery that several drugs, given intracavernosally, can induce erection in impotent men.

Until recently, acetylcholine was thought to be the primary peripheral neurotransmitter mediating erection. Experimental evidence now suggests that this is unlikely. There are a variety of more potent erectogenic substances found in the penis. These include vasoactive intestinal polypeptide (VIP), endothelium-derived relaxing factor (EDRF), and prostaglandins.

The role of adrenergic mechanisms has also been clarified recently: noradrenaline, released from sympathetic nerves, helps to maintain the flaccid state of the penis. Noradrenaline activates alpha-adrenoceptors on cavernosal and vascular smooth muscle, causing contraction of the supplying arterioles and cavernosal muscle. This restricts the corporal space, allowing minimal blood accumulation in the penis. Thus, the flaccid state of the non-erect penis is tonically maintained, at least in part, by an adrenergic mechanism (detumesence of the penis after ejaculation also involves adrenergically-mediated contraction of erectile smooth muscle). Blockade of this peripheral mechanism by alpha-blocking drugs, such as phenoxybenzamine, can thus cause erection (Brindley 1983). There may also be a sympathetic *erectile pathway* involved in mediating psychogenic stimuli for erection. The postganglionic fibres of this pathway, however, are cholinergic rather than adrenergic.

In addition to alpha-blockers, papaverine and prostaglandin E1 induce erection after intracavernous injection. They act directly on penile smooth muscle and are more effective than alpha-blockers. All three drugs can be used diagnostically, to help differentiate impotence of vascular origin from that of other causes (see Ch. 8). Therapeutically, these drugs can only help men with nonvascular causes for their impotence, since their action depends on an adequate blood supply to erectile tissue.

The central nervous system pharmacology of sexual function is also discussed in this chapter. Centrally-acting dopamine agonists can induce erection in man, while peptides, including oxytocin, cause erection in experimental animals when infused intracerebrally. Therapeutic claims have been made for the orally administered alpha$_2$-adrenoceptor blocker, yohimbine, and the opioid receptor blocker, naltrexone. It is likely that the effects of these drugs are centrally mediated. Many centrally acting drugs cause impotence; an understanding of how they do so can help the clinician select an alternative treatment without this side effect.

Before considering specific drugs any further, a brief outline of basic autonomic nervous system pharmacology is presented.

THE PHARMACOLOGY OF THE AUTONOMIC NERVOUS SYSTEM

The anatomical organizaton of the autonomic nervous system is decribed in Chapter 3. Centrally located preganglionic cells have axons which project to peripheral autonomic ganglia where they synapse with postganglionic neurones. The neurotransmitter at these sites is acetylcholine, regardless of whether they belong to the sympathetic or the parasympathetic division. Acetylcholine receptors on postganglionic cells are of the nicotinic subtype. This is in contrast to the muscarinic subtype found at neuroeffector junctions.

The peripheral transmitter released at the effector organ is different in sympathetic and parasympathetic divisions. At sympathetic postganglionic neuroeffector junctions the transmitter is generally noradrenaline (thus adrenergic); at parasympathetic postganglionic junctions it is usually acetylcholine (thus cholinergic). There are, however, important exceptions to this. Some postganglionic sympathetic fibres are cholinergic, as in the case of the sympathetic pathway for erection. Furthermore, there is evidence of the existence of nonadrenergic, noncholinergic autonomic neurotransmission involving peptides, GABA and other substances. Erection is again a case in point: the postganglionic fibres of the parasympathetic erectile pathway involve a nonadrenergic, noncholinergic mechanism (Ottsen et al 1984).

Another relatively new concept in neurotransmission is *cotransmission*: a second neurotransmitter, or a substance that modulates neurotransmission (neuromodulator), is released from the nerve terminal along with the 'classical' neurotransmitter (Lundberg 1981). This may occur in the control of erection when VIP and acetylcholine may be coreleased.

Noradrenaline receptors are called adrenoceptors. There are two main types: alpha-adrenoceptors and beta-adrenoceptors. These are further subtyped, for example, into alpha$_1$- and alpha$_2$-adrenoceptors. Alpha$_2$-adrenoceptors, as well as being pharmacologically distinct from alpha$_1$- adrenoceptors, are often located on the presynaptic nerve terminal, while alpha$_1$- adrenoceptors are located postsynaptically. The presynaptic adrenoceptors act as 'autoreceptors'. This means that when they are activated by noradrenaline, they have an inhibitory action on further noradrenaline release from the presynaptic nerve. Thus, a drug that blocks presynaptic alpha$_2$-adrenoceptors enhances noradrenergic neurotransmission through

that synapse, while a drug that blocks alpha$_1$-adrenoceptors inhibits such transmission.

Cholinergic mechanisms in erection

In normal sexual activity, erection is produced by activation of sacral parasympathetic pathways. However, muscarinic cholinergic transmission is not the main peripheral mechanism: postganglionic transmission is predominantly nonadrenergic, noncholinergic (NANC). At present, vasoactive intestinal polypeptide (VIP) is thought to be the most likely NANC transmitter. Acetylcholine, however, is still thought to be involved in the peripheral control of penile tumescence.

The results of research on acetylcholine's role in the control of erection are conflicting and it remains unclear whether muscarinic cholinergic transmission is important or not. Some investigators have found that muscarinic blockade with atropine partially inhibits erection induced by nerve stimulation in animals (Sjorstrand & Klinge 1979; Andersson et al 1984), while others have found it to have no effect (Dorr & Brody 1967; Henderson & Roepke 1933; Creed et al 1988). In a study of normal male volunteers, atropine had no effect on erection induced by erotic films or mechanical vibration (Wagner & Brindley 1980). Furthermore, intracavernosal injection of atropine does not inhibit erection (Brindley 1986).

Studies of acetylcholine's effect in vivo, on a variety of species, have also been contradictory. Injection of acetylcholine intravenously or into the aorta and penile artery had no erectile effect, while intracavernosal acetylcholine elicited a partial response in one animal study (Andersson et al 1987). In a human study, intracavernosal neostigmine (a cholinergic agent) had no effect (Brindley 1986). These findings suggest that many textbooks and clinical reports have overemphasized the significance of muscarinic transmission in the pharmacology of erection and have wrongly implicated anticholinergic drug effects in impotence.

Despite the uncertain effects of atropine and cholinergic agents on erection, it is evident from studies using a variety of other techniques that cholinergic muscarinic neurotransmission does occur in the human corpus cavernosum (Polak et al 1981; Gu et al 1983; Blanco et al 1986; Godec & Bates 1984; Lincoln et al 1987). What, if any, is its role in erection? A recent hypothesis has been that cholinergic nerves, rather than having a direct effect on the corpus cavernosum, modulate other neuroeffector systems (Saenz de Tejada et al 1988). Muscarinic receptors on noradrenergic nerve terminals have been identified in autonomic pathways (Burnstock 1986; Hedlund et al 1984). Their activation inhibits the release of noradrenaline. There is evidence suggesting that this might occur in the control of erection: atropine enhances adrenergically induced sinusoidal muscle contraction in vitro (Saenz de Tejada et al 1988). In addition to an inhibitory influence on the adrenergic control of smooth muscle tone, cholinergic modulation of peptidergically mediated relaxation of sinusoidal muscle may also occur.

A second site of cholinergic action is vascular endothelium: in addition to direct neural mechanisms for erection, there are substances released from the local endothelium that relax cavernosal smooth muscle. Acetylcholine facilitates the release of such a factor from arterial and cavernosal endothelium and may thus be indirectly involved in facilitating erection (Fig. 5.1).

Finally, a study by Stief et al (1989) will be described because it illustrates empirically the complex role of cholinergic transmission in erection. Intracavernous injections of increasing doses of acetylcholine (0.5 to 500 micrograms) were given to 10 monkeys. To differentiate between nicotinic (ganglionic) and muscarinic (parasympathetic postganglionic) effects, acetylcholine was likewise administered after a nicotinic blocker (trimethaphan camsylate) and a muscarinic blocker (atropine) alone or sequentially. The findings were that acetylcholine induced a dose-dependent, triphasic erectile response: an initial tumescence phase followed by contraction and a subsequent second phase of tumescence. Atropine reduced, but did not abolish, the erectile response to acetylcholine. Only after combined nicotinic and muscarinic blockade was the erectile response to acetylcholine completely abolished. These pharmacological findings suggest that earlier experiments may have yielded apparently conflicting data because of inadequate experimental design. Histological staining for acetylcholinesterase in five additional monkeys that had not received acetylcholine showed dense staining within the cavernous erectile tissue and around the cavernous arteries.

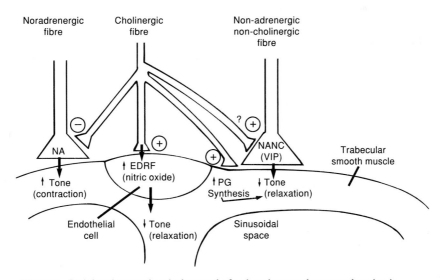

Fig. 5.1 Peripheral neurochemical control of trabecular muscle tone: relaxation is associated with erection, contraction with flaccidity and detumescence. NA noradrenaline; EDRF endothelium-derived relaxing factor; PG prostaglandin; NANC nonadrenergic, noncholinergic; VIP vasoactive intestinal polypeptide; ⊕ excitatory effect; ⊖ inhibitory effect; ↑ increases; ↓ decreases.

Alpha-adrenoceptors and sexual function

Activation of alpha-adrenoceptors on cavernosal and vascular smooth muscle tonically maintains muscular contraction, restricting bloodflow into the corporal space, and thus keeps the penis in a state of flaccidity. For erection to occur this mechanism must be antagonized. In theory, there are several ways this could happen. There may be central inhibition of the thoracolumbar adrenergic output; inhibition of peripheral alpha-adrenergic neuromuscular activity by endogenous substances such as prostaglandins, peptides or acetylcholine (discussed below) or simply increased opposing activity of erectogenic pathways. In addition to peripheral alpha-adrenoceptors, central alpha-adrenoceptors are involved in sexual pharmacology; these will be discussed in turn.

Intracavernosal alpha-adrenoceptor blockers

Non-selective alpha-antagonists, such as phenoxybenzamine and phentolamine, induce a marked increase in penile tumescence, often amounting to erection, when injected intracavernosally. This effect can be seen in both normal subjects and in men with neurogenic impotence (Brindley 1983, 1986). Non-selective alpha-adrenoceptor antagonists have also been shown to relax the cavernous muscle of several species in vitro (Klinge & Sjostrand 1977). Alpha-agonists, such as metaraminol, on the other hand, cause detumescence of the erect penis when injected intracavernosally (Brindley 1983, 1986) and several sympathomimetic agents cause contraction of cavernous smooth muscle in vitro (Carati et al 1985). In vitro studies all suggest that the contraction of smooth muscle seen with these agents is due to activation of a homogenous population of postsynaptic alpha-adrenoceptors (Adaikan & Karim 1981; Hedlund & Andersson 1985; Saenz de Tejada et al 1989).

While it is thus clear that alpha-adrenoceptors on cavernous muscle play an important role in regulating penile tumescence, until recently it was unclear whether these were $alpha_1$- or $alpha_2$-adrenoceptors. Although yohimbine, a fairly selective $alpha_2$-adrenoceptor antagonist, is reported to improve potency when taken orally, the evidence overall favours the view that postsynaptic $alpha_1$-, rather than $alpha_2$-adrenoceptors, mediate the tonic contraction of the vascular and trabecular smooth muscle responsible for the flaccid state of the penis. Any effect that yohimbine might have on erection is unlikely to be mediated by $alpha_2$-blockade in erectile tissue, since idazoxan, which is as potent as yohimbine and is more selective for the $alpha_2$-adrenoceptor, does not have this effect when injected intracavernosally (Brindley 1986). Evidence from in-vitro pharmacological studies also suggests that $alpha_1$-adrenoceptors have the predominant role (Christ et al 1990).

Alpha-blockers are less effective inducers of erection in impotent men than drugs that act directly on smooth muscle, such as papaverine and prostaglandin E1. Phentolamine is therefore often combined with papaverine in the treatment of impotence, allowing a reduction in the dose of papaverine. In theory, this diminishes the risk of priapism from papaverine, but there are no data proving that it does. Alpha-blockers alone are effective in some men with impotence.

Another drug that may act on penile alpha-receptors is trazodone hydrochloride. This is an antidepressant drug which, when taken orally, has led to improvement of erectile dysfunction in impotent men and the development of prolonged erections or priapism in potent men (Lal et al 1990). In the anaesthetized rabbit, intracavernosal trazodone and its major metabolite m-chlorophenyl-piperazine (m-CPP) produced full penile erection in three-quarters of animals studied (Azadzoi et al 1990). In 13 men intracavernosal trazodone caused tumescence but not full penile erection. Mean intracavernosal pressure was 28.2 +/- 5.8 mmHg with trazodone, while intracavernosal papaverine or papaverine and phentolamine resulted in a significantly higher pressure of 58 +/- 18 mmHg. Administration of alpha-adrenoceptor agonists, but not normal saline, resulted in complete detumescence of trazodone-induced erection in the animal studies (Azadzoi et al 1990).

The $alpha_1$-adrenoceptor agonist, methoxamine, has also been studied for its effects on sexual behaviour and penile reflexes in rats. It was found to inhibit reflex erectile responses, but to facilitate ejaculation (Clarke et al 1987). It was without effect in tests of motivation. In man, the $alpha_1$-

adrenoceptor agonist, metaraminol, taken systemically, has been found to cause an initial shrinkage of the flaccid penis followed, after about 12 hours, by sustained penile enlargement, lasting for many hours (Brindley & Murphy — unpublished data). This secondary tumescence may be a rebound phenomenon reflecting rapid downregulation of alpha$_1$-adrenoceptors with metaraminol treatment and subsequent reduction in adrenergically-mediated penile smooth muscle tone once the drug is cleared from the system.

Alpha-adrenoceptor agonists have recently been found useful in urological surgery: for example, in controlling erections during transurethral surgery (McNicholas et al 1989) or preventing nocturnal erections after penile surgery (Johansen et al 1989).

Oral alpha$_2$-adrenoceptor blockers

Yohimbine hydrochloride blocks the alpha$_2$-adrenoceptor at both presynaptic and postsynaptic sites. Presynaptic adrenoceptors, when activated by noradrenaline, inhibit further release of noradrenaline from the presynaptic nerve. Thus, blockade of the presynaptic autoreceptor increases noradrenergic activity. In male rats, yohimbine stimulates copulatory behaviour, while clonidine, an alpha$_2$-adrenoceptor agonist, inhibits it (Clarke et al 1984; Smith et al 1987a). Furthermore, yohimbine reverses the inhibition of sexual activity seen in rats after clonidine treatment. It is therefore likely that some of yohimbine's stimulant effects on sexual behaviour are mediated by its central alpha$_2$-adrenoceptor blocking effect (Clarke 1985a).

Yohimbine's effects on the sexual function of rats are of two types: effects on sexual 'motivation', and effects on genital reflexes. 'Motivation' in this context refers to the frequency with which the male rat mounts a receptive female. Yohimbine increases mounting behaviour in sexually active rats (Clarke et al 1984). This effect is seen despite anaesthetization of the genitals. It also stimulates copulatory behaviour in sexually inactive (Clarke et al 1984) and castrated male rats (Clarke et al 1985b). These findings have been interpreted as evidence that central alpha$_2$-adrenoceptors modulate sexual motivation.

Genital reflexes can be examined independently of sexual arousal, using tests that are conducted outside the context of sexual behaviour (ex copula). Relatively low doses of two alpha$_2$-adrenoceptor antagonists (idazoxan and yohimbine) have been shown to increase the frequency of erections in such tests. Idazoxan did so significantly, while yohimbine showed a non-significant trend in the same direction (Smith et al 1987b). Idazoxan is a more selective alpha$_2$-adrenoceptor blocker than yohimbine at central and peripheral receptors (Doxey et al 1983; Freedman & Aghajanian 1984; Dabire 1986). Unlike yohimbine it is devoid of activity at receptors other than adrenoceptors (Dabire 1986). At higher doses both drugs inhibited erections. This inhibition occurred at doses which have stimulatory effects on sexual arousal/motivation. Similar biphasic responses and diverging effects on different components of sexual behaviour have been described for drugs acting on other neurotransmitter systems (Stefanick et al 1982; Clarke et al 1983; Mas et al 1985).

There is evidence that yohimbine's central effects are not solely the result of alpha$_2$-antagonism (Smith et al 1987a). For example, idazoxan selectively antagonizes alpha$_2$-adrenoceptors on rat central neurones and its selectivity for alpha$_2$- over alpha$_1$-adrenoceptors is markedly superior to yohimbine's (Freedman & Aghajanian 1984), yet unlike yohimbine, it does not increase mounting behaviour after genital anaesthetization. We do not know what other systems are involved in yohimbine's effects on sexual function.

There have been several recent claims that yohimbine improves erectile function in men with impotence (Reid et al 1987; Morales et al 1987; Riley et al 1989; Susset et al 1989; Sonda et al 1990) (see Ch. 10). The outcome measures in these clinical trials have relied on patients' subjective reports of improvement. Where improvement has been reported, little attempt has been made to specify which components of sexual function have been affected. These are not necessarily shortcomings from the clinical point of view, but they make pharmacological interpretation difficult.

There are few objectively collected data on yohimbine's effect on erectile function. Danjou et al (1988) did a double-blind, placebo-controlled, laboratory study in which yohimbine was administered intravenously to 10 healthy male volunteers while penile circumference was monitored using plethysmography, with and without erotic visual stimulation. Yohimbine did not affect penile diameter, nor did it affect the physiological response to erotic stimuli. This was in contrast to the effect of the dopamine agonist, apomorphine, which induced erection and potentiated the visually-induced response (apomorphine is discussed in detail below).

There have been no published clinical trials on the effect of idazoxan, a more selective alpha$_2$-adrenoceptor blocker, in impotence. In normal men, idazoxan promotes pleasant penile sensations, and increases the amount by which the penis elongates in response to a standard rating procedure (Murphy & Brindley — unpublished study). This rating procedure has a psychological element, i.e. introspection, to decide whether pleasant penile sensations are occurring and how strong they are, and a mechanical element, i.e. pinching the glans. We do not know whether the drug augments a psychogenic response, a reflex response, or both. Augmentation of either, however, could be of therapeutic value in some patients. The effects of alpha$_2$-antagonism could be the result of idazoxan acting peripherally in the penis, or in the brain or spinal cord. The drug crosses the blood–brain barrier (Lewis et al 1988) and may thus act centrally. It is known, on local administration of larger doses than we used, to have no significant action on penile smooth muscle (Brindley 1986), but this does not exclude the possibility of a local action on penile sensory nerve endings.

It is difficult to explain how an alpha$_2$-antagonist might enhance penile sensation. Sensory impulses from the glans are transmitted by the dorsal nerve of the penis, a division of the pudendal nerve. In rats and cats the dorsal nerve of the penis also contains efferent autonomic fibres that arise in the sympathetic chain ganglia (Booth et al 1986) and it is possible, although the anatomical evidence is not conclusive, that such efferent projections occur in humans. It has been suggested that these autonomic efferents may modulate the sensitivity of afferent receptors (de Groat & Steers 1988), a phenomenon described at other cutaneous sites (Walin et al 1976).

Vasoactive intestinal polypeptide

Vasoactive intestinal polypeptide (VIP) is a 28 amino acid polypeptide found in highest concentration in the gut and genitourinary tract. It causes vasodilation and smooth-muscle relaxation, effects which make VIP a candidate neurotransmitter in penile erection.

Elevated concentrations of VIP have been found in penile venous blood during erection in men (Virag et al 1982); VIP relaxes adrenergically contracted cavernosal smooth muscle in vitro (Steers et al 1984; Hedlund 1985; Adaikan et al 1986) and causes slight tumescence in vivo (Ottsen et al 1984). In an animal model designed to examine the role of VIP in erection, its effects were reported as similar to those from electrostimulation of the cavernous nerve: VIP increased arterial flow, decreased venous flow, and induced sinusoidal relaxation (Juenemann et al 1987).

VIP, however, does not appear to hold as much therapeutic promise as other smooth muscle relaxants. In a double-blind, placebo-controlled clinical trial of the intracavernosal injection of VIP in 24 men with erectile dysfunction of diabetic, neurogenic and psychogenic etiology, VIP caused a significant increase in penile length and circumference, but only a slight non-significant increase in rigidity (Roy et al 1990). None of the patients achieved penile rigidity adequate for intercourse.

VIP may nevertheless play an important role in the pathophysiology of impotence. VIP-immunoreactive fibres innervate arterial, arteriolar and non-vascular smooth muscle in penile erectile tissue (Polak et al 1981; Gu et al 1983). Gu et al (1984) have compared erectile tissue obtained during surgery for impotence with tissue from men with normal erectile function, but undergoing gender reassignment operations. They found that almost all the impotent men had fewer VIP nerves than controls, regardless of the cause of impotence, suggesting that VIP fibre loss may be secondary to other causes. The lack of VIP nerves was most obvious where impotence was severe or of long duration. This neuronal depletion was, however, not specific to VIP fibres and may have been part of a more generalized loss of neural elements in the penis. Nevertheless, most of the fibres related to blood vessels contain VIP immunoreactivity.

VIP fibres follow the same anatomical course as cholinergic fibres, and ultrastructural examination of human penile tissue shows that VIP-containing vesicles are colocalized with other vesicles that probably contain acetylcholine (Polak et al 1981; Steers et al 1984; Gu et al 1983). In the rat, VIP has been identified in pelvic ganglion cell bodies that have cholinergic projections to the penis (Dail et al 1986).

VIP is also found in sympathetic, as well as parasympathetic, postganglionic fibres at various sites in the autonomic nervous system, where again there is evidence that it is a cotransmitter with acetylcholine (Lundberg 1981, Burnstock 1986). VIP can also stimulate sexual behaviour in rats, suggesting that it may also play a role in the central control of sexual behaviour (Gozes et al 1989).

Other peptides acting in the periphery

Several other peptides have been identified in cavernous nerve fibres, of which substance P and neuropeptide Y (NPY) look the most likely candidates for a physiological role (Gu et al 1983; Adrian et al 1984). Like VIP, substance P has an inhibitory effect on cavernosal muscle, but is found in smaller concentration and is localized mainly in nerves around the corpuscular receptors beneath the epithelium of the glans penis, rather than in relation to vascular or trabecular smooth muscle (Gu et al 1983). NPY has both direct and indirect vasoconstrictor actions and is found in high concentrations in the penis (Adrian et al 1985). It is thought to have a role in detumescence of the penis (Wespes 1988). It will no doubt be the focus of future research.

Local chemical mechanisms

Endothelium-derived relaxing factor(s)

The vasodilatory effect of acetylcholine has been shown to require the presence of the vascular endothelium (Furchgott & Zawadzki 1980; Furchgott 1988). This indicates that the relaxation of arterial smooth muscle may not be mediated by mus-

carinic neuromuscular junctions, but rather by endothelium-derived relaxing factor(s) (EDRF). Acetylcholine also relaxes contracted strips of human cavernosal smooth muscle in vitro, and there is evidence that this, too, depends on an intact endothelium (Saenz de Tejada et al 1988). EDRF evokes smooth-muscle cell relaxation by activating guanylate cyclase and thus increasing the production of intracellular 3',5'-cyclic guanosine monophosphate (GMP) (Palmer et al 1987, 1988). Research on the chemical identity of this factor suggests that it is nitric oxide. Sodium nitroprusside, which is a vasodilatory and erectogenic drug, has a similar action. There is also a possibility that there is more than one EDRF (Vanhoutte 1987).

A study of cavernosal tissue from diabetic men with impotence has suggested that impairment of this endothelium-mediated mechanism may be involved in the impotence associated with diabetes (Saenz de Tejada et al 1989). It is possible that the erectile difficulties accompanying hypertension and arteriosclerosis may also result, in part, from damage to the endothelium.

Prostaglandins

Intracavernosal injection of prostaglandin E1 (PGE1) elicits erection in normal and many impotent men. It has thus been used as an alternative to papaverine, in both the diagnosis and treatment of impotence. There have been a number of therapeutic trials of PGE1 and several studies comparing the efficacy and adverse effects of PGE1 with papaverine and papaverine/phentolamine mixtures. The results suggest that PGE1 is at least as effective as, if not superior to, papaverine for inducing erection in non-vasculogenic impotence (Stackl et al 1988; Sarosdy et al 1989; Beretta et al 1989; Lee et al 1989; Earle et al 1990; Schrey 1990). Of more clinical significance, the adverse effects that limit papaverine's use have rarely occurred with PGE1 (see Ch. 11).

The clinical effects of PGE1 suggest that prostaglandins may be physiologically involved in erection. There is further evidence of this. Human cavernosal tissue can synthesize various prostaglandins in vitro, including large amounts of prostacyclin (PGI2) (Jeremy et al 1986b; Roy et al

1989). Like PGE1, prostacyclin is a potent vasodilator. Furthermore, prostacyclin synthesis in penile tissue can be stimulated by cholinergic (muscarinic) agonists (Jeremy et al 1986a). Not surprisingly, these findings have led to speculation that prostacyclin is involved in erection.

In contrast to the relaxing effect of PGE1 and prostacyclin on cavernosal smooth-muscle, PGF2 (alpha) causes contraction and initiates rhythmic activity, while PGE2 causes contraction at low doses and relaxation at high doses (Roy et al 1989). Since tissue concentrations of prostaglandins depend upon the rate of degradation as well as synthesis, the activity of the enzyme prostaglandin 15-hydroxydehydrogenase, which differentially inactivates PGE1, PGE2 and PGF1 (alpha), may play a role in the control of erection (Roy et al 1988).

More direct evidence of locally synthesized prostaglandins having a role in erection comes from pharmacological studies of isolated human erectile tissue (HET). HET is obtained from the vascular sinusoids of the corpus cavernosum of men undergoing surgery for impotence. Maintained in an organ bath at 37°C, HET preparations show spontaneous myotonic oscillations. The effect of adding drugs to the organ bath on these muscular contractions can then be studied. The drug indomethacin inhibits the synthesis of prostaglandins, by inhibiting the enzyme cyclo-oxygenase. Studies by Christ et al (1990) have shown that the myotonic oscillations are related to the generation and release of a stable endogenous substance. Since indomethacin and other agents that inhibit the cyclo-oxygenase pathway also inhibit the myotonic oscillations, it seems that a prostaglandin or a related compound (a thromboxane) is the endogenous substance (Christ et al 1990).

PGE1, in addition to relaxing cavernosal smooth muscle, inhibits the alpha-adrenergic mechanism which tonically contracts this muscle and maintains the flaccid non-erect state of the penis (Adaikan & Ratnam 1988). Thus it has a dual erectogenic action.

Papaverine

Papaverine was the first drug to be injected intracavernosally to treat impotence (Virag 1982).

It is still the most widely used drug for this purpose, although several other drugs have similar effects (Brindley 1986). Clinical aspects of papaverine treatment are discussed in Chapter 11.

Papaverine hydrochloride is the salt of a benzylisoquinoline alkaloid, produced either from opium or synthetically. It has a direct relaxant effect on smooth muscle, regardless of its innervation. In the penis, it relaxes vascular and trabecular smooth muscle, mimicking the autonomically mediated vascular events that occur during normal erection. These result from effects on the biochemical pathways that regulate tension in smooth muscle.

Its action, only partially understood, involves inhibition of oxidative phosphorylation and blocking of cyclic adenosine monophosphate phosphodiesterase (Poch & Kukovetz 1971). Smooth muscle cell calcium exchange is also altered and this may be mediated by cyclic GMP (Krall et al 1988). There is no evidence of any neurotransmitter receptor mediated mechanism.

Central neurotransmitter mechanisms and sexual behaviour

Before neuropeptides were recognized, experimental studies of central neurotransmission in sexual behaviour concentrated on serotonergic and dopaminergic systems (see Everitt 1983 for review). Most studies use the copulatory behaviour of the rat as a model. This has the advantage of being stereotyped and quantifiable. For example, the number of rats mounting receptive females after treatment with a particular drug can be compared with the number that mount after a sham treatment. The oversimplified conclusion often drawn from this research is that dopamine facilitates, and serotonin inhibits sexual behaviour. While still dogmatically asserted in textbooks and journal articles, this thesis ignores the observation that drugs acting on these systems may inhibit one component of sexual behaviour and enhance another, rather than having a general effect. Central noradrenergic mechanisms have received less attention than dopaminergic mechanisms, but it is clear from research on the role of central alpha$_2$-adrenoceptors dicussed above that they have an important role.

An increasing number of neuropeptides are being shown to have roles in regulating behaviour, including sexual behaviour. Two of these, oxytocin and ACTH, induce penile erection when injected into specific brain regions. These substances are not, however, specifically involved in sexual function. Their actions depend on their interaction with other factors, including environmental context and gonadal steroids, as well as having different effects at different sites in the brain. Oxytocin, for example, is also involved in the neural systems underlying maternal and other social affiliative behaviours.

Central dopaminergic mechanisms

The dopamine agonist, apomorphine, causes erection in man. Subcutaneous or intramuscular injection of a low dose of the drug is followed, within 20 minutes, by penile tumescence. This is not accompanied by sexual arousal, and often amounts to only a partial erection. It occurs in most normal volunteers examined in the laboratory (Lal et al 1984; Danjou et al 1988; Murphy & Brindley — unpublished data).

Double-blind studies of dopamine agonists are confounded by the frequent occurrence of nausea and other introceptive cues. However, in a study described as double-blind and placebo-controlled, apomorphine was give to 10 healthy volunteers. Penile circumference was monitored using plethysmography and subjective sexual arousal was self-assessed. Data were collected before, during and after a stimulation session during which 50 erotic slides were shown to the subjects. Apomorphine induced an erection starting from the fourth minute post-injection, and potentiated the response to erotic slides. Self-assessment showed increased tumescence and rigidity without modifications of sexual arousal (in the same study yohimbine had no effect on any of the variables measured) (Danjou et al 1988).

Unfortunately, in the author's experience, the clinical use of apomorphine is limited by the high incidence of nausea and vomiting. Nausea occurs in most cases at the dose needed to produce partial erection. At slightly higher doses, vomiting occurs and erection is unlikely to occur. The frequency of nausea also casts doubt on the claims of studies purporting to be double-blind. Attempts to attenuate nausea by pretreatment with the peripheral dopamine antagonist antiemetic, domperidone, makes little difference to nausea (Murphy — unpublished data).

In animal studies, apomorphine has a biphasic effect on erection, with lower doses facilitating and high doses inhibiting erection in freely moving rats. This biphasic effect is also seen when penile reflexes are tested (Pehek et al 1988). Haloperidol, a centrally-acting dopamine antagonist, blocks these effects, while domperidone, a dopamine antagonist which does not cross the blood–brain barrier, has no effect.

Similarly, in man domperidone does not prevent apomorphine from inducing erection, indicating that apomorphine is having its erectogenic effect at central receptors. Until recently two main types of dopamine receptor, D_1 and D_2, were distinguished on pharmacological grounds. The D_2 subtype is found on the presynaptic nerve terminal, as well as on postsynaptic neurones. The presynaptic receptor functions as an autoreceptor: its activation by dopamine leads to a reduction of further dopamine release from the presynaptic neurone and thus reduced dopaminergic transmission. There is evidence that dopamine agonists induce erection through their actions on dopamine D_2 autoreceptors. This would explain the biphasic effects of apomorphine, which preferentially stimulates D_2 autoreceptors at low doses and D_1 postsynaptic receptors at higher doses. Also, dopamine agonists, more selective for D_2 autoreceptors than apomorphine, cause penile erections in rats. Such erections are accompanied by stretching, yawning and sedation, all considered typical signs of central dopamine autoreceptor stimulation (Ferarri et al 1988).

These studies raise the possibility that erection occurs when dopaminergic transmission is reduced, rather than enhanced. This is likely to involve a particular set of dopaminergic fibres rather than dopaminergic systems generally. In the last few years, several novel dopamine receptors have been distinguished by molecular biological strategies (Civelli et al 1991). This opens the way for the development of more specific drugs that may have more specific actions on sexual function.

There are several well defined dopaminergic

fibre systems in the brain: the striatal system, the mesolimbic and mesocortical systems, and the hypothalamic tuberoinfundibular system, which regulates prolactin secretion. However, it is a less studied group of neurones, belonging to the incertohypothalamic system, that seem to be involved in mediating the effects of dopamine agonists on erection. The evidence for this comes from microinjection studies in the rat. Injection of apomorphine into the paraventricular nucleus (PVN), which contains dopaminergic cells of the incertohypothalamic system, elicits erection, while injection into neighbouring structures does not (Melis et al 1987). Apomorphine-induced erection is blocked by dopamine blockers, but also by agents that block oxytocin receptors. This suggests that apomorphine's effect depends on oxytocin release. Microinjection of oxytocin into the PVN also induces erection (Melis et al 1986) and while this effect is also prevented by oxytocin receptor blockade, it is not prevented by dopamine blockade. Thus, it seems that dopaminergic neurones activate oxytocinergic neurones in the PVN of the hypothalamus, which act through oxytocin receptors to produce erection (further details of the neuroanatomy of this system are discussed in Ch. 4).

Naloxone potentiates apomorphine-induced penile erections in rats, suggesting an opiate–dopamine receptor interaction in this response. Atropine, on the other hand, blocks them, suggesting a cholinergic–dopaminergic interaction (Berendsen & Gower 1986). Atropine's effect on apomorphine-induced erections must occur in the central nervous system, since it is not seen with methylatropine, which selectively blocks peripheral muscarinic receptors.

The therapeutic potential of dopamine agonists is unclear. Lal et al (1987, 1989) report that apomorphine induced full erection in 17 out of 28 men with impotence. Some of these men also reported improved potency with low doses of the oral dopamine agonist, bromocriptine (2.5 to 3.75 mg daily). Lal et al (1989) thus suggest that apomorphine be used as a test to detect impotence responsive to treatment with bromocriptine. Their positive outcome with bromocriptine, however, was obtained in a small group (6 patients out of 9 reported subjective improvement) using non-

blind ratings. Previous studies of bromocriptine in impotence have had negative results (Ambrosi et al 1977; Cooper 1977; Pierini et al 1981). Perhaps it works in selected cases. Among the impotent men who have responded, a few have had serum prolactin levels above the standard upper limit of normal, but not in the accepted range of pathological hyperprolactinaemia (HPRL) (Lal et al 1987). Since dopamine tonically inhibits prolactin release, the slight elevation of prolactin might reflect a central dopaminergic dysfunction in these men. Of further interest, mild elevations of prolactin are thought to be stress-related and may thus provide a lead to understanding the neurobiological correlates of psychogenic impotence.

When impotence is due to pathological hyperprolactinaemia, bromocriptine is effective in restoring sexual function rapidly. It is not clear whether it does this through lowering prolactin levels or directly through its effect on neural structures involved in sexual function. Hyperprolactinaemia also causes hypogonadism, which could contribute to the impotence. However, hypogonadism is not the main cause of impotence: recovery of potency with bromocriptine treatment occurs before gonadal function normalizes (Buvat et al 1985). Furthermore, testosterone replacement, without bromocriptine, is ineffective in such cases.

Treatment for Parkinson's disease with levodopa (a dopamine precursor) has often been noted to improve sexual performance. This benefit has been attributed by some to improved mobility or a general effect on mental state. Studies of levodopa in impotence have produced conflicting results (Pierini et al 1981; Benkert et al 1972). Erections have also been reported as a side effect of treatment with pergolide, a dopamine agonist used in Parkinson's disease (Lees & Stern 1981; Jeanty et al 1984).

Serotonin (5-HT)

A decrease in brain serotonin (5-hydroxytryptamine or 5-HT) levels can be achieved by inhibiting serotonin synthesis with parachlorophenylalanine (pCPA). The effect on male rats is a dramatic increase in sexual activity (Tagliamonte et al 1969; Whalen & Luttge 1970; Ahlenius et al 1971).

Drugs that increase central serotonergic neuro-transmission, on the other hand, depress sexual activity (Ahlenius et al 1980). These findings are the opposite of the results obtained by manipulating brain catecholamines, particulaly dopamine (Everitt 1983). It has thus been hypothesized that catecholamines exert a stimulatory influence, while serotonin exerts an inhibitory influence in the neural control of male rat sexual behaviour (Gessa & Tagliamonte 1974). However, it remains unclear how specific to sexual behaviour these neuronal systems are. The cerebral cortex and the limbic system are extensively innervated by ascending projections from serotonergic neurones in the brain-stem raphe nuclei. Serotonin pathways regulate many behaviours and affective states, including sleep, appetite, anxiety and aggression. The influence of 5-HT on this wide range of behaviours is mediated by its interaction with three families of receptors, although more are likely to be discovered. These receptors differ in their binding affinities for selective ligands, their receptor–effector coupling mechanisms, and the functions they regulate. The main types of 5-HT receptor are called 5-HT_1, 5-HT_2 and 5HT_3. 5-HT_1 is further subdivided into 4 types denoted by the subscripts A-D. Little is yet known of the sites at which sexual behaviour is modulated. The sexual responses seen with drugs acting on 5-HT systems may be a reflection of effects on general behavioural arousal.

Spinal serotonergic receptors appear to be involved in modulating penile reflexes. In rats, pharmacological stimulation of these receptors suppresses erection, while simultaneously facilitating seminal emission (Mas et al 1985). But findings are conflicting: serotonin agonists have also been shown to induce erection in both man and the rhesus monkey after intravenous injection (Horby Petersen et al 1988; Szele et al 1988). As with other neurotransmitter receptors, there are several subtypes of serotonin receptor. The erectogenic effect of serotonin agonists appears to be mediated by 5-HT_2 receptors in the central nervous system (Szele et al 1988).

Clinically, drugs that act on serotonergic mechanisms dramatically affect orgasm, rather than erection. Clomipramine, an antidepressant that increases synaptic concentrations of serotonin, abolishes orgasm in both men and women, but the mechanism for this is unclear (Monteiro et al 1987; Murphy 1987). The widely prescribed antidepressant and 5-HT reuptake inhibitor, fluoxetine, and the illicitly used drug 'ecstasy' (methylenedioxymethamphetamine or MDMA), a potent 5-HT agonist taken for its euphoriant effects, both impair orgasm and ejaculation. MDMA users report enhancement of the sensuous aspects of sex, despite inhibition of orgasm.

Opioid systems and sexual function

Endogenous opioid peptides (EOPs) are involved in the regulation of male sexual behaviour. Opiate drugs, β-endorphin and an enkephalin analogue all cause a specific, naloxone-reversible, inhibition of copulatory behaviour when administered acutely to male rodents (McIntosh et al 1980; Murphy 1981; Meyerson 1981; Pellegrini-Quarantotti et al 1979). In other words, stimulation of opioid receptors disrupts copulatory behaviour at doses which do not affect other motor or social behaviours.

The opioid antagonist, naloxone, given alone, has had more variable effects on copulation. Some have found no effect and others have described facilitatory effects in sexually active rats (McIntosh et al 1980; Myers & Baum 1979; Wu & Noble 1986; Pfaus & Gorzalka 1987). Naloxone has also induced copulation in rats normally sexually inactive (Gessa et al 1979).

In experimental tests for reflex erectile responses and seminal emission, morphine reduced the proportion of animals showing erections in a dose-related fashion. Seminal emission was more sensitive to morphine inhibition than erectile responses, since it was virtually suppressed by all the doses of morphine tested. Naloxone, given alone, had little effect in most doses, although a significant decrease in the display of erection was observed with the lowest dose. These results indicate that, in addition to the effects of opiates on sexual drive, their acute effects on genital reflexes could play a role in the sexual dysfunction associated with opiate intake (Gomez-Marrero et al 1988).

By contrast, studies of penile reflexes in rats treated chronically with morphine found that erectile ability was relatively well preserved, suggesting that the decline in sexual behavior induced by chronic morphine is primarily due to a failure of sexual arousal, and not of erectile ability (Clark et al 1988).

In a study using anaesthetized male cats, naloxone caused penile erection in 5 of 11 experiments (Domer et al 1988). The erections rapidly followed the drug's injection by 30 seconds to 4 minutes, and their duration was 5 to 36 minutes. Morphine, given either before or after the naloxone, made no difference to these erections, suggesting that the relevant opioid receptors are not of the same type as those for morphine (there are several different types of opioid receptor; morphine acts mainly through the μ-subtype). Domer et al (1988) suggested that the erections resulted from removal of tonic opioid-mediated inhibition of reflex mechanisms in the spinal cord or sacral parasympathetic ganglia.

In monkeys, opiate antagonists have been reported to have either no effect or to inhibit sexual behaviour (Meller et al 1980; Glick et al 1982; Abbot et al 1984). In healthy men, the acute effects of opioid antagonists have varied, but include a report of spontaneous penile erections following naltrexone 50 mg orally (Mendelson et al 1979). In a double-blind cross-over study of naloxone's effect on the sexual responses of normal male volunteers, intravenous naloxone attenuated the pleasure experienced with arousal and at orgasm, but had no effect on erection (Murphy et al 1990). Naloxone also inhibited oxytocin release at orgasm.

The combination of naloxone with yohimbine has been reported to cause sustained and full erection in healthy voluteers (Charney and Heninger 1986). A high dose of naloxone (1 mg/kg) alone induced partial erection in 3 of 6 volunteers, while yohimbine alone had no effect. The combination was associated with full erection, lasting for at least 60 minutes in all 6 subjects. There was no effect on sexual drive, but the combination caused marked anxiety, the extent of which would limit clinical application. This synergistic effect of the combination of opioid receptor and alpha₂-adrenergic receptor blockade suggests an important functional relationship between central opioid and noradrenergic systems in erection.

The orally administered opioid antagonist, naltrexone, has been reported to have a therapeutic effect in impotence (see Ch. 10). This clinical study relied on subjective reports of improvement rather than objective measures.

The chronic use of opiates is associated with a generalized attrition of sexual function with loss of desire, impotence and anorgasmia (Cushman 1972; DeLeon & Wexler 1973; Greenberg 1984). These features are, however, part of a broad picture of psychophysiological disturbance and tell us little about the direct role of endogenous opioid peptides (EOP) in sexual function or sexual dysfunction.

Other centrally-acting neuropeptides: oxytocin and ACTH

Oxytocin is a nonapeptide synthesized in the neurones of the paraventricular nucleus (PVN) and supraoptic nucleus of the hypothalamus. It is released into the circulation from nerve terminals in the neurohypophysis (posterior pituitary gland) during sexual activity in men (Murphy et al 1987). Its function in this setting is unknown, but it may be related to ejaculation rather than erection, since oxytocin receptors are found on genital tract smooth muscle. Oxytocin is also thought to be a central neurotransmitter or neuromodulator. One of its central actions is to induce erection on injection into the PVN, a property it shares with apomorphine (see p. 63).

There is pharmacological evidence that the central oxytocin receptors mediating the expression of penile erection are similar to those present in the uterus (Argiolas et al 1989a). Oxytocin receptors in the PVN appear to be located on oxytocinergic neurones, where they are excitatory. In other words, oxytocinergic activity stimulates further oxytocinergic activity, suggesting a positive feedback loop. This positive feedback mechanism is important for the neurosecretory bursts that underlie the secretion of oxytocin into the blood, but the role of such a mechanism in the control of erection has not been examined.

In addition to its erectogenic action in the PVN, oxytocin can also provoke erection if injected bilaterally into the hippocampus. This is a site known to contain a relatively dense population of oxytocin receptors that modulate hippocampal output. This effect is not seen at other sites in the brain apart from the PVN.

Adrenocorticotrophic hormone (ACTH), injected into the cerebral ventricles, also causes erection. This occurs along with other behaviours (grooming, stretching, yawning and inhibition of food intake). It was believed that oxytocin's erectogenic effect was mediated by ACTH release (or release of an ACTH-derived peptide) from hypothalamic opiomelanotropinergic neurones. This now appears unlikely because oxytocin remains effective after depletion of hypothalamic opiomelanocorticotropin-derived peptides (this is achieved by neonatal treatment with monosodium glutamate, which depletes hypothalamic opiomelanocorticotropin-derived peptides without altering their pituitary and circulating concentration) (Argiolas et al 1989b).

Tolerance develops to the behavioural effects of ACTH during continuous infusion in rats, and is associated with increased hypothalamic levels of beta-endorphin (Vergoni et al 1989). Also, hypophysectomy prevents the erectile response to ACTH (Argiolas 1987). In other words, the pituitary gland plays a role in the expression of the erectile response induced by ACTH. It also plays a permissive role in oxytocin-induced erection (Argiolas et al 1989b).

DRUGS THAT CAUSE ERECTILE DYSFUNCTION

Anti-hypertensives

Anti-hypertensive drugs are frequently blamed for causing impotence. There are several types of anti-hypertensive drug, each with a different pharmacological action. The two most frequently used first-line drugs are thiazide diuretics and beta-blockers. Alpha-blockers, calcium channel antagonists, and angiotensin converting enzyme (ACE) inhibitors are also widely used. An old treatment for hypertension was the use of ganglion blockers — drugs that block neurotransmission through both sympathetic and parasympathetic autonomic ganglia. Since erection depends on autonomic nerve impulses reaching erectile tissue, these drugs usually caused impotence. However, they are seldom used today.

Methyldopa interferes with noradrenaline synthesis and adrenergic transmission in peripheral and central neurones. It is still used to treat hypertension, particularly in the elderly. Its main effect on sexual function is loss of libido (Kolodny et al 1979). Most of the newer antihypertensive drugs are also thought to cause impotence. ACE inhibitors such as captopril, and nifedipine are possible exceptions (Kostis 1988; Croog et al 1988). Many anti-hypertensives also interfere with ejaculation. It is not clear how these newer drugs interfere with erection, or what predisposes some men more than others to this effect. Many patients with hypertension have arterial disease which can cause impotence per se. In some cases, an anti-hypertensive drug may precipitate impotence because the blood supply to the penis is already diminished (but sufficient to allow erection) until the drug aggravates the problem by reducing blood pressure. There is evidence that untreated hypertensive men without impotence have subclinically reduced penile blood flow. Karacan et al (1989) studied erectile haemodynamics during nocturnal penile tumescence in drug-free hypertensive patients with and without erectile dysfunction, and normotensive controls without erectile problems. Penile blood flow during rapid eye movement sleep differed significantly among all 3 study groups: normotensive controls had the highest amplitudes, hypertensive patients without erectile problems had lower values and hypertensives with erectile complaints had the lowest values. They concluded that their measurements in hypertensive men without erectile complaints indicate subclinical signs of developing vasculogenic erectile dysfunction.

A clinical study by Bulpitt et al (1976) found that impotence was reported significantly more often in hypertensives on treatment than it was in normal controls (25% vs. 7%). Untreated hypertensives reported impotence in 17%, a frequency that was not statistically significantly different from either of the other two groups.

Impotence is unlikely to be the result of simply lowering blood pressure. Some drugs are more likely to cause impotence than others, suggesting other pharmacological mechanisms are involved. This is clinically important, because drug-induced impotence may be alleviated by switching to a drug with dissimilar mechanisms, allowing potency to recover while maintaining control of the patient's blood pressure.

Thiazide diuretics have been shown to cause impotence more frequently than beta-blockers in a Medical Research Council (MRC) trial of treatment of mild hypertension (MRC Working Party 1981 & 1985). This trial was designed to examine the effect of drug treatment on the rate of strokes, coronary events and death. Patients were randomized to one of three groups: bendrofluazide, propranolol or placebo. 9000 men entered the study, which was single-blind and based in general practice. Impotence was the commonest reason for withdrawal from active treatment and was significantly more common with bendrofluazide than with propranolol. Compared with the placebo, the difference was significant at the $p < 0.001$ level for both drugs. It is difficult to ascribe much meaning to this last figure in a single-blind design, since doctors are unlikely to attribute impotence to a placebo. On the other hand, they are more likely to blame the drug when other causes may be operating. However, the difference between the two drugs is unlikely to be the consequence of the study design. The mechanism by which bendrofluazide causes impotence is not known. In most of those affected by impotence, erectile function recovered within a few weeks of stopping bendrofluazide.

Suzuki et al (1988) compared the effects of 4 antihypertensive drugs on sexual function in 156 men, using a self-report questionnaire at 1–4 weeks of treatment and after one year. The drugs were a thiazide (trichloromethiazide), a beta-blocker (atenolol), an ACE inhibitor (captopril), and a calcium channel antagonist (nifedipine). Daily drug treatment was preceded by a 2–4 week period of placebo during which only 5% of the hypertensive patients complained of some sexual disturbance. After 1–4 weeks of antihypertensive therapy there was an increase in the reporting of sexual dysfunction with all drugs except captopril. Patients on atenolol or trichloromethiazide complained of both erectile and ejaculatory problems, while those on nifedipine complained mainly about problems with ejaculation. In the case of atenolol, serum levels of both testosterone and follicular stimulating hormone were decreased and there was mild elevation of oestradiol. But given what

we know about the relationship between testosterone and erectile function (see Ch. 3), the hormonal changes are unlikely to have played a significant role in the impotence. At 1 year, only patients taking atenolol still reported an increase in sexual dysfunction.

Other clinical studies have also incriminated beta-blockers in impotence (Riley 1980; Croog et al 1988). Propranolol may be more likely than other beta-blockers to cause impotence and some individuals may be especially vulnerable to it (Riley 1980; Rosen et al 1988). Although beta-adrenoceptors are present in the corpus cavernosum, little is known of their physiological significance (Hedlund & Andersson 1985). Intracavernosal injection of propranolol does not prevent erection in normal subjects, making it unlikely that beta-blockers cause impotence by blocking receptors in erectile tissue (Brindley 1986).

Alpha-blockers also lower blood pressure, but seem not to cause impotence (Pentland et al 1981; Riley & Riley 1983). Indeed, as discussed previously, their effect on penile smooth muscle when injected intracavernosally is to induce relaxation, and therefore they might be expected to improve potency. Alpha blockade can, however, cause failure of ejaculation (Pentland et al 1981).

There is little clinical information on the effect of calcium channel blockers on erection. There is a case report of a calcium channel blocker causing impotence (Luderschmidt 1987). By contrast, intracavernosal injection of the calcium channel blocker, verapamil, induces erection (Brindley 1986). There is also a case report of nifedipine causing erection in a previously impotent man (Rayner et al 1988). Other antihypertensive vasodilators, including hydralazine and prazosin, have also been reported to cause priapism (Rubin 1968).

The effects of calcium channel blockers on isolated human penile erectile tissue taken from men with normal erectile function has been investigated (Fovaeus et al 1987). They were found to inhibit electrically induced contractions of the trabecular muscle. They also inhibited contractions induced by noradrenaline. Since the flaccid state of the penis is dependent on contraction of muscle in erectile tissues, and this is mediated mainly by neuronally released noradrenaline stimulating alpha-adrenoceptors, these data are compatible with calcium channel blockers having an erecto-genic effect. However, the plasma levels obtained during systemic treatment are unlikely to be high enough to have this effect.

In contrast to the effect of calcium channel blockers on erectile tissue, they have been shown to prevent apomorphine- and oxytocin-induced penile erection and yawning in male rats (Argiolas et al 1989a). This suggests that calcium channels are involved in other, possibly central, processes mediating erection.

Clonidine is an alpha$_2$-agonist used to treat hypertension and has been reported to cause impotence (Smith & Talbert 1986). It is not clear whether it does so by a peripheral or a central effect.

Pinacidil is an antihypertensive vasodilator thought to act through the opening of potassium channels. Its action on isolated human corpus cavernosum is to abolish spontaneous contractile activity and relax preparations precontracted by noradrenaline and to inhibit contractions induced by electrical field stimulation of nerves (Holmquist et al 1990). It is yet to be tested clinically in humans, but tests on monkeys have shown that it induces erection (Giraldi & Wagner 1990).

Nitrates are used to treat ischaemic heart disease, rather than hypertension, but like some of the drugs discussed above, they cause vasodilatation. Topical glyceryltrinitrate causes penile arterial dilatation in impotent men, measured by ultrasound (Heaton et al 1990). They also cause relaxation of adrenergically contracted strips of human penile tissue taken from impotent men (Heaton 1989). The clinical potential of nitrates still needs to be assessed. One study suggests that nitroglycerin patches applied to the skin of the penile shaft may benefit patients with moderate erectile disturbances (Claes & Baert 1989). There is, however, a risk of the drug being absorbed through the vaginal wall of the partner and causing severe headache (Talley & Crawley 1985).

Antidepressants

These drugs are widely used to treat depression and anxiety disorders. They act by increasing synaptic concentrations of noradrenaline and serotonin. There are two main groups: those that inhibit the reuptake of monoamines into the pre-synaptic neurone (tricyclics and related compounds), and those that inhibit the breakdown of monoamines in the presynaptic neurone by inhibiting the enzyme, monoamine oxidase (monoamine oxidase inhibitors — MAOIs).

As with antipsychotic drugs, there are numerous case reports of these drugs causing impotence, but few systematically collected data. In a controlled study of patients treated with either imipramine or phenelzine, neither drug increased the frequency of erectile problems as assessed by questionnaire (Harrison et al 1986). There are case reports suggesting that both of these drugs can, however, cause impotence (Greenberg 1965; Rabkin et al 1984). Other antidepressants reported to have caused impotence include amitriptyline (Lipsedge et al 1971; Hekimian et al 1978), amoxapine (Hekimian et al 1978), protriptyline (Vaisberg 1974), tranylcypromine (Simpson et al 1965), and clomipramine (Wooton & Bailey 1975). Since clomipramine prevents orgasm in almost all cases, impotence may arise secondarily in its case (Monteiro et al 1987). In most of the reports, erectile difficulties have usually occurred within the first few weeks of treatment and cease on stopping the drug or with dose reduction.

Since these drugs increase peripheral as well as central adrenergic neurotransmission, they may cause erectile difficulties by enhancing the adrenergically-mediated contraction of erectile smooth muscle. Most antidepressants are also anticholinergic, and although muscarinic blockade alone does not interfere with erection, it may aggravate the difficulty of increased adrenergic control.

Antidepressants may lead to an improvement in erectile function in some men. This can be the result of improvement in the patient's mental state, but in the case of one antidepressive, trazodone, it appears to be a more direct action. It has led to both improvement of erectile dysfunction in impotent men and the development of prolonged erections or priapism in potent men (Lal et al 1990; Bardin & Krieger 1990). Like other drugs that cause priapism, trazodone probably does so by blocking peripheral alpha-adrenoceptors. Imipramine has also been observed to induce erection in horses in a nonsexual context (McDonnell et al 1987). Erection typically occurred within 10 minutes of injection, continued intermittently for

1 to 2 hours, and was associated with masturbation. Imipramine has numerous effects on different neurotransmitter systems, but mainly it inhibits the reuptake of serotonin and noradrenaline from central synapses. However, it is not at all clear how it induces erection in horses.

Antipsychotic drugs (neuroleptics)

These agents are used to treat and prevent relapses of psychotic illness. Their antipsychotic action results from their blockade of central dopamine D_2 receptors. Most of the commonly prescribed agents also antagonize dopamine D_1 receptors, acetylcholine muscarinic receptors and alpha-adrenoceptors. Almost all of these drugs have been reported to cause erectile problems, however there is no good systematic research on the incidence of this. Esimates of the prevalence of erectile difficulties in patients on antipsychotics vary between 23% and 54% (Segraves 1989).

There are several mechanisms by which antipsychotic drugs could cause erectile dysfunction. It follows from the preceding discussion of dopamine agonists, that dopamine D_2 blockade is a likely cause. Sulpiride is an antipsychotic agent selective for dopamine D_2 receptors and it causes impotence (Weizman et al 1985). It also prevents apomorphine-induced erections in rats (Melis et al 1987) and normal volunteers (Nair et al 1982). In patients, however, impotence might also be the result of hyperprolactinaemia, which also results from dopamine D_2 blockade. Impotence with antipsychotics may be dose-related and recovery has been reported following dose reduction (Anath 1974; Weizman et al 1985).

Antipsychotics may also diminish libido and can interfere with ejaculation through their anti-adrenergic effect. Indeed, they have been used with the aim of reducing libido in men with deviant sexual behaviour (Tennet et al 1974). In a double-blind, placebo-controlled study of low dose benperidol and chlorpromazine in such men, neither drug had any effect on erection (Tennet et al 1974). However, the doses used were lower than those used to treat psychosis.

Alcohol

Surveys have shown that alcohol may enhance sexual enjoyment, presumably by disinhibiting feelings and behaviour, particularly in women (Bancroft 1987, p. 608). However, many men reported the converse: alcohol reduced their enjoyment. Acute intoxication is frequently described as a cause of erectile failure, but it is not clear what the mechanism for this effect is. It is generally assumed that alcohol has a direct pharmacological inhibiting effect on genital responses above the blood alcohol concentration of 0.04 g/100 ml (Bancroft 1987). Morlet et al (1990) have examined the effect of alcohol in normal volunteers on nocturnal penile tumescence (NPT). NPT was monitored in 11 subjects over three consecutive nights. On the third night, volunteers drank alcohol, achieving blood alcohol concentrations of 0.154 g/100 ml. Alcohol had no effect on the size, duration or number of erections.

Additional experiments using pelvic nerve stimulation were performed in dogs. Alcohol had no effect on the magnitude or duration of corpus cavernosal pressure changes produced by nerve stimulation, nor was the latent period from stimulation to erection affected. Mean blood alcohol levels were 0.327 g/100 ml in the dogs. These results were taken as evidence that the inhibition of erection after a bout of alcohol is not due to a suppression of the underlying spinal mechanisms, but may be the result of effects on perceptual or cognitive sexual mechanisms (Morlet et al 1990). It is important to realize, however, that NPT may not be a good model for erections occurring in the sexual context and that different neural pathways are likely to be involved. Alcohol could thus be acting on central neural mechanisms involved in these erections, and this would not be apparent in the above experiments.

Using another model, apomorphine-induced erections in rats, alcohol did suppress erection in a dose dependent manner (Heaton & Varrin 1991). Two possible mechanisms of action were suggested: alcohol may interfere with dopaminergic receptor mechanisms, or alcohol may alter a second neurotransmitter/neuropeptide more directly responsible for the production of apomorphine-induced erection, possibly oxytocin.

Chronic heavy drinking of alcohol can affect erectile function through its effects on several different organ systems, including the nervous system, endocrine system and the liver. In addition, the psychological consequences of alcohol dependence, such as depression, low self-esteem and marital conflict, can also add to sexual problems. Peripheral neuropathy occurs in alcoholism and can involve the sensory fibres of the dorsal nerve of the penis and pudendal nerve, resulting in diminished tactile sensation and impairment of the reflex mechanism for erection. The autonomic fibres to erectile tissue can also be damaged by alcohol (Novak & Victor 1974). There is no detectable abnormality in adrenoceptor mechanisms in impotence associated with alcoholism (Creed et al 1989).

Benzodiazepines

Benzodiazepines are widely used to treat anxiety. Their use is diminishing since it became clear that they frequently lead to dependency and severe withdrawal effects. They act in the central nervous system by binding to an unusual kind of receptor, known as the benzodiazepine-GABA receptor complex (GABA is gamma-aminobutyric acid, a widely distributed inhibitory neurotransmitter in the CNS). There is evidence that stimulation of GABA receptors in the lumbosacral spinal cord inhibits erectile reflexes in rats (Bitran et al 1988; Leipheimer & Sachs 1988).

Effects on sexual function are uncommon with benzodiazepines. In a large trial comparing various anxiolytic drug side effects, impotence occurred only in patients treated with chlorazepate and lorazepam, and was infrequent (Newton et al 1986). Diazepam was, however, associated with decreased libido. There has also been a case report of chlordiazepoxide causing impotence. Chlordiazepoxide also inhibits apomorphine-induced erections in rats (Gower et al 1986). In apparent contradiction to this, chlordiazepoxide has been found to enhance penile reflexes (Martino et al 1987).

Nicotine

Cigarette smoking has been associated epidemiologically with impotence (Jeremy et al 1986). Experimental studies suggest that nicotine's vaso-constrictor effect may play a causal role. Gilbert et al (1986) examined the effect of nicotine on 42 male cigarette smokers, aged 18 to 44 years. Subjects were randomly assigned to high-nicotine, low-nicotine or control groups and were shown a series of erotic films while their penile diameters, heart rates, and finger pulse amplitudes were continuously recorded by a polygraph. Subjects in the smoking groups smoked relatively high-nicotine (0.9 mg) or very low-nicotine (0.002 mg) cigarettes prior to watching the last two films, while control subjects ate candy. Smoking two high-nicotine cigarettes in immediate succession significantly decreased the rate of penile diameter change relative to the other conditions. These effects were not seen after a single cigarette was smoked. High-nicotine cigarettes also caused significantly more vasoconstriction, as measured by finger pulse amplitude than did low-nicotine cigarettes, which did not differ from control conditions.

Cigarette smoke extracts also inhibit methacholine-stimulated prostacyclin secretion in a dose dependent way. As previously discussed, prostacyclin is a vasodilator and is thought to be a local mediator of erection (see p. 61). Thus, the inhibition of its secretion by cigarette smoke may be a mechanism accounting for the above observations (Jeremy et al 1986).

Smoking has also been shown to inhibit papaverine-induced erection. Glina et al (1988) tested 12 patients' responses to intracavernous injections of 100 mg papaverine hydrochloride on two occasions. On the second occasion, the papaverine test was performed after the patient smoked 2 cigarettes. With the first test, all men obtained a full erection, compared to only 4 in the second. The average intracavernous pressures were 85.8 and 53.5 mmHg, respectively ($p < 0.01$). It is therefore important to note that cigarette smoking may cause false negative results in the papaverine diagnostic test (Glina et al 1988).

Drugs with anti-androgenic effects

As discussed in Chapter 3, many elements of sexual behaviour have been shown to be androgen-dependent. However, in men with normal gonadal function there is no correlation between circulating testosterone levels and erectile function. Furthermore, the levels of testosterone required for optimal and basal function remain elusive.

There are several different types of anti-androgenic agent. Some are used for their anti-androgenic effect, as for example in the treatment of carcinoma of the prostate. Others are not used as anti-androgens, and their effect on the endocrine system is a side effect. Drugs in the latter group include cimetidine, digoxin and metoclopramide; it has not been shown for any of these drugs that their anti-androgenic effects cause impotence (Bancroft 1987).

Cyproterone acetate is an anti-androgen used in the treatment of sex offenders. It reduces sexual interest and activity, but does not impair the erectile response to erotic films (Bancroft et al 1974). Medroxyprogesterone acetate (MPA) has also been used in sex offenders. In a laboratory study of MPA, there was a significant reduction in the report of arousal to erotic stimuli, but 'genital arousal' decreased only slightly. Nocturnal penile tumescence was significantly decreased during MPA administration and appeared to be related to decreases in total testosterone (Wincze et al 1986). The effects of both these drugs resemble the effects of hypogonadism (see Ch. 3).

Flutamide is a nonsteroidal pure anti-androgen which acts by inhibiting the uptake and/or binding of dihydrotestosterone (DHT) to the target cell receptor. DHT is one of testosterone's two main metabolites; the other, oestradiol, is unaffected by flutamide. It is therefore notable that flutamide does not cause impotence when given alone (Warren et al 1990). This suggests that oestradiol may be the more important metabolite in maintaining erectile function. This is compatible with evidence from animal studies showing that the nerve cells of the MPOA aromatize testosterone to oestradiol, which then stimulates the cellular processes leading to activation of male copulatory behaviour (Watson et al 1989). Flutamide is indicated in combination with an LHRH agonist in the treatment of metastatic (stage D2) prostate cancer. This combination causes loss of libido and impotence, but this is due to the LHRH agonist (Warren et al 1990). Flutamide has also been used, with success, to treat patients with urinary obstruction caused by benign prostatic hypertrophy and was noted not to cause impotence (Stone 1989).

Buserelin is a synthetic gonadotrophin-releasing hormone (GnRH) analogue which produces a short phase of stimulation followed by a selective inhibition of secretion of pituitary gonadotrophins, resulting in 'medical castration'. It is used in the palliative treatment of advanced prostatic cancer and advanced male breast cancer and can, but does not always, cause impotence and/or loss of libido (Roila 1989; Doberauer et al 1988).

Hypolipidaemic agents

The isobutyric acid derivatives, gemfibrozil and fenofibrate, are used to reduce serum triglyceride and cholesterol levels in patients with hyperlipidaemia unresponsive to dietary restriction. They are indicated in men under the age of 55 in the prevention of coronary artery disease and cause impotence in a small number of cases (Blane 1987; Pizarro et al 1990; Bain et al 1990). The mechanism of this is unknown.

Drugs and priapism

Priapism is defined as a persistent painful erection that cannot be relieved by sexual intercourse or masturbation. If untreated, priapism subsides spontaneously, but may take several days to do so. Impotence is a frequent complication. In almost half of all cases, priapism is idiopathic. Drug-induced priapism acounts for almost a third of cases. Other causes include sickle cell anaemia, leukaemia and other haematological diseases, malignancy and trauma.

Drugs which cause priapism include antipsychotic drugs (especially phenothiazines), trazodone, antihypertensives (mainly prazosin) and heparin. Intracavernosal injection of papaverine for impotence has become an important cause. With the exceptions of papaverine and heparin, alpha-adrenergic blockade is the likely mechanism for drug-induced priapism. In these cases treatment with an alpha-agonist, such as metaraminol, can reverse the priapism. Priapism is a urological emergency and surgery may be necessary if drugs do not work (see Banos et al 1989 for review).

SUMMARY

The peripheral neurotransmitter mechanisms controlling erection have still not been fully elucidated. Transmission is predominantly nonadrenergic noncholinergic (NANC), with VIP playing a main role in this. Acetylcholine is indirectly involved in facilitating erection. It does so by modulating other neuroeffector systems and facilitating the release of a smooth muscle relaxant from the vascular endothelium, EDRF (nitric oxide).

Inhibition of erection occurs through activation of alpha-adrenoceptors on cavernosal and vascular smooth muscle. This tonically maintains muscular contraction. Alpha$_1$-adrenoceptors have the predominant role.

The clinical effects of PGE1 suggest that prostaglandins may be physiologically involved in erection, and human cavernosal tissue produces large amounts of the potent vasodilatory prostacyclin. Furthermore, prostacyclin synthesis in penile tissue can be stimulated by cholinergic (muscarinic) agonists.

The dopamine agonist, apomorphine, causes erection in man. Its action is on the central nervous system, probably in the hypothalamus. In rats, oxytocin and ACTH also induce penile erection when injected into the PVN of the hypothalamus. Endogenous opioid peptides probably play an inhibitory role in the central pathways mediating erection, while central alpha$_2$-adrenoceptor mechanisms are involved in arousal mechanisms rather than erection. Serotonergic and GABAergic spinal systems are thought to play a role in erection, but the data on them are conflicting.

Table 5.1 Drugs that cause impotence.

Drug	Suggested mechanisms	Comments
Antihypertensives	Several possible mechanisms; reduction of blood pressure per se may be sufficient cause in some	
Thiazides	Unknown	Cause impotence more often than beta-blockers
Beta-blockers	May be a central effect	
Methyldopa	Disrupts adrenergic transmission by interfering with noradrenaline synthesis	Reduces desire as well
Sympathetic blocking drugs	Disrupt sympathetic nerve supply by depleting postganglionic fibre of noradrenaline	Rarely used today
Antidepressants		
Tricyclics	Unclear — not only an anti-cholinergic effect; possibly central	Dose related
MAOIs	Unknown	
Antipsychotics	Dopamine blockade; hyperprolactinaemia	Dose related
Antiandrogens	Block effects of androgens on hormone-sensitive neural components	May be secondary to loss of desire
Barbiturates	General depressant effect	
Hypolipidaemic agents		
Gemfibrozil and fenofibrate	Unknown	

REFERENCES

Abbot D, Holman S, Berman M, Neff D, Goy R 1984 Effects of opiate antagonists on hormones and behaviour of male and female rhesus monkeys. Archives of Sexual Behaviour 13: 1–25

Aboseif S R, Breza J, Bosch R J, Benard F, Stief C G, Stackl W, Lue T F, Tanagho E A 1989 Local and systemic effects of chronic intracavernous injection of papaverine, prostaglandin El and saline in primates. Journal of Urology 142(2): 403–408

Adaikan P G, Ratnam SS 1988 Pharmacology of penile erection in humans. Cardiovascular Interventive Radiology 11(4): 191–194

Adrian T E, Gu J, Allen J M, Takemoto K, Polak J M, Bloom S R 1984 Neuropeptide Y in the human genital tract. Life Science 35: 2643–2648

Ahlenius S, Heimann M, Larsson K 1971 Mating behaviour in the male rat treated with p-chlorophenylalanine methyl ester alone and in combination with pargyline. Psychopharmacology 20: 383–388

Ahlenius S, Larsson K, Svensson L 1980 Further evidence for an inhibitory role of 5-HT in male rat sexual behaviour. Psychopharmacology 68: 217–220

Andersson P O, Bloom S R, Mellander S 1984 Haemodynamics of pelvic nerve induced penile erection in the dog: possible mediation by vasoactive intestinal polypeptide. Journal of Physiology 350: 209–224

Argiolis A, Melis M R, Gessa G L 1986 Oxytocin: an extremely potent inducer of penile erection and yawning in male rats. European Journal of Pharmacology 130: 264–373

Argiolas A, Melis M R, Mauri A, Gessa G L 1987 Paraventricular nucleus lesion prevents yawning and penile erection induced by apomorphine and oxytocin but not by ACTH in rats. Brain Research 421(1–2): 349–352

Argiolas A, Melis M R, Fratta W, Mauri A, Gessa G L 1987 Monosodium glutamate does not alter ACTH- or apomorphine-induced penile erection and yawning. Pharmacology, Biochemistry and Behaviour 26(3): 503–507

Argiolas A, Melis M R, Gessa G L 1989a Calcium channel inhibitors prevent apomorphine- and oxytocin-induced penile erection and yawning in male rats. European Journal of Pharmacology 166(3): 515–518

Argiolas A, Melis M R, Mauri A, Gessa G L 1989b Oxytocin-induced penile erection and yawning in male rats: effect of neonatal monosodium glutamate and hypophysectomy. Psychopharmacology (Berlin) 97(3): 383–387

Argiolas A, Melis M R, Stancampiano R, Gessa G L 1989 Penile erection and yawning induced by oxytocin and related peptides: structure-activity relationship. Peptides 10(3): 559–563

Azadzoi K M, Payton T, Krane R J, Goldstein I 1990 Effects of intracavernosal trazodone hydrochloride: animal and human studies. Journal of Urology 144(5): 1277–1282

Bain S C, Lemon M, Jones A F 1990 Gemfibrozil-induced impotence. Lancet 336(8727): 1389 [letter]

Balon R, Ramesh C, Pohl R 1989 Sexual dysfunction associated with diazepam but not with clonazepam. Canadian Journal of Psychiatry 34(9): 947–948 [letter]

Bancroft J, O'Carroll R, McNeilly A, Shaw R W 1984 The effects of bromocriptine on the sexual behaviour of hyperprolactinaemic men: a controlled case study. Clinical Endocrinology 21: 131–137

Banos J E, Bosch F, Farre M 1989 Drug-induced priapism: Its aetiology, incidence and treatment. Medical Toxicology and Adverse Drug Effects 4(1): 46–58

Beretta G, Zanollo A, Ascani L, Re B 1989 Prostaglandin El in the therapy of erectile deficiency. Acta Europa Fertility 20(5): 305–308

Bitran D, Miller S A, McQuade D B, Leipheimer R E, Sachs B D 1988 Inhibition of sexual reflexes by lumbosacral injection of a GABA agonist in the male rat. Pharmacology, Biochemistry and Behaviour 31(3): 657–666

Brindley G S 1982 Cavernosal alpha-blockade: a new technique for investigating and treating erectile impotence. British Journal of Psychiatry 143: 332–337

Brindley G S 1985 Pathophysiology of erection and ejaculation. In: Whitfield H N & Hendry W F (eds) Textbook of genito-urinary surgery. Churchill Livingstone, Edinburgh

Brindley G S 1986 Pilot experiments on the actions of drugs injected into the human corpus cavernosum penis. British Journal of Pharmacology 87: 495–500

Burnstock G 1986 The changing face of autonomic neurotransmission. Acta Physiologica Scandinavica 126: 67–91

Buvat J, Lemaire A, Buvat-Herbaut M, Fourlinnie J, Racedot A, Fossati P 1985 Hyperprolactinaemia and sexual function in men. Hormone Research 22: 196–203

Carani C, Scuteri A, Marrama P, Bancroft J 1990 The effects of testosterone administration and visual erotic stimuli on nocturnal penile tumescence in normal men. Hormones and Behaviour 24(3): 435–441

Charney D S, Heninger G R 1986 Alpha$_2$-adrenergic and opiate receptor blockade: synergistic effects on anxiety in healthy subjects. Archives of General Psychiatry 43: 1037–1041

Christ G J, Maayani S, Valcic M, Melman A 1990 Pharmacological studies of human erectile tissue: characteristics of spontaneous contractions and alterations in alpha-adrenoceptor responsiveness with age and disease

in isolated tissues. British Journal of Pharmacology 101(2): 375–381

Civelli O, Bunzov J R, Grandy D K, Zhou Q Y, Van Tol H M 1991 Molecular biology of the dopamine receptors. European Journal of Pharmacology 207: 277–286

Claes H, Baert L 1989 Transcutaneous nitroglycerin therapy in the treatment of impotence. Urology International 44(5): 309–312

Clark J T, Gabriel S M, Simpkins J W, Kalra S P, Kalra P S 1988 Chronic morphine and testosterone treatment: effects on sexual behavior and dopamine metabolism in male rats. Neuroendocrinology 48(1): 97–104

Clark J T, Smith E R, Davidson J M 1984 Enhancement of sexual motivation in male rats by yohimbine. Science 225: 847–849

Cocores J A, Miller N S, Pottash A C, Gold M S 1988 Sexual dysfunction in abusers of cocaine and alcohol. American Journal of Drug and Alcohol Abuse 14(2): 169–173

Creed K E, Carati C J, Adamson G M, Callahan S M 1989 Responses of erectile tissue from impotent men to pharmacological agents. British Journal of Urology 63(4): 428–431

Creed K E, Carati C J, Keogh E J 1988 Autonomic control and vascular changes during penile erection in monkeys. British Journal of Urology 61(6): 510–505

Croog S H, Levine S, Sudilovsky A, Baume R M, Clive J 1988 Sexual symptoms in hypertensive patients. A clinical trial of antihypertensive medications. Archives of Internal Medicine 148(4): 788–794

Cushman P 1972 Sexual behaviour in heroin addiction and methadone maintenance. New York State Journal of Medicine 72: 1261–1265

Dabire H 1986 Idazoxan: a novel pharmacological tool for the study of alpha$_2$-adrenoceptors. Journal of Pharmacology (Paris) 17: 113–118

Dail W G, Moll M A, Weber K 1983 Localization of vasoactive intestinal polypeptide in penile erectile tissue and in the major pelvic ganglion of the rat. Neuroscience 10: 1379–1386

Dail W G, Minorsky N, Moll M A, Manzanares K 1986 The hypogastric nerve pathway to penile erectile tissue: histochemical evidence supporting a vasodilator role. Journal of the Autonomic Nervous System 15: 341–349

Danjou P, Alexandre L, Warot D, Lacomblez L, Puech A J 1988 Assessment of erectogenic properties of apomorphine and yohimbine in man. British Journal of Clinical Pharmacology 26(6): 733–739

DeLeon G, Wexler H 1973 Heroin addiction: its relation to sexual behaviour and sexual experience. Journal of Abnormal Psychology 81: 36–38

Domer F R, Wessler G, Brown R L, Matthews A 1988 Effects of naloxone on penile erection in cats. Pharmacology, Biochemistry and Behaviour 30(2): 543–545

Dorr L D, Brody M J 1967 Hemodynamic mechanisms of erection in the canine penis. American Journal of Physiology 213: 1526–1531

Doxey J C, Roach A G, Smith C F C 1983 Studies on RX781094: a selective, potent and specific antagonist of alpha$_2$-adrenoceptors. British Journal of Pharmacology 78: 489–505

Earle C M, Keogh E J, Wisniewski Z S, Tulloch A G, Lord D J, Watters G R, Glatthaar C 1990 Prostaglandin El therapy for impotence; comparison with papaverine. Journal of Urology 143(1): 57–59

Everitt B J 1983 Monoamines and the control of sexual behaviour. Psychological Medicine 13: 715–720

Ferrari F, Mangiafico V, Tartoni P, Tampieri A 1988 Imidazole and yohimbine antagonize hypomotillty, penile erection, stretching and yawning induced in rats by BHT 920, a selective dopamine autoreceptor agonist. Pharmacology Research Communications 20(9): 827–837

Fovaeus M, Andersson K E, Hedlund H 1987 Effects of some calcium channel blockers on isolated human penile erectile tissues. Journal of Urology 138(5): 1267–1272

Freedman J E, Aghajanian G K 1984 Idazoxan (RX 781094) selectively antagonizes alpha$_2$-adrenoceptors on rat central neurones. European Journal of Pharmacology 105: 265–272

Furchgott R F 1984 The role of endothelium in the responses of vascular smooth muscle to drugs. Annual Review of Pharmacology and Toxicology 24: 175–197

Gessa G L, Tagliamonte A 1974 Role of brain monoamines in male sexual behaviour. Life Sciences 14: 425–436

Gessa G, Paglietti E, Pellegrini-Quarantotti B 1979 Induction of copulatory behaviour in sexually inactive rats by naloxone. Science 204: 203–205

Gilbert D G, Hagen R L, D'Agostino J A 1986 The effects of cigarette smoking on human sexual potency. Addiction Behaviour 11(4): 431–434

Giraldi A, Wagner G 1990 Effects of pinacidil upon penile erectile tissue, in vitro and in vivo. Pharmacology and Toxicology 67(3): 235–238

Glick B, Baughman W, Jensen J and Phoenix C 1982 Endogenous opiate systems and primate reproduction: inability of naloxone to induce sexual activity in rhesus males. Archives of Sexual Behaviour 11: 267–275

Glina S, Reichelt A C, Leao P P, Dos-Reis J M 1988 Impact of cigarette smoking on papaverine-induced erection. Journal of Urology 140(3): 523–524

Gomez Marrero J, Feria M, Mas M 1988 Stimulation of opioid receptors suppresses penile erectile reflexes and seminal emission in rats. Pharmacology, Biochemistry and Behaviour 31(2): 393–396

Gower A J, Berendsen H H, Broekkamp C L 1986 Antagonism of drug-induced yawning and penile erections in rats. European Journal of Pharmacology 122(2): 239–244

Greenberg A 1984 Effects of opiates on male orgasm. Medical Aspects of Human Sexuality 18: 207–210

Gu J, Polak J M, Probert L et al 1983 Peptidergic innervation of human male genital tract. Journal of Urology 130: 386–391

Gu J, Lazarides M, Pryor J P et al 1984 Decrease of vasoactive intestinal polypeptide in the penises from impotent men. Lancet ii: 315–318

Heaton J P 1989 Synthetic nitrovasodilators are effective, in vitro, in relaxing penile tissue from impotent men: the findings and their implications. Canadian Journal of Physiology and Pharmacology 67(1): 78–81

Heaton J P, Morales A, Owen J, Saunders F W, Fenemore J 1990 Topical glyceryltrinitrate causes measurable penile arterial dilation in impotent men. Journal of Urology 143(4): 729–731

Heaton J P, Varrin S 1991 The impact of alcohol ingestion on erections in rats as measured by a novel bioassay. Journal of Urology 145(1): 192–194

Hedlund H, Andersson K E 1985 Effects of some peptides on isolated human penile tissue and cavernous artery. Acta Physiologica Scandinavica 124: 413–419

Henderson V E, Roepke M H 1933 On the mechanism of erection. American Journal of Physiology 106: 441–448

Holmquist F, Andersson K E, Hedlund H 1990 Effects of pinacidil on isolated human corpus cavernosum penis. Acta Physiologica Scandinavica 138(4): 463–469

Horby-Petersen J, Nielsen F C, Schmidt P F 1988 Penile tumescence after injection of a serotonin antagonist (ketanserin). British Journal of Urology 62(3): 277–278

Jeremy J Y, Mikhailidis D P, Dandona P 1986a Muscarinic stimulation of prostacyclin synthesis by the rat penis. European Journal of Pharmacology 123(1): 67–71

Jeremy J Y, Morgan R J, Mikhailidis D P, Dandona P 1986b Prostacyclin synthesis by the corpora cavernosa of the human penis: evidence for muscarinic control and pathological implications. Prostaglandins and Leukotrienes Medicine 23(2–3): 211–216

Jeremy J Y, Mikhailidis D P, Thompson C S, Dandona P 1986c The effect of cigarette smoke and diabetes mellitus on muscarinic stimulation of prostacyclin synthesis by the rat penis. Diabetes Research 3(9): 467–469

Johansen L V, Kirkeby H J, Kiil J 1989 Prevention of erection after penile surgery. A double–blind trial of intracavernous noradrenaline versus placebo. Urology Research 17(6): 393–395

Juenemann K P, Lue T F, Luo J A, Jadallah S A, Nunes L L, Tanagho E A 1987 The role of vasoactive intestinal polypeptide as a neurotransmitter in canine penile erection: a combined in vivo and immunohistochemical study. Journal of Urology 138(4): 871–877

Karacan I, Salis P J, Hirshkowitz M, Borreson R E, Narter E, Williams R L 1989 Erectile dysfunction in hypertensive men: sleep-related erections, penile blood flow and musculovascular events. Journal of Urology 142(1): 56–61

Kostis J B 1988 Angiotensin converting enzyme inhibitors II. Clinical use. American Heart Journal 116 (6 Pt. 1): 1591–1605

Krall J F, Fittingoff M, Rajfer J 1988 Characterization of cyclic nucleotide and inositol 1, 4, 5-trisphosphate-sensitive calcium-exchange activity of smooth muscle cells cultured from the human corpora cavernosa. Biology of Reproduction 39(4): 913–922

Lal S, Ackman D, Thavundayil J X, Kiely M, Etienne P 1984 Effect of apomorphine, a dopamine receptor agonist, on penile tumescence in normal subjects. Progress in Neuro-Psychopharmacology and Biological Psychiatry 8: 695–699

Lal S, Laryea E, Thavundayil J X et al 1987 Apomorphine-induced penile tumescence in impotent patients — preliminary findings. Progress in Neuro-Psychopharmacology and Biological Psychiatry 11: 235–242

Lal S, Tesfaye Y, Thavundayil J X et al 1989 Apomorphine: clinical studies on erectile impotence and yawning. Progress in Neuro-Psychopharmacology and Biological Psychiatry 13: 329–339

Lal S, Rios O, Thavundayil J X 1990 Treatment of impotence with trazodone: a case report. Journal of Urology 143(4): 819–820

Lee L M, Stevenson R W, Szasz G 1989 Prostaglandin E1 versus phentolamine/papaverine for the treatment of erectile impotence: a double-blind comparison. Journal of Urology 141(3): 549–550

Lewis C J, Havler M E, Humphrey M J, Lloyd–Jones J G, McCleavy M A, Muir N U, Waltham K 1988 The pharmacokinetics and metabolism of idazoxan in the rat. Xenobiotica 18: 519–532

Lundberg J M 1981 Evidence of coexistence of vasoactive intestinal polypeptide (VIP) and acetylcholine in neurones of cat exocrine glands. Morphological, biochemical and functional studies. Acta Physiologica Scandinavica [suppl.] 496: 1–57

Lundberg J M, Hedlund B, Bartfai T 1982 Vasoactive intestinal polypeptide enchances muscarinic ligand binding in cat submandibular salivary gland. Nature 295: 147–149

Lydiard R B, Howell E F, Laraia M T, Ballenger J C 1987 Sexual side effects of alprazolam. American Journal of Psychiatry 144(2): 254–255 [letter]

McIntosh T, Vallano M, Barfield R 1980 Effects of morphine, beta-endophin and naloxone on catecholamine levels and sexual behaviour in the male rat. Pharmacology, Biochemistry and Behaviour 13: 435–41

McNicholas T A, Thomson K, Rogers H S, Blandy J P 1989 Pharmacological management of erections during transurethral surgery. British Journal of Urology 64(4): 435–6

Martino V, Mas M, Davidson J M 1987 Chlordiazepoxide facilitates erections and inhibits seminal emission in rats. Psychopharmacology (Berlin) 91(1): 85–89

Mas M, Zahradnik M A, Martino V, Davidson J M 1985 Stimulation of spinal serotonergic receptors facilitates seminal emission and suppresses penile erectile reflexes . Brain Research 342: 128–134

Melis M R, Ariolis A, Gessa G L 1986 Oxytocin-induced penile erection and yawning: sites of action in the brain. Brain Research 398: 259–265

Melis M R, Ariolis A, Gessa G L 1987 Apomorphine-induced penile erection and yawning: sites of action in the brain. Brain Research 415: 948–104

Meller R, Keverne E, Herbert J 1980 Behavioural and endocrine effects of naltrexone in male talapoin monkeys. Pharmacology, Biochemistry and Behaviour 13: 663–668

Mendelson J, Ellingboe J, Kuenhle J, Mello N 1979 Effects of naltrexone on mood and neuroendocrine function in normal adult males. Psychoneuroendocrinology 3: 231–236

Meyerson B 1981 Comparison of the effects of beta-endorphin and morphine on exploratory and socio–sexual behaviour in the male rat. European Journal of Pharmacology 69: 453–463

Morales A, Condra M, Owen J, Surridge D H, Fenemore J, Harris C 1987 Is yohimbine effective in the treatment of organic impotence? Journal of Urology 137: 1168

Morlet A, Watters G R, Dunn J, Keogh E J, Creed K E, Tulloch A G, Lord D J, Earle C M 1990 Effects of acute alcohol on penile tumescence in normal young men and dogs. Urology 35(5): 399–404

Morley J E, Flood J F, Silver A J 1990 Opioid peptides and aging. Annals of the New York Academy of Science 579: 123–132

Murphy M R 1981 Methadone reduces sexual performance and sexual motivation in the male Syrian golden hamster. Pharmacology, Biochemistry and Behaviour 14: 561–567

Murphy M R 1987 Down-regulation of post-synaptic serotonin receptors as a mechanism for clomipramine-induced anorgasmia. British Journal of Psychiatry 151: 704

Murphy M R, Seckl J R, Burton S, Checkley S A, Lightman S L 1987 Changes in oxytocin and vasopressin secretion during sexual activity in men. Journal of Clinical Endocrinology and Metabolism 65: 738–741

Murphy M R, Seckl J R, Checkley S A, Lightman S L 1990 Naloxone inhibits oxytocin release at orgasm in man. Journal of Clinical Endocrinology and Metabolism 71(4): 1056–1058

Murray F T, Cameron D, Ketchum C 1984 Return of gonadal function in men with prolactin-secreting pituitary tumors. Journal of Clinical Endocrinology and Metabolism 59: 79–85

Myers B, Baum M 1980 Facilitation of copulatory performance in male rats by naloxone: effects of hypophysectomy, 17-estradiol, and luteinizing-hormone releasing hormone. Pharmacology, Biochemistry and Behaviour 12: 365–370

Nagulesparen M, Ane V, Jenkins J C 1978 Bromocriptine treatment of males with pituitary tumors, hyperprolactinemia and hypogonadism. Clinical Endocrinology 9: 73–80

Ottsen B, Wagner G, Virag R, Fahrenkrug J, 1984 Penile erection: possible role for vasoactive intestinal polypeptide as a neurotransmitter. British Medical Journal 288: 9–11

Palmer R M J, Ferrige A G, Moncada S 1987 Nitric oxide release accounts for the biological activity of endothelium-derived relaxing factor. Nature 327: 524–526

Pehek E A, Thompson J T, Eaton R C, Bazzett T J, Hull E M 1988 Apomorphine and haloperidol, but not domperidone, affect penile reflexes in rats. Pharmacology, Biochemistry and Behaviour 31(1): 201–208

Pellegrini-Quarantotti B, Paglietti E, Bonanni A, Petta M, Gessa G 1979 Naloxone shortens ejaculation latency in male rats. Experientia 35: 524–525

Pfaus J G, Gorzalka B B 1987 Opioids and sexual behaviour. Neuroscience and Biobehavioural Reviews 11: 1–34

Pizarro S, Bargay J, D'Agosto P 1990 Gemfibrozil-induced impotence. Lancet 336(8723): 1135 [letter]

Polak J M, Gu J, Mina S, Bloom S R 1981 Vipergic nerves in the penis. Lancet ii: 217–219

Reid K, Morales A, Harris C, Surridge D H C, Condra M, Owen J, Fenemore J 1987 Double blind trial of yohimbine in treatment of psychogenic impotence. Lancet i: 421–423

Riley A J, Goodman R E, Kellet J M, Orr R 1989 Double blind trial of yohimbine hydrochloride in the treatment of erectile inadequacy. Journal of Sexual and Marital Therapy 4: 17–26

Roila F 1989 Buserelin in the treatment of prostatic cancer. Biomedical Pharmacotherapy 43(4): 279–285

Rosen R C, Kostis J B, Jekelis A W 1988 Beta-blocker effects on sexual function in normal males. Archives of Sexual Behaviour 17(3): 241–255

Roy A C, Adaikan P G, Sen D K, Ratnam S S 1989 Prostaglandin 15-hydroxydehydrogenase activity in human penile corpora cavernosa and its significance in prostaglandin-mediated penile erection. British Journal of Urology 64: 1180–182

Roy J B, Petrone R L, Said S I 1990 A clinical trial of intracavernous vasoactive intestinal peptide to induce penile erection. Journal of Urology 143(2): 302–304

Sachs B D, Leipheimer R E 1988 Rapid effect of testosterone on striated muscle activity in rats. Neuroendocrinology 48(5): 453–458

Saenz de Tejada I, Blanco R, Goldstein I et al 1988 Cholinergic neurotransmission in human corpus cavernosum I. Responses of isolated tissue. American Journal of Physiology 254: H459–H467

Saenz de Tejada I, Goldstein I, Azadzoi K, Krane R J, Cohen R A 1989 Impaired neurogenic and endothelium-mediated relaxation of penile smooth muscle from diabetic men with impotence. New England Journal of Medicine 320(16): 1025–1030

Sarosdy M F, Hudnall C H, Erickson D R, Hardin T C, Novicki D E 1989 A prospective double-blind trial of intracorporeal papaverine versus prostaglandin El in the treatment of impotence. Journal of Urology 141(3): 551–553

Scharf M B, Mayleben D W 1989 Comparative effects of prazosin and hydrochlorothiazide on sexual function in hypertensive men. American Journal of Medicine 86(lB): 110–112

Schramek P, Dorninger R, Waldhauser M, Konecny P, Porpaczy P 1990 Prostaglandin El in erectile dysfunction: efficiency and incidence of priapism. British Journal of Urology 65(1): 68–71

Schramek P, Waldhauser M 1989 Dose-dependent effect and side-effect of prostaglandin El in erectile dysfunction. British Journal of Clinical Pharmacology 28(5): 567–571

Schrey A 1990 Prostaglandin El injection in erectile dysfunction. Current diagnostic and therapeutic possibilities. Fortschr Med 108(30): 577–580

Segraves R T 1989 Effects of psychotropic drugs on human erection and ejaculation. Archives of General Psychiatry 46: 275–284

Siad S I 1981 VIP overview. In: Bloom S R, Polak J M (eds) Gut hormones, 2nd edn. Churchill Livingstone, Edinburgh p 379–384

Sjostrand N O, Klinge E 1979 Principal mechanisms controlling penile retraction and protrusion in rabbits. Acta Physiologica Scandinavica 106: 199–214

Smith E R, Lee R E, Schnur S L, Davidson J M 1987a Alpha₂-adrenoceptor antagonists and male sexual behaviour: I. Mating behaviour. Physiology and Behaviour 41: 7–14

Smith E R, Lee R E, Schnur S L, Davidson J M 1987b Alpha₂-adrenoceptor antagonists and male sexual behaviour: II. Erectile and ejaculatory reflexes. Physiology and Behaviour 41: 7–14

Sonda L P, Mazo R, Chancellor M B 1990 The role of yohimbine for the treatment of erectile impotence. Journal of Sex and Marital Therapy 16(1): 15–21

Stackl W, Hasun R, Marberger M 1988 Intracavernous injection of prostaglandin El in impotent men. Journal of Urology 140(1): 66–68

Steers W D, McConnell J, Benson G 1984 Anatomical localization and some pharmacological effects of vasoactive intestinal polypeptide in human and monkey corpus cavernosum. Journal of Urology 132: 1048–1053

Stief C, Benard F, Bosch R, Aboseif S, Nunes L, Lue T F, Tanagho E A 1989 Acetylcholine as a possible neurotransmitter in penile erection. Journal of Urology 141(6): 1444–1448

Susset J G, Tessier C D, Wincze J, Bansal S, Malhotra C, Schwacha M G 1989 Effect of yohimbine on erectile impotence: a double-blind study. Journal of Urology 141: 1360–1363

Suzuki H, Tominaga T, Kumagai H, Saruta T 1988 Effects of first-line antihypertensive agents on sexual function and sex hormones. Journal of Hypertension (suppl.) 6(4): S649–651

Swanson L W, Sawchenko P E 1983 Hypothalmic integration: organization of the paraventricular and supraoptic nuclei. Annual Review of Neuroscience 6: 269–324

Szele F G, Murphy D L, Garrick N A 1988 Effects of fenfluramine, m-chlorophenylpiperazine, and other serotonin-related agonists and antagonists on penile erections in nonhuman primates. Life Sciences 43(16): 1297–1303

Tagliamonte A, Tagliamonte P, Gessa G L, Britishodie B B 1969 Compulsive sexual activity induced by p-chlorophenylalanine in normal and pinealectomized rats. Science 166: 1433–1435

Talley J D, Crawley I S 1985 Transdermal nitrate, penile erection, and spousal headache. Annals of Internal Medicine 103: 804 [letter]

Vergoni A V, Poggioli R, Facchinetti F, Bazzani C, Marrama D, Bertolini A 1989 Tolerance develops to the behavioural effects of ACTH-(1–24) during continuous i.c.v. infusion in rats, and is associated with increased hypothalamic levels of beta-endorphin. Neuropeptides 14(2): 93–98

Virag R, Ottesen J, Fahrenkrug J, Levy C, Wagner G 1982 Vasoactive intestinal polypeptide release during penile erection in man. Lancet ii: 1166

Wagner G, Brindley G S 1980 The effect of atropine and beta-blockers in human penile erection: a combined pilot study. In: Zorgniotti A W, Ross G (eds) Vasculogenic impotence. Charles C Thomas, Springfield, Illinois, p 77

Wespes E, Schiffmann S, Gilloteaux J, Schulman C, Vierendeels G, Menu R, Pelletier G, Vaudry H, Vanderhaeghen J J 1988 Study of neuropeptide Y-containing nerve fibers in the human penis. Cell and Tissue Research 254(1): 69–74

Wincze J P, Bansal S, Malamud M 1986 Effects of medroxyprogesterone acetate on subjective arousal, arousal to erotic stimulation, and nocturnal penile tumescence in male sex offenders. Archives of Sexual Behaviour 15(4): 293–305

Wu F M, Noble R J 1986 Opiate antagonists and copulatory behaviour of male hamsters. Physiology and Behaviour 38: 817–825

Assessment of erectile dysfunction

6. The clinical interview

Alain Gregoire

As in most other areas of medical practice, the history remains the most crucial part of the investigation of erectile dysfunction. The wide range of investigative techniques now available in this area sometimes lulls clinicians into a false sense of security that the diagnosis will be reached by arranging tests, even in the absence of a detailed history. Such an approach is expensive and detrimental to the doctor–patient relationship; it subjects patients to unnecessary procedures and may result in inappropriate or inadequate treatment. This applies as much to therapists who, for various reasons, may choose to ignore physical factors, as it does to surgeons who fail to give attention to psychological ones.

The aim of the history is to assess not only the dysfunction, but its impact on the patient and his relationships. Inevitably, this interaction between the clinician and the patient (and his partner) provokes a number of processes which the clinician should be aware of. These include the development of a therapeutic relationship between clinician and patient, provision of education and information and facilitation of communication about sensitive topics. Thus it is not simply *what* you ask about but how you do so which will determine the quality and accuracy of your assessment. Furthermore, some of these processes may in themselves have a positive therapeutic impact.

AIMS OF THE ASSESSMENT INTERVIEW

The primary aim of the patient in consulting the clinician is usually to obtain treatment to alleviate the dysfunction. He will also have a secondary interest in an adequate explanation of why the problem has occurred. It should not, however, be assumed that this is always the case. Some men have other motives for their consultations. They may be seeking help wlth some other, even more embarrassing or stigmatizing problem, such as transvestism. Some patients may only be attending from a sense of duty or on the insistence of their partners, without any real desire to achieve

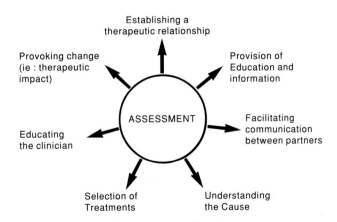

Fig. 6.1 The aims of the assessment interview.

change. Occasionally this occurs when the man is involved in another sexual relationship in which he is not impotent and he only attends to prevent his partner becoming suspicious over his apparent lack of concern.

Thus one crucial aim of the interview is to establish clearly why the patient is seeking help. Also implicit in the patient's aim of getting his problem treated is that he has identified the problem correctly. In fact, this is often not the case. Men commonly present for treatment of loss of erections when in fact they are experiencing premature ejaculation with a consequent physiological loss of tumescence. Clear identification of the problem is crucial to the establishing of goals which patient and partner would like to achieve through treatment.

Notwithstanding these qualifications, the primary aim of the clinician is to gain the information needed to provide the most effective treatment approach. It is often assumed that this aim is synonymous with that of establishing the aetiology. This is not so: although aetiology clearly plays a role in determining treatment choice, many other factors are involved. Thus understanding the causes of the problem is a distinct aim in itself which not only assists in treatment choice but satisfies the patient's need for explanation and, not least, the academic interests of the clinician.

As mentioned above, it is inevitable that the assessment interview will initiate the therapeutic relationship and may provoke beneficial (or indeed detrimental) change. The able clinician will use his skills to maximize the benefits of these processes.

The methods of achieving these aims will now be considered in terms of the informational content of the assessment as well as the context in which the interview is carried out.

THE CONTEXT OF THE INTERVIEW

The first contact

The earliest contact between patient and clinic is usually postal, in the form of the appointment letter, or by telephone. Although this contact seems trivial to clinic staff, it produces important first impressions for the patient. Whatever the nature of the clinic, it is desirable that a positive,

encouraging attitude be portrayed in this initial contact. This is neither difficult nor time consuming: appointment letters should be clear, informative and welcoming. It is helpful to give some indication of what the patient should expect (e.g. if he may be kept waiting, how long he will be seen for, whom/what sort of clinician he will be seeing) and any request the clinic may have (e.g. inviting the partner, if there is one, to attend).

In this sensitive and personal area of health care, it is important to train secretaries and receptionists to be sensitive to the patient's embarrassment. Telephone enquiries, within the time available, should be answered in a clear, informative and non-judgemental manner. Staff answering telephone enquiries or making appointments should be able to inform patients of the services available, general clinic policies and waiting lists. In the private sector, details of costs and policies on payment of bills should also be clearly explained.

The image conveyed in such first contacts can have important effects on the proportion of patients who eventually attend clinics.

Pre-assessment questionnaires

Many practitioners in this field ask patients to fill in questionnaires before being seen. These are normally sent to the patient for completion at home. This has the advantage of giving the clinician some idea of the nature of the problem. In the ideal setting of a multidisciplinary clinic, this may be useful in determining who would be the most appropriate person to see the patient. This can, of course, save valuable time for both the patient and the services. Filling in questionnaires can also help the patient to formulate clearly in his mind the nature of his difficulties. It can also reassure him that the clinic is well used to dealing with the sensitive issues which he may be fearful of talking about.

The information gained from this procedure can also be used for clinical audit, providing basic information on the clinic population and, more significantly, a baseline against which progress can be measured. This is obviously useful both clinically and for research purposes. A number of standardized questionnaires have been used in this way and some clinics devise their own to meet their particular needs. Several instruments measuring various aspects of sexuality and relationships are described in Chapter 7.

Pre-assessment questionnaires also have some disadvantages which lead some workers to decide against their use. Some patients describe being put off by having to answer very personal questions before seeing anyone face to face. Foreign patients or those with poor literacy will feel intimidated. Patients who are unable to understand some of the questions may have a similar reaction. This may lead to patients being put off attending.

The clinic environment

Just as the adequacy of lighting and the condition and sterility of instruments are of direct concern to surgeons in operating theatres, the clinic environment should be of concern to practitioners dealing with sexual problems. Clinics in hospitals should be well signposted to spare patients the embarrassment of having to ask the way. Receptionists should have a separate area away from the waiting room to take patients' details and answer their queries in privacy. For consultations, it seems obvious that private, relatively soundproof rooms with space enough for clinician and two partners are a basic requirement. Clinicians should ensure that they are not interrupted while conducting interviews.

Time

Because of the high demand for the often limited services in this area, time is usually a scarce commodity. However, the temptation to minimize time spent on taking a history should be balanced against the time, effort and money lost in carrying out avoidable tests and inappropriate treatments. Time spent in preparation is seldom wasted!

It is usually possible, in the course of one hour, to obtain a good history which fulfils all or most of the aims which have been discussed. Although this is less than the time advocated by some clinicians, it is in practice much more time than is available in many general urology clinics. This suggests that such clinics are not an appropriate setting for dealing with such problems. In addi-

tion to simple time requirements, the need for an eclectic approach makes the specialist, multi-disciplinary clinic the optimum setting for the management of erectile problems (Gregoire 1990).

The time available for the interview and its scope should be made clear to the patient/couple so that they can anticipate the pace and allow themselves enough time to raise matters of particular concern.

It is essential, whenever possible, to see both the man and his partner if he has one. However, it is important that in addition to being seen together, each partner be interviewed individually. This permits an open and frank discussion of the views of each partner on the nature and causes of the problem. Each partner's reaction to the problem may be crucial to their responses to intervention. Many views and feelings which are not secrets as such are unspoken because of fears of hurting the partner's feelings. However, some items of information disclosed in individual interviews *are* secrets — for example, past or current affairs or homosexual inclinations.

A commonly employed scheme is to see a couple together initially for 10 minutes or so. This time is used to provide an introduction and to obtain an outline of the history. Each partner is then seen alone, starting usually with the man (i.e. the one who has presented with the problem). He is seen for 20–30 minutes, after which time his partner is seen for 10–20 minutes. The remaining time is used by the clinician to sum up his findings, and give a brief explanation about the problem. The choices available at this stage (further investigations, treatments) should then be discussed. Although some patients are able to make rapid decisions about what they want to do next, some need time to think through the options and discuss them with their partners.

Confidentiality

From the first contact with the patient it should be made clear to him that any information he gives will be kept confidential. However, two areas of difficulty may arise in this respect. One relates to the ethical duty which doctors have to society, which may override the duty of confidentiality to the individual patient. This might include situations such as the disclosure of rape, violence or sex with underage children. Fortunately, difficulties in this area arise only very rarely.

The second, more common, area of difficulty arises when disclosures about affairs or more significant secrets are made during individual interviews. The moral issues in such situations are not the proper concern of clinicians or therapists. However, there may be considerable implications for the success of interventions. Sex therapy is contraindicated if either partner is currently involved in another relationship. It is important therefore that such information be elicited. This will only happen if confidentiality in the individual interviews is assured. Each partner should be specifically asked to indicate any information which he or she does not want revealed to the spouse.

Some therapists feel that collusion with one or both partners in such secrets makes therapy impossible and therefore avoid the issue by not carrying out individual interviews. My view is that this is even more of a collusion as it does not ever give the partners an opportunity to admit to having secrets. Considerable time may also be wasted engaging patients in treatments doomed to failure because of major problems occurring in addition to the superficial ones elicited.

Starting the interview

The importance of putting the patient/couple at ease has already been stressed. The interview room should not be arranged in too formal a manner, such as a doctor and patient on each side of a desk reminiscent of the media image of doctor–patient relationships. Seating should be at the same height and comfortable enough to sit in for the duration of the interview!

Before asking the patient in, the clinician should acquaint himself with whatever information is available about him. This means reading referral letters, past notes, screening questionnaires and checking on details such as age and marital status. In the all important first encounter with the patient, the clinician will then be able to greet him by name, welcome his partner and introduce him or herself. At this stage it is useful for the interviewer to summarize what he knows about the patient so far, for example by describing the contents of the referral letter. This reassures the patient that the clinician knows what the consultation is about and begins to establish that this is a safe place to talk about sensitive personal issues. However, this is usually not the best time to launch into a detailed examination of the presenting problem.

Another way of starting the interview is to describe the purpose of this consultation and the way in which it will be carried out, i.e. joint and individual interviews, timing, what will be discussed and what information or decisions will be forthcoming at the end. Patients can be relieved of a good deal of embarrassment and reluctance to discuss sexual matters by the clinician explaining that most people find it very difficult to talk about such things but that it gradually becomes easier.

During this initial phase, the clinician should be observing the responses of patient and partner. Both what they say and how they say it will provide him with a preliminary guide on how to conduct the interview most efficiently. With highly anxious or embarrassed patients it is usually best to spend more time on relatively non-embarrassing topics before questioning about the sexual problem. A calm reassuring approach will be particularly important. Sometimes one partner appears to be a reluctant attender. This situation is usually evident from an early stage — the person will usually avoid eye contact with interviewer and partner, may tut or look away whilst the partner is speaking or stare at the partner in an expectant or sometimes frankly hostile manner. He or she will need to be encouraged and engaged in a manner which reassures them that their attendance and their point of view is as important as their partner's. In the individual interviews, this issue will need to be raised with both partners and the clinician should plan to allocate more time than usual to interview the reluctant party.

Note taking

It is advisable, and from the time point of view usually essential, to take notes during the course of the interview. Deferring note taking to the end of the consultation is time consuming and likely to be less accurate. As the patient may feel he is not always receiving your undivided attention, it is advisable to briefly explain the need for record keeping and of course the confidentiality of the notes. The less experienced interviewer should be aware that detailed note taking can become a displacement activity engaged in to avoid eye contact and distract from anxiety or embarrassment. This sort of behaviour should be consciously and actively controlled as it can be detrimental to the relationship with the patient.

Interviewing technique

Clinicians lacking experience in the field of human sexuality often feel uncomfortable asking about details of sexual activity. Unfortunately this is a neglected area of many professional training courses, despite being officially recognized as an area of need (Fisher et al 1988; Royal Commission on Medical Education 1968). In this situation, as much as in any other task, anxiety will hamper performance. This may express itself in a lack of eye contact with the patient, bluntness in the discussion and unwillingness to probe into detail, and even surprise or disapproval at information revealed. In addition to these relatively subtle signs of anxiety, most clinicians are able to recall experiencing facial flushing, perspiration and even hand tremor when seeing patients in the early stages of their training.

Confidence in trainees or clinicians new to this field can be effectively and rapidly enhanced by providing basic, brief education into the range of human sexual behaviour, coupled with an opportunity to experience sexual history-taking through observation, video recordings or role playing. An understanding of some basic interviewing techniques will greatly increase the clinician's efficiency in eliciting the history.

It is best to start a line of questioning with open ended questions. These will elicit the patient's own description of the situation. This gives essential information on his attitudes, emotions and understanding. Furthermore, it allows the patient to volunteer what is often vital information which might otherwise take a long time to elicit or indeed might never be uncovered. Examples of open ended questions include 'What is your view of the problem?' or 'What effects has this had on your general relationship?'.

The patient's answers to open questions, both what was and what was not said, will point to specific areas needing further enquiry. In addition, answers in the patient's own words inform the clinician of the vocabulary that they feel able to use. Descriptive terms used by patients vary from idiosyncratic and obscure euphemisms to well researched medical terminology. Either way, it is important that the clinician establish exactly what patients mean by the terms they use. In general it is advisable for the clinician, in a non-patronizing way, to explain the meaning of the terms he uses and to stick to them, rather than attempting to adopt the variety of terms used by each of his patients.

At this stage, closed questions can be employed. These should not be confused with leading questions, which must be avoided wherever possible. Closed questions limit the answer to yes or no; for example, 'Can you get a full erection during masturbation?'. Leading questions suggest an answer; for example, 'Don't you think you are a bit old to expect a reliable erection?' This question is also an example of a judgemental reflection, which is likely to alienate the patient and make further progress with an accurate assessment impossible.

When the interviewer feels unsure of the accuracy of his understanding it is useful to summarize this, seeking the patient's/couple's comments. For example, 'Am I right in thinking that your difficulties with erections began about three years ago, ... that before that you had never had any difficulties with erections at all, ... and that things have got gradually worse so that you now can not get any erections, even slight ones, at any time at all?' It may also be necessary, at times, to ask patients to clarify by discussing specific examples, which will verify that answers to closed questions are accurate.

Doctor : Can you tell me a little more about your difficulties?
Mr A.H.: Well, I just can't get an erection at all.
Doctor: Do you mean during intercourse, or at other times?
Mr A.H.: Never. So now we can't have sex anymore.
Doctor: Do you ever get erections during the night or when you wake up in the morning?
Mr A.H.: No, not now.
Doctor: Can you tell me the last time you had an erection in the morning?

Mr A.H.: It must be at least two weeks ago.
Doctor: And when did you last have intercourse?
Mr A.H.: Not since Saturday.
Doctor: Did you have a firm erection then?
Mr A.H.: Yes — but it has not worked properly since
           then.

In addition to facilitating and controlling the gathering of information by verbal techniques, there are also nonverbal means of achieving this. Facial expression, eye contact and posture are highly effective ways of expressing concern (and lack of concern!). Positive 'body language', including leaning towards the individual, smiling, making eye contact and using hand movements can provide non-verbal prompts to encourage the taciturn patient.

With the garrulous patient, non-verbal messages are less effective and often counterproductive. The best method of retaining control here is to tactfully explain that although what is being said is important, the interviewer may be obliged to interrupt in order to cover all the important points in the limited time available. Patients respect such a statement more than being ignored, seeing the doctor tapping his pen on the desk or being interrupted without explanation. With such patients, the clinician may be obliged to restrict his use of open ended questions.

After taking the history it is important (as every clinical exam. candidate knows) to always ask patients a final general question such as, 'Is there anything else which you think may be important that we have not discussed?' It is surprising how often unexpected relevant information is proffered at this stage.

THE CONTENT OF THE INTERVIEW

In this section, I will attempt to provide a comprehensive discussion of the areas which need to be considered in the assessment. This does not imply that all the issues discussed must be covered for each individual — the detailed content of each assessment is tailored by the clinician according to the circumstances. Nevertheless, the clinician should work within the framework of an assessment routine which suits him. Recommendations regarding the organization of joint and individual interviews are discussed above (p. 83). Within

these interviews, it is useful to follow a scheme which covers all the topics which need considering. Some clinicians simply use a mental list, others prefer to use preprinted assessment schedules, prepared to varying levels of detail. Formal standardized interviews exist but are mainly used in research, where flexibility needs to be exchanged for standardization. (Questionnaires and rating scales are discussed in Ch. 7.)

In working through the schedule proposed below, bear in mind the goals of the interview discussed earlier, i.e. to establish:

1. What is the patient seeking?
2. What is the nature of the problem?
3. What are the causes of the problem?
4. What is the best further management?
5. Finally, although less relevant to the content, to achieve some therapeutic impact.

In considering the cause of a patient's difficulties, it is essential to follow an aetiological model to prevent either confusion or oversimplification. One of the most useful, proposed by Hawton (1985) divides aetiological factors into predisposing, precipitating and perpetuating factors (Table 6.1).

Factors falling into these three categories may be 'psychological or physical'. It is essential to be aware that the term 'psychological or physical' does not imply a concept of mutual exclusivity between psychological or physical causes for a man's dysfunction. Organic and psychogenic factors should be considered not on each end of a bipolar axis, as is assumed in so much of the contemporary literature, but as two orthogonal dimensions. Before discussing content, let us consider the ways in which information about erectile dysfunction and associated factors are organized in current classification systems.

Classification systems

The two most widely used diagnostic systems for the classification of mental disorders are the DSM-III, produced by the American Psychiatric Association, and the World Health Organization's International Classification of Diseases (ICD 9, soon to be replaced by ICD 10). Although the DSM-IIIR and ICD 10 (draft) both attempt to

Table 6.1 Psychological causes of sexual dysfunction. (Modified from Hawton 1985, by permission of Oxford University Press.)

Predisposing factors
Restrictive upbringing
Traumatic early sexual experiences
Disturbed family relationships
Early insecurity in psychosexual role
Inadequate sexual information
Socially withdrawn personality type

Precipitating factors
Reaction to organic factors
Discord in the general relationship
Ageing
Infidelity
Unreasonable expectations
Depression and anxiety
Dysfunction in the partner
Traumatic sexual experience
Random failure

Maintaining factors
Performance anxiety
Anticipation of failure
Guilt
Loss of attraction between partners
Poor communication between partners
Discord in the general relationship
Fear of intimacy
Impaired self-image
Inadequate sexual information; sexual myths
Restricted foreplay
Psychiatric disorder

reduce diagnostic variability and discrepancies by giving clear and detailed criteria for each diagnostic category, their success in achieving this aim is considerably less with the disorders of sexual functioning than with psychiatric disorders such as schizophrenia and depression. This is partly because the definitions are brief and therefore lack both specificity and detail.

DSM-III classifies all sexual dysfunctions as 'psychosexual disorders', specifically excluding disorders of organic origin. Erectile failure is classified under 'inhibited sexual excitement' and defined as 'recurrent and persistent inhibition of sexual excitement during sexual activity manifested by partial or complete failure to obtain or maintain an erection until completion of the sexual act' which must occur in combination with 'a clinical judgement that the individual engages in sexual activity that is adequate in focus, intensity and duration'.

The draft version of ICD 10 classifies erectile dysfunction as 'failure of genital response' in men (F52.2), under the main heading of 'Sexual dysfunction' (F52). Dysfunction with organic aetiology is admitted, and the possibility of mixed aetiology is recognized, an improvement over ICD 9 and DSM-III.

For the research worker or clinician specifically interested in classification of erectile problems, both these classification systems are severely inadequate on several counts:

a. They do not take account of the complex interaction between organic and psychological aetiological factors.
b. They are too imprecise in the definition of what constitutes a problem in terms of persistence, duration and severity.
c. Crucial to any conceptualization of sexual disorders is an understanding of the degree to which a patient or couple perceives the disorder as a problem. This is not considered by either of these systems.

To overcome some of these problems, Schover et al (1982) have developed a problem orientated diagnostic system specifically for sexual dysfunctions. A much greater degree of specificity about the nature of the problem is achieved by having a larger number of mutually exclusive categories, described in much greater detail than in the above systems. Furthermore, categorization is achieved by a description of behaviour as well as cognitions and affect but not through aetiological influences. The disorders are listed under five axes: desire, arousal, orgasm, coital pain and dissatisfaction with frequency. A sixth axis allows the listing of qualifying information including marital distress, sexual preferences and other relevant psychological or physical disorders. Erectile problems are listed under axis II (see Table 6.2). Categorization on this axis is further qualified by indicating whether the problem has been lifelong or not, whether it is the presenting complaint of the patient, and whether it is global (i.e. occurring with different partners or with different types of stimulation) or situational (i.e. occurring only with certain partners or with certain types of stimulation).

The main criticism which can be directed against this classification system is that it does not contain adequate information about the aetiology

Table 6.2   Axis II from the Multiaxial Problem-Orientated System (Schover et al 1982).

Arousal phase
Decreased subjective arousal
Difficulty achieving erections
Difficulty maintaining erections
Difficulty achieving and maintaining erections
Decreased subjective arousal and difficulty achieving erections
Decreased subjective arousal and difficulty maintaining erections
Decreased subjective arousal and difficulty achieving and maintaing erections
Decreased physiological arousal, female
Decreased physiological arousal, male
(L vs. N) (G vs. S) (P)

Notes: L vs. N indicates lifelong vs. not lifelong; G vs. S: global vs. situational; P: presenting complaint.

of the erectile dysfunction which, as advances are made in our understanding and ability to investigate, is another essential part of the description. In recognition of this, Benkert et al (1985) have developed a classification system with 7 axes and six sub-types (see Table 6.3). Unfortunately, in a commendable attempt to cover more ground, the authors have lost some of the specificity of description which was achieved by Schover et al. Another problem is that although the authors acknowledge the possibility of combined physical and psychological aetiologies, they have ranked 'organic disorders' above other physical conditions and psychiatric disorders above psychosocial conditions. It is not clear why the authors have done so, since they clearly acknowledge the multifaceted complexity of aetiological processes.

Table 6.3   The Multiaxial Classification System proposed by Benkert et al 1985.

Multiaxial description of sexual dysfunction
Axis A: Description of the syndrome
Axis B: Description of the course
Axis C_1:   Description of relevant organic diseases
Axis C_2:   Description of relevant laboratory findings
Axis D_1:   Description of relevant psychiatric disorder
Axis D_2:   Description of relevant psychosocial stressors
Axis E: Description of medication

Classificatory system for sexual dysfunction
Subtype Ia: Organic disorder
Subtype Ib: Physical conditions
Subtype IIa: Psychiatric disorder
Subtype IIb: Psychosocial conditions
Subtype III: Pharmacological conditions
Subtype IV: Cryptogenic disorder

As classification systems become more complex in an attempt to match the developments in our understanding of erectile dysfunction, they begin to look more and more like clinical descriptions. It is inevitable that no classification system will ever be ideal, and potential users will always have to select the one which best meets their particular needs. For example, a survey of the prevalence of erectile dysfunction in a normal population requires a classification system which includes all men with a clearly defined level of symptoms, irrespective of aetiological factors. However, research of treatment outcome in clinic populations requires systems which give reliable details on both the severity and all relevant aetiological factors.

Transcultural issues

Sexual attitudes and behaviours are amongst the most culturally determined aspects of the human condition. Any attempt to understand and provide help for difficulties arising in this area demands an awareness of the more important sexual norms operating in the patient's culture. However, this must be coupled with a sense of the individual's variation within his culture, as well as the alterations which occur as different cultures integrate (d'Ardenne 1987; Bhugra & Cordle 1988).

The presenting problem

A clear picture of the exact nature of the problem needs to be established. It is not enough to assume that the referral letter or the patient's complaint is accurate. The most common example of misunderstandings which arise in this way is of the man who complains of loss of erections during intercourse but who, in fact, is losing his erection secondary to premature ejaculation. Precise details regarding current erectile functioning are essential.

In a study by Segraves et al (1987), 18 questions were assessed for their ability to discriminate organic from psychogenic aetiology. The adequacy of early morning erections was found to be the most sensitive and specific predictor of organic aetiology. Only 2 other questions also discriminated between organic and psychogenic to a statistically significant degree both of which involved the adequacy of masturbating the non-coital erections. The authors point out that there are two conditions in which these questions might provide misleading answers. The 'pelvic steal' syndrome can occur in the presence of full early morning and non-coital erections. It is only with thrusting that diversion of blood to the buttocks and thigh muscles produces loss of erection. In hyperprolactinaemia, also, the answers to the above question may suggest psychogenic impotence.

Some patients find it difficult to describe the quality of their erections and others appear to have an 'all or none' concept, in which anything but a full erection counts as none at all. It is useful, therefore, for the clinician to offer some sort of understandable scale. Although many patients give a score out of 10 or use percentages, the individual variations in scoring render such figures meaningless. I recommend offering a scale such as:

- full as ever before
- full enough to penetrate with
- some swelling but not enough for penetration
- only very slight swelling
- absolutely no swelling at all

Patients also frequently confuse quality with duration of erection, such that full erections which disappear on attempted penetration are considered to count as none at all.

Thus, carefully distinguishing quality and duration, specific enquiries about erections in the following situations should be made: early morning, with sexual partner(s), (foreplay, penetration), during masturbation, and with erotic fantasies or literature. The very common presentation of loss of erections on attempted penetration, or very soon after, strongly suggests that the problem is related to anxiety. This is the moment when the erection becomes essential and many men clearly describe a peak of anxiety about loss of erection at this time. As discussed in Chapter 2, the effects of anxiety on sexual function are probably idiosyncratic. It is thus only fair to assume an anxiety effect if the appropriate emotional or somatic symptoms are described by the patient at a time when erectile failure occurs.

Certain cognitions are commonly associated with anxiety in this situation (Barlow 1986). For example, patients on attempting penetration may become preoccupied with the thought that they will lose their erection. In heightened states of anxiety, patients who suffer from phobias and panic attacks commonly experience 'catastrophic thoughts'. This also occurs in some patients with erectile failure, for example, 'I am going to lose my erection again and she will leave me' or, 'She will laugh at me because I can't even keep my erection'. Unfortunately, such cognitions make it almost impossible to maintain arousal, and coupled with the physiological effects of anxiety lead to loss of erection. This only serves to reinforce the thought on any subsequent attempt that failure is inevitable.

Documenting the occurrence of such cognitions not only confirms the presence of sexual anxiety but suggests that a cognitive therapy element in the treatment may prove beneficial. It is worth remembering, particularly in older men, that loss of erection after penetration may also result from a reduction in physical penile stimulation.

Other sexual difficulties

In up to a third of couples presenting with a sexual problem, the partner is also experiencing a sexual dysfunction. The interactions between different dysfunctions experienced by a couple are usually complex, with no simple causal or consequential relationships (Fig. 6.2). Thus erectile dysfunction may result in the man's partner becoming generally dissatisfied and unresponsive to advances which in turn leads to frustration or anorgasmia. In some cases, partners become overtly hostile or seek other sexual relationships. Equally, erectile failure can also be precipitated by the partner's low sexual interest, hostility, lack of arousal or anorgasmia.

Various organic pathologies are suggested by the presence of additional sexual symptoms in the man. Loss of desire commonly accompanies erectile failure in men with low testosterone levels. Failure of ejaculation may indicate neurological pathology.

The development of the problem

Precipitating and perpetuating factors, both physical and psychological, can be established or at

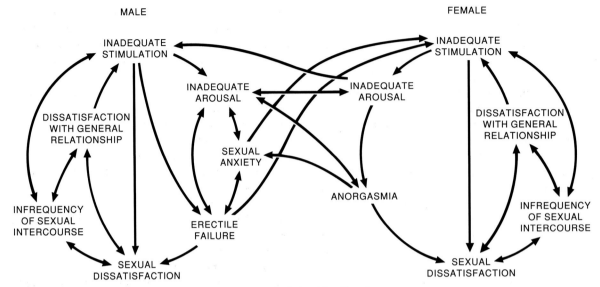

Fig. 6.2 The complex interactions of sexual and general relationship effects between partners.

least suggested though a clear understanding of the history of the problem.

1. *Onset*:
   — Sudden onset suggests precipitation by *an event* (physical, e.g. trauma or drug induced; or psychological, e.g. discovery of infidelity).
   — Gradual onset suggests *a process* (again physical, e.g. peripheral vascular disease; or psychological, e.g. deterioration in marital relationship).

2. *Course*:
   — Intermittent erectile dysfunction virtually excludes significant organic pathology, whereas continuous erectile inadequacy occurring in all situations strongly suggests some organic pathology.
   — Conditions which lead to improvement or deterioration may suggest both aetiological factors and therapeutic possibilities. For example, advice about reducing alcohol consumption or smoking, both of which are known to adversely affect erectile function, may be particularly important in some individuals (Farkas & Rosen 1976; Morlet et al 1990; Forsberg et al 1979; Juenemann et al 1987). Advice to improve psychological factors may also be suggested, such as not attempting intercourse late at night when the couple are too tired to spend time getting aroused.

3. *The couple's response*:
   Problems which have considerable impact on people's lives inevitably lead to change in the way they think and behave. These changes usually consist of a mixture of adaptive and maladaptive responses. In this context adaptive responses include increasing sexual stimulation, greater communication between partners and seeking information and explanation. Maladaptive responses, such as withdrawing from any sexual contact or blaming the partner, can perpetuate the problem and become issues which will need to be dealt with in their own right.

Sexual behaviours and attitudes

Some knowledge of a couple's sexual attitudes and behaviours is essential to an adequate understanding of any sexual problem. In this area of history taking, the clinician must steer a careful course between the gathering of information which will be useful for diagnosis and treatment, and interrogation about details which are of no direct relevance to management, and which could be perceived by some patients as professional voyeurism.

Factors which are often relevant to management are listed below.

- Does the couple engage in sexual behaviour which provides adequate physical and psychological stimulation?
- Consider the amount of time spent on foreplay and whether the types of behaviours engaged in are too restricted.
- Does the man or his partner have any unrecognized sexual preferences or inclinations, such as fetishism, transvestism or homosexual preference?
- Are negative cognitions or emotions interfering with sexual behaviours or the pleasure derived from them?
- Feelings of anger, guilt, anxiety or depression can all interfere significantly with the arousal process. Such thoughts and emotions can arise from the current situation or past experiences.

The general relationship

The full assessment of a marital relationship requires considerable skill and time. As it is not practical to attempt this in the current context, the clinician must restrict his enquiry to areas which have specific significance to the aetiology or management of erectile dysfunction. Clinicians should be cautious in ascribing cause and effect in interactions between sexual and marital problems. There is no doubt that marital disharmony can precede sexual dysfunction and vice versa (Gurman & Kniskern 1981). By the time couples are seen in sexual problems clinics, however, a two way, circular process has usually been established (LoPiccolo & Friedman 1985). In a study of the relationship between marital dissatisfaction and sexual dysfunction, Rust et al (1988) found a much closer link in men than in women. Furthermore, impotence and premature ejaculation played a much larger part in marital discord than did female anorgasmia or vaginismus.

The special considerations relating to men who have no current relationship are discussed in Chapter 15.

1. The quality of the current relationship can be briefly assessed by asking about how a couple get on with each other and probing into affection or love for each other, pleasure in each other's company, common interests and social activities. An important indication is the amount of time that a couple spend together. The results of these enquiries may suggest that starting marital or relationship therapy is appropriate before attempting any sort of treatment for the erectile dysfunction.

2. Communication in the general relationship permits the couple to function cohesively and to tackle problems jointly. Good communication is more about quality than quantity: couples who talk to each other a lot about the weather and what to eat for meals are not communicating about issues central to their relationship or personal needs. Although usually inextricably linked to the quality of the general relationship, poor communication between partners can in itself lead to treatment failure.

3. Commitment to the relationship. The interaction between commitment to the future of the relationship and its quality is often of vital importance to attitudes towards the sexual relationship. Couples may stay together *despite* a poor relationship for a number of reasons, including religious or moral beliefs, children, financial interests or even fear of physical harm. In such situations, a satisfactory sexual relationship would be surprising. Attempting to improve the sexual relationship by concentrating on the erectile problem would be inappropriate and possibly even damaging.

At the opposite end of the spectrum are couples who may consider separation because of the sexual problem, despite an apparently good general relationship. In such couples, sex is usually important to one or both partners and they tend to be well motivated about treatment which they often seek at a relatively early stage.

Couples with a longstanding poor relationship who are seeking treatment for impotence in an attempt to combat their thoughts of separation can make better use of the limited time left by seeking therapy either to mend the relationship or assist in reducing the trauma of the separation (Rice 1989).

Personal and family history

Predisposing factors to the later development of

erectile problems may emerge from even brief enquiry into the patient's past. Experience of sexual, physical and emotional abuse may be revealed by the patient, sometimes for the first time. However, a lengthy analysis of the patient's past experiences and development is unlikely to have any specific effect on his future management. Furthermore, a controlled examination of sexual histories in 100 couples with sexual dysfunction and 100 non-dysfunctional controls revealed no significant differences between frequencies of what are often supposed to be pathogenic past events (Heiman et al 1986). This suggests that one should be cautious before ascribing any aetiological significance to past events.

Limited time is better spent assessing the patient's situation when the problem started and at the present time. The following areas are particularly relevant:

1. Employment: hours, regularity (do partners work opposite shifts?), work satisfaction and security.
2. Housing: quality, security, privacy.
3. Financial worries.
4. Any other recent stressful events, such as bereavement or serious illness in the family.

The medical history

This should concentrate on the presence or absence of any disorders or symptoms which are associated with impaired vascular, neurological or hormonal functioning. The patient should be asked if he has ever had any of the following disorders. If so, is he receiving treatment and is the doctor aware of his erectile dysfunction? In a patient whose presentation suggests the presence of organic factors, it is worth also enquiring about suggestive symptoms.

1. Peripheral vascular disease:
   - high blood pressure
   - heart attack
   - angina
   - claudication (severe pain in legs on walking)
   - cold extremities
   - blackouts
2. Diabetes:

- family history of diabetes
- altered sensation in legs/feet
- polyuria (frequent urination)
- frequent infections
3. Neurological disorders:
   - multiple sclerosis
   - spinal injury
   - spinal or brain surgery
4. Hormonal/endocrine abnormalities
5. Genital abnormality, disease or surgery.

In all these areas, the interviewer should try to establish what investigations have been carried out, the severity of the problem, whether the patient is obtaining adequate treatment, and whether he is complying with it.

Psychiatric history

Disturbances of sexual desire and sexual behaviour are associated with disorders such as anxiety, depression, mania and schizophrenia. However, there is no clear evidence from controlled studies (e.g. Matthew & Weinman 1982) of any association between impaired erectile function and these disorders. Unfortunately, this does not apply to the drugs used to treat them.

The presence of a psychiatric disorder may make some patients difficult to treat. The acutely ill psychiatric patient and those with significant chronic impairment only rarely present for treatment. Currently well patients who suffer from acute psychotic episodes should only be treated after consultation with their psychiatrist. Their dysfunction may relate to antipsychotic medication which could be altered. Furthermore, their mental state during acute episodes of illness may create problems with certain treatments, for example manic patients who experience hypersexuality might misuse intracavernosal injections, increasing the dose or the frequency.

Depression is not uncommon in sexual dysfunction clinics although the relationship between mood and sexuality is a variable and two-way process. Furthermore, impairment of erectile function has been described in patients on antidepressants (see Ch. 5). Confusion arises from the fact that there are some patients whose dysfunction relates to episodes of depression and improves on antidepressant treatment. Others can become mildly depressed as a result of erectile failure, and show improvement in mood if sexual functioning is restored. However, patients presenting with anything but very mild psychiatric symptoms should undergo a full psychiatric assessment.

Treatment history

The influence of various drugs on erectile function has been discussed in Chapter 5. In deciding whether any drug should be suspected of causing a patient's dysfunction, the clinician should consider the following questions (Bancroft 1989):

— Have effects on erection been described?
— Is there a clear temporal association between when the drug is taken and when the problem occurs?
— Is the effect very specific, e.g. loss of stimulated erections only, with normal ejaculation and libido?
— Can the effect be explained by the drug's known pharmacological actions?

Details of alcohol and tobacco consumption should always be obtained. Their effects are described in Chapter 5.

Contraception

Preventing unwanted pregnancy is a major consideration during the reproductive years. Worries about risk of pregnancy, methods of contraception or indeed effects of the methods themselves can affect function. For some men, fear that the contraception method (if any) will fail, interferes with arousal. Good family planning management and reassurance must be included in their treatment package and may cure their problem.

The reduction in stimulation produced by condoms is blamed for loss of erections in many men. Others also find them a psychological 'turn off'. Again, good contraceptive advice may prove to be treatment enough.

Couples who have not had intercourse for some time because of dysfunction commonly cease to use contraception at all. They should be advised to arrange a suitable method before starting treatment, seeking contraceptive advice if necessary.

Motivation

During the course of the interview, the clinician should try to assess the patient's (and partner's) desire to see change and their motivation to go through the treatment being contemplated. There is no perfect treatment for impotence — all have their pros and cons and current evidence suggests that motivation and realistic expectations are key factors in successful outcome for both psychological and physical treatments (Hawton & Catalan 1986; Berg et al 1984).

Motivation can only be assessed accurately if the couple base their views on accurate information about the advantages and disadvantages of the treatment method. The provision of adequate information about the treatment options thus becomes an essential component of a complete assessment interview. Such information can be provided verbally during the interview, or time can be saved by giving patients handouts describing available treatments before or after they are seen.

THE ASSESSMENT OF PROGRESS AND OUTCOME

This chapter is mainly concerned with the assessment which takes place prior to treatment. Nevertheless, it would be incomplete without some reference to the assessment of progress and outcome. Although this forms the basis of clinical audit and outcome research, it is a frequently neglected issue. Retrospective assessments of change, by patient or clinician (e.g. 'Are things better than before treatment started?'), are notoriously unreliable (Barlow et al 1984). Prospective assessment can only be accomplished through careful planning which involves two stages: first, defining the goal of treatment, and secondly, selecting the method of recording.

The goal will define the content of the assessment. In general, the appropriate goal for men with erectile dysfunction is the restoration of sexual *satisfaction* in addition to simply improving erections. 'Satisfaction' in addition to 'functioning' implies that the assessment will consider not only *physiological response* (e.g. quality of erections) and *behaviour* (e.g. frequency of intercourse) but also *cognitive state* (e.g. 'I am no longer an impotent man') and *emotional state* (e.g. pleasure from the sexual relationship).

Methods of recording progress.

The principle methods of recording are listed in Table 6.4.

The most commonly used method in clinical practice is the clinical interview. Although the most flexible and adaptable to individual situations, the lack of standardization can produce incomplete and incomparable data. Reliability can be increased by also interviewing the partner about change at each follow-up.

Physiological recordings (e.g. NPT, snap gauges) are sometimes quoted in research. These methods,

Table 6.4 Methods of recording.

Clinical interview
Standardized interview
Physiological recordings
Self-report questionnaires and rating scale
Information from partner (interview or questionnaire)

discussed in detail in Chapter 9, are relatively insensitive to change and give little useful information on erectile dysfunction during sexual activity.

The other methods of assessment, namely standardized interviews, questionnaires and rating scales, provide more reliable and replicable measures of progress in both clinical and research settings. These are discussed in the next chapter.

SUMMARY

In taking the history, the clinician should bear in mind that the interview is the foundation for the subsequent relationship with the patient. Psychological and physical aetiological factors are not mutually exclusive. Their presence and interactions should be considered. The principle aims of the interview are to understand aetiology and select appropriate further investigations or treatment. Assessment should not cease once these aims have been achieved. Progress and outcome assessment are essential to both research and good clinical practice.

REFERENCES

Bancroft J 1989 Human sexuality and its problems, 2nd edn. Churchill Livingstone, Edinburgh

Barlow D H 1986 Causes of sexual dysfunction: the role of anxiety and cognitive interference. Journal of Consulting and Clinical Psychology 54(2): 140–148

Barlow D H, Hayes S C, Nelson R O 1984 The Scientist Practitioner. Pergamon, Oxford

Benkert O, Maier W, Holsboer F 1985 Multiaxial classification of male sexual dysfunction. British Journal of Psychiatry 146: 628–632

Berg R, Mindus P, Berg G, Gustafson H 1984 Penile implants and erectile impotence: outcome and prognostic indicators. Scandinavian Journal of Urology and Nephrology 18: 277–282

Bhugra D, Cordle C 1988 A case control study of sexual dysfunction in Asian and non–Asian couples 1981–1985. Sexual and Marital Therapy 3(1): 71–76

d'Ardenne P 1987 Sexual dysfunction in a transcultural setting: assessment, treatment and research. Sexual and Marital Therapy 1: 23–34

Diagnostic and statistical manual of mental disorders 1980 American Psychiatric Association, Washington D C

Farkas G M, Rosen R 1976 Effect of alcohol on elicited male sexual response. Journal of Studies on Alcohol 37(3): 265–272

Fisher W A, Grenier G, Watters W W, Lamont J, Cohen M, Askwith J 1988 Students' sexual knowledge, attitudes toward sex and willingness to treat sexual concerns. Journal of Medical Education 63: 379–385

Forsberg L, Gustavii B, Hojerback T, Olsson A M 1979

Impotence, smoking and B-blocking drugs. Fertility and Sterility 31: 589

Gregoire A 1990 Physical vs. psychological: a need for an integrated approach. Sexual and Marital Therapy 5(2): 103–104

Gurman A S, Kniskern D P 1981 Handbook of family therapy. Brummer, Mazel, New York

Hawton K 1985 Sex therapy. A practical guide. Oxford University Press, Oxford

Hawton K, Catalan J 1986 Prognostic factors in sex therapy. Behaviour Research and Therapy 24(4): 377–385

Heiman J R, Gladue B A, Roberts C W, LoPiccolo J 1986 Historical and current factors discriminating sexually functional from sexually dysfunctional married couples. Journal of Marital and Family Therapy 12(2): 163–174

Juenemann K P, Lue T F, Luo J A, Benowitz N L, Abozeid M, Tanagho E A 1987 The effect of cigarette smoking on penile erection. Journal of Urology 138: 438–447

LoPiccolo J, Friedman J 1985 Sex therapy: an integrative model. In: Lynn S, Garske J (eds) Contemporary psychotherapies: models and methods. C.E. Merrill, New York

Mathew R J, Weinman M L 1982 Sexual dysfunctions in depression. Archives of Sexual Behaviour 11(4): 323–328

Morlet A, Watters G R, Dunn J, Keogh E J, Creed K E, Tulloch A G, Lord D J, Earle C M 1990 Effects of acute alcohol on penile tumescence in normal young men and dogs. Urology 35(5): 399–404

Rice D G 1989 Marital therapy and the divorcing family. In: Textor M (ed) The divorce and divorce therapy handbook. Jason Aronson, Northval, N J

Royal Commission on Medical Education (1968) H M

Stationery Office, London

Rust J, Golombok S, Collier J 1988 Marital problems and sexual dysfunction: how are they related? British Journal of Psychiatry 152: 629–31

Schover L R, Friedman J M, Weiler S J, Heiman J R, LoPiccolo J 1982 Multiaxial problem-orientated system for sexual dysfunctions: an alternative to DSM-III. Archives of General Psychiatry 39: 614–619

Segraves K A, Segraves R T, Schoenberg H W 1987 Use of sexual history to differentiate organic from psychogenic impotence. Archives of Sexual Behaviour 16(2): 125–137

7. Questionnaires and rating scales

Alain Gregoire

Reviewers of outcome research in sex therapy (Reynolds 1977; Wright et al 1977; Cole 1985) and of more recent treatments (Gregoire 1992) are unanimous in recommending the use of standardized, validated instruments for the measurement of outcome in future research. The need for such recommendations reflects the all too common methodological inadequacy of the research so far carried out: much of the published data lack information on validity and reliability and are generally not replicable.

In clinical practice, there are a number of situations in which questionnaires and rating scales can be used to great advantage. The use of pre-assessment packages has been described on p. 82. Until recently, the better quality instruments were also rather long, which limited their usefulness as repeated progress measures (Conte 1983). The development of shorter, more user-friendly scales may therefore have a significant impact in this area. Despite the obvious need for such instruments, their development is still in its infancy. Much work still needs to be done to establish validity and provide normative data for these instruments.

The increase in choice and quality of techniques for the physiological assessment of erectile function may tempt researchers and clinicians alike to neglect the use of questionnaires and rating scales, which have been criticized for their subjective nature. This attitude is critically flawed in that it denies the subjective nature of the sexual experience and of sexual dysfunction. Although erectile failure is probably the most tangible of the sexual dysfunctions, it continues to elude precise objective definition. The experienced clinician knows very well that what constitutes dysfunction for one person may be normality to another. Attempts to construct objective definitions, such as 'inability to achieve an erection for adequate penetration on 75% of occasions' (Masters & Johnson 1970), are methodologically important in the definition of samples in research, but are also merely the imposition of the researchers' arbitrary and subjective judgement. Thus in the clinical situation, and in research that wishes to yield clinically useful information, patients' subjective views and experiences are central to the assessment of erectile function.

Advantages of standardized instruments

1. The application of standardized instruments yields information which is comparable both within individuals at different times as well as between individuals or groups. Some comparability is also possible between different studies which use the same instruments, either in similar groups of patients for replication or in other groups to provide comparative information.
2. Questionnaires and rating scales, when appropriately selected, can provide additional and more detailed information to complement that elicited in the clinical interview. This is particularly useful when the clinician perceives a need for assessment in an area in which he does not possess specialist skills. For example, screening for depression or anxiety disorders can be effectively carried out using a rapidly completed self-rating scale, such as the Hospital Anxiety and Depression Scale (see p. 102).
3. Questionnaires and rating scales also have

obvious practical advantages. They can save time for researcher and clinician alike. Self-rating scales can also be administered by post, although care must be taken in this situation that clear instructions are included.

4. The use of self-rating scales also carries an educational and therapeutic benefit. Reading the questions may reassure patients that they are not the only ones to experience such difficulties and thinking about their responses may facilitate a more realistic and objective analysis of their problem. Because there is a frequent tendency for patients to forget how bad things were once improvement has been made, they may fail to appreciate progress and become disillusioned with treatment. This is particularly so with lengthier treatments, such as sex therapy. This counter-therapeutic process can be prevented, or even reversed, by demonstrating positive change using the ratings made by patients as they have progressed through treatment.

It is appropriate to remind ourselves that the word *instrument* is a well chosen one: these scales and questionnaires are only as good as the professional who uses them. An understanding of the purpose and population for which they are designed and some knowledge about their limitations is essential. This will allow sensible selection of the most appropriate instrument and a more accurate interpretation of the results. Finally, it is the responsibility of the professional administering self-rating questionnaires to ensure that the patient understands clearly how he should go about answering them.

INSTRUMENTS FOR QUANTIFYING SEXUALITY AND SEXUAL DYSFUNCTIONS

In a thorough review of self-report techniques for assessing sexual functioning, Conte (1983) selects two inventories as being particularly appropriate for clinical use. These are the Sexual Interaction Inventory (LoPiccolo & Steger 1974) and the Derogatis Sexual Function Inventory (Derogatis 1975, 1978). These two instruments, together with the more recently developed Golombok &

Rust Inventory of Sexual Satisfaction (Rust & Golombok 1985), will be described in turn.

Sexual Interaction Inventory (SII)

This inventory was designed to measure various aspects of sexual functioning as well as sexual satisfaction in heterosexual relationships.

Male and female partners separately rate the answers to 102 questions on a six point rating scale. An 11 scale profile for each person is derived from the responses and comparisons of scores can be made both between partners and between different stages of treatment. The reported results using the instrument indicate acceptable test/retest reliabilities of the scales and good internal consistency. Validity is demonstrated by significant correlations between the scales and global ratings of sexual satisfaction. Nine of the scales significantly differentiated dysfunctional from normal couples.

The reliability, validity and usefulness of the scales was strongly criticized by McCoy & D'Agostino (1977), who failed to replicate the original findings. In his review of this critique, Conte rightly points to a number of problems with the data on which it is based. He therefore rejects the criticism as premature on several grounds and concludes that the SII would appear to be 'a generally useful instrument for clinical assessment of the sexual adjustment and sexual satisfaction of heterosexual couples' (Conte 1983). In view of the limited data available on this scale, this conclusion may itself be somewhat premature.

The main disadvantages of the SII are its length and effective limitation to individuals who are currently in sexual relationships.

The Derogatis Sexual Functioning Inventory (DSFI)

This much longer inventory of 258 items has a more wide ranging orientation than the SII. It provides scores on ten subtests as well as a measure of the global level of functioning, referred to as the sexual functioning index (SFI). One of the 10 subtests is not directly related to sexual functioning but considers a range of psychological symptoms including anxiety, depression and somatization.

Test/retest reliability and internal consistency appear to be good on most of the subtests. Information on external validity is at present limited.

As with the SII, its emphasis on current functioning allows it to demonstrate change and it has the additional advantage of being applicable to individuals with or without partners. However, it is a lengthy instrument which takes a considerable time to complete and for this reason has a rather limited usefulness when repeated measures are required.

The Golombok & Rust Inventory of Sexual Satisfaction (GRISS) Table 7.1

This more recent instrument has been specifically devised for use with heterosexual men and women suffering from sexual dysfunction. It has the very considerable advantage over the previous two questionnaires of being considerably shorter and therefore taking less time to complete and score.

There are two questionnaires, one for men and one for women, with 28 items, each rated on a 5 point scale. The responses provide results on 12 subscales as well as a global score. The 12 subscales are based on diagnostic dimensions, including impotence, premature ejaculation, infrequency, dissatisfaction and avoidance.

Good results are presented for split half reliabilities for both the male and female scales. Validation carried out using comparisons with therapist ratings of severity and diagnosis provided evidence of good convergent and discriminant validity. The mean scores on male and female scales are reactive to treatment effects.

For clinicians and researchers seeking a scale which provides information on diagnosis and severity of sexual dysfunctions, and which is sensitive to change, this is currently the instrument of choice. It has the great advantage of being relatively short and considerable efforts have been made in its validation.

Use of inventories to differentiate psychogenic from organic aetiology

The expense and limited availability of physiological tests such as NPT and cavernosometry, as well as their diagnostic limitations, has led to a search for inventories which might discriminate between organic and psychogenic aetiologies. Specifically designed scales and pre-existing scales have been evaluated for this purpose. Findings concerning discriminating questions in the assessment interview are discussed on p. 88. Most of the work done on pre-existing inventories has concentrated on the Minnesota Multiphasic Personality Inventory (MMPI) and the Deragotis Sexual Functioning Index (DSFI).

Results on the MMPI from 10 subjects were used by Beutler et al (1975) to develop two decision rules intended to discriminate psychogenicity from organicity. Cases which met the defined criteria, which involved a) an elevation on one or more clinical scales of the MMPI, and b) an elevation on the masculinity–feminity scale, were considered to be psychogenic. All others were considered to be organic.

Application of these rules to a subsequent sample of 22 subjects produced 90% accuracy of discrimination. Efforts to replicate this study by Marshall et al (1980) produced quite different results. Indeed, they found that the patients with organic dysfunction showed higher levels of psychological disturbance on the MMPI than did the subjects with psychogenic dysfunction.

Table 7.1 The four questions from the impotence subscale of the Golombok & Rust Inventory of Sexual Satisfaction (GRISS). Reproduced by kind permission of NFER–Nelson

	Never	Hardly ever	Occasionally	Usually	Always
Do you become easily sexually aroused?	N	H	O	U	A
Do you fail to get an erection?	N	H	O	U	A
Do you get an erection during foreplay with your partner?	N	H	O	U	A
Do you lose your erection during intercourse?	N	H	O	U	A

They concluded, not surprisingly, that such gross inconsistencies in results eliminated the MMPI as a useful instrument for assessing the aetiology of erectile dysfunction.

A number of subsequent studies have confirmed these negative findings (Staples et al 1980; Marshall et al 1981; Saypol et al 1983; Martin et al 1983). If one considers the nature of the MMPI, which was developed in an effort to measure relatively stable 'trait' features, it may not be so surprising that it fails to identify accurately psychological features associated with what is usually a 'state' condition. Although the concept of impotence has frequently been associated with certain, usually negative, personality features (see Ch. 1), there has never been any positive evidence for this. Using the MMPI, Robiner et al (1982) found a wide variety of personality types, but found that 'no discernable configuration of MMPI scales could be identified, that, if found, might have suggested an impotent personality type'.

Significant differences in scores on the DSFI between men with clear organic impotence and men with psychogenic impotence have been reported by Derogatis et al (1976). The authors suggest that it gives the inventory clinical predictive value. This conclusion, based simply on significant associations between diagnosis and scores, was probably overoptimistic. Segraves et al (1981) were unable to differentiate significantly men with organic impotence from those with psychogenic dysfunction on the basis of DSFI scores.

A number of other inventories, specifically developed for the purposes of discriminating organic from psychogenic cases, have yielded similarly poor or inconsistent results (El-Senousi 1964). As pointed out by Conte (1986), this failure is probably due to a conceptual inaccuracy in which psychological and organic factors are perceived on either end of a single continuum. Thus any attempt to construct a scale based on this premise is doomed to failure. Efforts would be far more effectively channelled into producing new scales, such as the one described in the next section. Alternatively, standardized and validated pre-existing scales for the measurement of psychological morbidity can be used, and physical morbidity identified separately. Particularly relevant psychological areas include depression, anxiety and marital disharmony. Suggestions for appropriate instruments which could be used in these areas are discussed below.

A checklist to assess organic and psychological factors

The checklist set out in Table 7.2, which first appeared in its original form in Cole and Dryden (1989), was designed to assist the clinician in assessing the contributions of the main causes of erectile loss, namely vasculogenic (V), neurogenic (N), hormonal (H), and psychogenic (P). This instrument has not been formally standardized or validated and is therefore not suitable for research use. However, it clearly has sufficient face validity for use in clinical settings.

The authors recommend that the scores for V, N, H, and P be totalled separately, scoring one point for each capital letter (i.e. P = 1, PP = 2). They state that a total V + N + H score greater than the P score suggests a significant organic component to the dysfunction, and that similar scores suggest a combination of physical and psychological aetiologies. The individual V, N or H scores provide a pointer to the nature of the organic factors which might be involved, if any.

Since the checklist can be completed in the presence of the patient in only two or three minutes, its use also provides an opportunity to discuss with him the various ways in which his erectile response may have been impaired and may help to structure the assessment interview. It is likely to prove a particularly useful tool for non-medically qualified therapists, providing them with important information on possible physical problems and reassuring their patients that such problems are not being ignored.

SCALES OF PSYCHOLOGICAL MORBIDITY AND MARITAL DISHARMONY

The use of self-rating scales to detect psychological and psychiatric morbidity has considerable advantages, particularly for non-psychiatrically trained practitioners. There is not only a saving in time but also, with a good scale, an increase in selectivity and specificity without the need for any

Table 7.2 Diagnostic Impotence Questionnaire (DIQ)

		P (24)	V (16)	H (8)	N (13)
	Maximum score:				
1. Has the presenting problem with erection always been present?	YES		V	H	N
2. Are good erections easily obtained in self-masturbation?	YES	P			
	NO		V	H	N
3. Are good, persistent morning erections regularly present, i.e. at least once a week?	YES	P			
4. Are there strong feelings of performance anxiety present, i.e. a fear of sexual failure, when intercourse is attempted?	YES	P			
5. Are there any known relevant health problems?	YES		V	H	N
6. Is erection lost immediately before or after penetration when intercourse is attempted, but not at other times?	YES	P			
7. Is erection lost with some partners but not with others?	YES	P			
8. Is erection lost in some situations but not in others with the same partner?	YES	P			
9. Has there been a recent loss of partner through divorce, bereavement or rejection?	YES	PP			
10. Was there a history of depression preceding the erectile loss?	YES	PP			
11. Is there a history of psychiatric problems requiring hospitalization?	YES	P			
12. Are there problems within the relationship (if any)?	YES	PP			
13. Are there serious lifestyle problems (e.g. work, money, housing, etc.)?	YES	P			
14. Does the patient have an over-anxious personality* and/or is obsessional (i.e. excessively tidy, clean, punctual and strict)?	YES	PP			
15. Was there a lot of stress and trauma in childhood?	YES	P			
16. Are rigid, traditional and moral attitudes a feature of the personality?	YES	PP			
17. Is there a history of homosexual behaviour or fantasy?	YES	P			
18. How old — aged over 60?	YES	P	V		
19. Are the sexual fantasies during masturbation unusual (e.g. sadistic, masochistic, fetishistic, etc.)?	YES	P			
20. Are there any physical clues, e.g. small testes, marked presence of breast tissue, loss of facial hair, female body shape?	YES			H	
21. When investigated, were abnormal hormone levels discovered?*	YES			HH	
22. Have any medicines containing hormones been prescribed recently?	YES			H	
23. Has any other medication, likely to cause a loss of erection, been prescribed?	YES		V		N
24. Have there been any recent major surgical operations in the pelvic region (other than a hernia)?	YES				NN
25. Have there been any injuries or operations on the back?	YES				N
26. Are there any difficulties experienced controlling urination?	YES	P			N
27. Is there a history of high blood pressure, heart disease or stroke?	YES		VV		N
28. Do specialized neurological (nerve) tests reveal any abnormalities?*	YES				NN
29. Is there a history of poor circulation, cold fingers or feet and, particularly, a cold penis?	YES		V		
30. Does the penis bend in the middle or change in colour on erection?	YES		V		
31. Has a programme of properly supervised sensate focus with a supportive partner been completed unsuccessfully?	YES		V	H	N

Table 7.2   Diagnostic Impotence Questionnaire (DIQ) (contd)

		P (24)	V (16)	H (8)	N (13)
Maximum score:					
32. Is a good erection obtained after an injection of papaverine into the penis?*	YES	P			N
	NO		VV		
33. Do specialized tests reveal problems with blood flow in the penis?*	YES		VV		
34. Is there a loss of erection on standing or changing position?	YES		V		
35. Is the blood pressure in the penis low?*	YES		V		

*A few of these questions can only be answered after the results of further investigations are available.

Possible causes: *Score:*
P = psychological   P =
V = blood supply   V =
H = hormonal   H =
N = nerve supply   N =

P : V + H + N ratio =

specialized training or experience. A number of self-rating scales exist.

The most commonly used is probably still the General Health Questionnaire (GHQ) developed by Goldberg (1978). The GHQ provides a score which relates to global morbidity and, by the use of a pre-defined cut off point, a measure of caseness. However, it does not provide any diagnostic information. It has been extensively validated in both hospital and general practice settings. It has a number of significant disadvantages in addition to its length. It has an emphasis on somatic symptoms, which gives it a low specificity with patients also suffering from physical illness. The elderly find it particularly difficult to complete. In addition, it is only sensitive to changing symptoms and may not detect chronic illness. These disadvantages are particularly significant when dealing with patients with erectile dysfunction, as many of these patients are in older age groups and are also suffering from physical disorders.

The Hospital Anxiety and Depression Scale (Zigmond & Snaith 1983) has considerable advantages over the GHQ, particularly in the assessment of patients with physical problems, including erectile dysfunction. It is a short questionnaire of 14 items, each rated on a 4 point scale and is very quick and simple to score (see Appendix 7.1). It not only gives information on severity and caseness but also differentiates the diagnoses of depression and anxiety disorder. It has been validated in both primary care settings (Wilkinson & Barczak 1988) and in hospital outpatient clinics (Zigmond & Snaith 1983). Its specificity and selectivity are as good, if not better, than the GHQ (Wilkinson & Barczak 1988).

Two particularly appropriate scales exist for the assessment of marital state in sexual dysfunction clinics.

1. The Locke–Wallis Marital Adjustment Test (Locke & Wallace 1959) consists of 15 items which are relatively easy and quick to complete and are the same for male and female partners. It is quite heavily orientated towards issues of communication and agreement within the relationship. The original data on it provide evidence of good reliability. Normative data are available on community samples (Oltmanns et al 1977) and on patients attending marital therapy clinics (O'Leary & Arias 1983; Turkewitz & O'Leary 1981). Discriminant validity and optimum cut-off scores are discussed by O'Leary & Arias (1987). The MAT has been the subject of criticism on conceptual and methodological grounds (O'Leary & Arias 1987; Rust et al 1986).

2. The Golombok & Rust Inventory of Marital State (GRIMS) (Table 7.3) is a more recent questionnaire which was psychometrically constructed for use in clinical and research

Table 7.3 Four questions from the Golombok & Rust Inventory of Marital State (GRIMS). Reproduced by kind permission of NFER–Nelson

	Strongly Disagree	Disagree	Agree	Strongly Agree
My partner is usually sensitive to and aware of my needs	SD	D	A	SA
There is always plenty of 'give and take' in our relationship	SD	D	A	SA
I no longer feel I can really trust my partner	SD	D	A	SA
I suspect we may be on the brink of separation	SD	D	A	SA

situations (Rust et al 1986). It is a companion scale to the GRISS (discussed above). It consists of 28 items, each rated on a 4 point scale, identical for male and female partners. Completion, scoring and interpretation are rapid.

The scale demonstrates good split half reliabilities for men and women. The information on validity is still relatively limited, although the original validation demonstrates significant differences in mean scores between groups of patients clinically selected for the presence or absence of marital problems and/or sexual problems. The usefulness and applicability of the GRIMS and the GRISS in the assessment of patients with sexual problems has been clearly demonstrated (Collier 1989).

SUMMARY

The use of standardized instruments to measure sexual function offers considerable advantages in both research and clinical practice, including the provision of reliable, replicable, detailed and complete data. The use of such scales can also carry educational and therapeutic benefits, both by inducing an analysis of the problem and by demonstrating change during treatment. Although several such scales are now available, they have only rarely been used in outcome research into sex therapy and the newer treatments for erectile dysfunction.

Scales can also be very useful in both the clinical and research situation to examine issues related to erectile dysfunction, such as marital satisfaction, mood and anxiety levels.

REFERENCES

Beutler L E, Karacan I, Anch A M, Salis P J, Scott F B, Williams R L 1975 MMPI and MIT discriminators of biogenic and psychogenic impotence. Journal of Consulting and Clinical Psychology 43: 899–903

Cole M 1985 Sex therapy — a critical appraisal. British Journal of Psychiatry 147: 337–351

Cole M, Dryden W 1989 Sex problems: your questions answered. Macdonald, London

Collier J L 1989 The use of the GRIMS and the GRISS in the assessment and outcome of sexual problems: are questionnaires of more value than a clinical interview? Sexual and Marital Therapy 4(1): 11–16

Conte H R 1983 Development and use of self-report techniques for assessing sexual functioning: a review and critique. Archives of Sexual Behaviour 12: 555–576

Conte H R 1986 Multivariate assessment of sexual dysfunction. Journal of Consulting and Clinical Psychology 54(2): 149–157

Derogatis L R 1975 Derogatis sexual functioning inventory. Clinical Psychometrics Research, Baltimore

Derogatis L R 1978 Derogatis sexual functioning inventory (Revised ed.). Clinical Psychometrics Research, Baltimore

Derogatis L R, Meyer J K, Dupkin C N 1976 Discrimination

of organic versus psychogenic impotence with the DSFI. Journal of Sex and Marital Therapy 2: 229–240

El-Senousi A, 1964 The male impotence test. Western Psychological Services, Los Angeles

Goldberg D 1978 Manual of the general health questionnaire. NFER, Windsor

Gregoire A 1992 New treatments for erectile impotence. British Journal of Psychiatry 160: 315–326

Locke H J, Wallace K M 1959 Short marital adjustment and prediction tests: their reliability and validity. Marriage and Family Living 21: 251–255

LoPiccolo J, Steger J 1974 The sexual interaction inventory: a new instrument for assessment of sexual dysfunction. Archives of Sexual Behaviour 3: 585–595

Marshall P, Delva N 1980 Differentiation of organic and psychogenic impotence on the basis of MMPI decision rules. Journal of Consulting and Clinical Psychology 48: 407–408

Marshall P, Morales A, Surridge D 1981 Unreliability of nocturnal penile tumescence recording and MMPI profiles in assessment of impotence. Urology 17(2): 136–139

Martin L M, Rodgers D A, Montague D K 1983 Psychometric differentiation of biogenic and psychogenic impotence. Archives of Sexual Behaviour 12: 475–485

Masters W, Johnson V 1970 Human sexual inadequacy.

Little, Brown, Philadelphia

McCoy N N, D'Agostino P A 1977 Factor analysis of the Sexual Interaction Inventory. Archives of Sexual Behaviour 6: 25–35

O'Leary K D, Arias I 1987 The influence of marital therapy on sexual satisfaction. Journal of Sexual and Marital Therapy 9(3): 171–181

O'Leary K D, Arias I 1983 Marital assessment in clinical practice. In: O'Leary K D (ed) Assessment of marital discord. Lawrence Erlbaum, Hillsdale, N J

Oltmanns T F, Broderick J E, O'Leary K D 1977 Marital adjustment and the efficacy of behaviour therapy with children. Journal of Consulting and Clinical Psychology 45(5): 724–729

Reynolds B S 1977 Psychological treatment models and outcome results for erectile dysfunction: a critical review. Psychological Bulletin 84(6): 1218–1238

Robiner W N, Godec C J, Cass A S, Meyer J J 1982 The role of Minnesota Multiphasic Personality Inventory in evaluation of erectile dysfunction. Journal of Urology 128: 487–488

Rust J, Bennun I, Crowe M, Golombok S 1986 The Golombok-Rust Inventory of Marital State (GRIMS). Sexual and Marital Therapy 1(1): 55–60

Rust J, Golombok S 1985 The Golombok-Rust inventory of sexual satisfaction (GRISS). British Journal of Clinical Psychology 24: 63–64

Rust J, Golombok S 1986 The GRISS: a psychometric

instrument for the assessment of sexual dysfunction. Archives of Sexual Behaviour 15(2): 157–165

Saypol D C, Peterson G A, Howards S S, Yazel J J 1983 Impotence: are the newer diagnostic methods a necessity? Journal of Urology 130: 260–262

Segraves R T, Schoenberg H W, Zarins C K, Knopf J, Camic P 1981 Discrimination of organic versus psychological impotence with DSFI: a failure to replicate. Journal of Sexual and Marital Therapy 7: 230–238

Staples R, Fisher I, Shapiro M, Martin K, Gonik P 1980 A re-evaluation of MMPI discriminators of biogenic and psychogenic impotence. Journal of Consulting and Clinical Psychology 48: 543–545

Turkewitz H, O'Leary K D 1981 A comparative outcome study of behavioural marital therapy and communication therapy. Journal of Marital and Family Therapy 7: 159–169

Wilkinson M J B, Barczak P 1988 Psychiatric screening in general practice: comparison of the general health questionnaire and the hospital anxiety depression scale. Journal of the Royal College of General Practitioners 38: 311–313

Wright J, Perreault R, Mathieu M 1977 The treatment of sexual dysfunction. Archives of General Psychiatry 34: 881–890

Zigmond A S, Snaith R P 1983 The Hospital Anxiety and Depression Scale. Acta Psychiatrica Scandinavica 67: 361–370

APPENDIX 7.1

The Hospital Anxiety and Depression Scale. The scores are given in the left column. Separate totals are derived for anxiety (A) and depression (D). Scoring figures should be put on a separate sheet from that given to the patient.

The Hospital Anxiety and Depression Scale

Doctors are aware that emotions play an important part in most illnesses. If your doctor knows about these feelings, he will be able to help you more.

This questionnaire is designed to help your doctor to know how you feel. Ignore the numbers printed on the left of the questionnaire. Read each item and <u>underline</u> the reply which comes closest to how you have been feeling in the past week.

Don't take too long over your replies; your immediate reaction to each item will probably be more accurate than a long thought out response.

1. I feel tense or 'wound up' :
   Most of the time
   A lot of the time
   From time to time, occasionally
   Not at all

2. I still enjoy the things I used to enjoy :
   Definitely as much
   Not quite so much
   Only a little
   Hardly at all

3. I get a sort of frightened feeling as if something awful is about to happen :
   Very definitely and quite badly
   Yes, but not too badly
   A little, but it doesn't worry me
   Not at all

4. I can laugh and see the funny side of things :
   As much as I always could
   Not quite so much now
   Definitely not so much now
   Not at all

5. Worrying thoughts go through my mind :
   A great deal of the time
   A lot of the time
   From time to time, but not too often
   Only occasionally

6. I feel cheerful :
   Not at all

Not often
Sometimes
Most of the time

7. I can sit at ease and feel relaxed :
   Definitely
   Usually
   Not often
   Not at all

8. I feel as if I am slowed down :
   Nearly all the time
   Very often
   Sometimes
   Not at all

9. I get a sort of frightened feeling like 'butterflies' in the stomach :
   Not at all
   Occasionally
   Quite often
   Very often

10. I have lost interest in my appearance :
    Definitely
    I don't take so much care as I should
    I may not take quite as much care
    I take just as much as ever

11. I feel restless as if I have to be on the move :
    Very much indeed
    Quite a lot
    Not very much
    Not at all

12. I look forward with enjoyment to things :
    As much as ever I did
    Rather less than I used to
    Definitely less than I used to
    Hardly at all

13. I get sudden feelings of panic :
    Very often indeed
    Quite often
    Not very often
    Not at all

14. I can enjoy a good book or radio or TV programme :
    Often
    Sometimes
    Not often
    Very seldom

Anxiety: score 0, 1, 2, 3 for Q. 7, 9
score 3, 2, 1, 0 for Q. 1, 3, 5, 11, 13
Depression: score 0, 1, 2, 3 for Q. 2, 4, 12, 14
score 3, 2, 1, 0 for Q. 6, 8, 10

8. Examination and basic investigations

John P. Pryor   Ian K. Dickinson

It is essential to diagnose the nature of any disturbance in order to offer the most effective form of treatment. It is usually possible to achieve this within one or two outpatient visits. During the first visit a complete history should be obtained (see Ch. 6), the patient examined and simple blood tests arranged. The history may suggest abnormalities which can be confirmed during the clinical examination, or which may require investigations on subsequent visits. A urologist considers it mandatory to examine the penis of all patients presenting with erectile dysfunction. He might, reluctantly, accept the proposition that this was unnecessary if the history clearly indicated a psychological problem and the patient was in agreement with this causation.

On the return visit, the results of those tests arranged during the first visit are discussed and it may be desirable to give a diagnostic intracavernous injection. On this basis it is possible to have a reasonable idea of the causation of the erectile dysfunction and any special investigations can then be organized if required.

GENERAL EXAMINATION

The patient may appear to be depressed or anxious and there may be evidence of a generalized metabolic disturbance such as anaemia, the stigmata of liver disease such as jaundice (rarely), spider naevi, liver palms or chronic renal failure. It is also important to look for the signs of endocrine dysfunction of the thyroid gland (e.g. alterations in pulse rate, hair loss, skin changes or eye signs) or of the pituitary or adrenal glands.

Examination of the genitalia

The normal pattern of male hair distribution should be noted and the possibility of gynaecomastia considered. The penis is examined for any abnormality that may be associated with erectile dysfunction (Table 8.1).

Painful conditions of the penis may cause impotence and the most common of these is phimosis (inability to retract the foreskin). This may be congenital in origin, but when acquired it is often secondary to diabetes. Rupture of a tight frenulum may be associated with brisk bleeding, particularly if the frenular artery is torn, but more often causes pain and ulceration. The latter may become chronic and a source of persistent discomfort. This condition is usually self-limiting but is otherwise overcome by a simple operation. It should be noted that a tight frenulum rarely causes a deformity of the penis during erection. Longstanding penile

Table 8.1 Penile abnormalities causing erectile dysfunction.

1. *Painful conditions*
   phimosis
   torn frenulum
   penile ulceration

2. *Curvature*
   hypospadias
   chordee without hypospadias
   congenital short urethra
   other congenital erectile deformities
   Peyronie's disease

3. *Abnormalities of size*
   absent penis
   micropenis — with or without hypospadias
   megapenis
      congenital
      lymphoedema

4. *Abnormalities associated with impaired erection*
   penile fibrosis following priapism
   Peyronie's disease
   abnormal blood supply
   abnormal cavernous muscle
   abnormal leakage of blood from the corpora

ulceration should always be regarded with suspicion for malignancy. If there is any doubt, a biopsy will need to be taken after excluding sexually transmitted diseases.

Erectile dysfunction may result from penile abnormalities causing deformity, the most common of which are those producing a curvature. Congenital abnormalities associated with hypospadias or the presence of ventral chordee (thickening) without hypospadias are easily detected. However, it is also important to remember that dorsal, lateral or ventral curvature on erection are not always associated with any visible or palpable clinical abnormality when the penis is examined in the flaccid state. In these conditions, there is an abnormality of the tunica albuginea and corpus cavernosus and the corpora do not expand uniformly. The condition characterized by a ventral erectile deformity is sometimes called a congenital short urethra, but in reality the urethra and corpus spongiosus are normal.

The most common erectile deformity is associated with Peyronie's disease. In this condition there is a palpable lump (plaque) which is usually situated on the dorsum of the penis. The plaque is composed of fibrous tissue which is less elastic than the normal tunica albuginea and does not stretch as much during erection. It should be noted that young men with a congenital deformity of less than 30° often suffer severe anxiety on account of their deformity and may even require surgical correction, whereas older men with a greater deformity will often consider surgical correction to be unnecessary. Any scars on the penis should be noted together with any thickening of the corpora cavernosa — following either direct trauma to the penis, injection of intracavernous drugs or priapism.

It is unusual for an abnormality of penile size to cause erectile dysfunction. Some patients with lymphoedema find that the penis is too large. In others, the penis may be absent (a congenital abnormality, or lost through accident or disease) or too small (congenital micropenis either as an isolated abnormality or associated with hypospadias or intersex) to permit vaginal penetration (Figs 8.1 & 8.2).

Testes of normal size and consistency are usually found to function normally, but when small they may be associated with hypogonadism. In these circumstances it is wise to check for gynaecomastia and the pattern of hair distribution. Testicular sensation may be diminished in lesions of the sympathetic nervous system.

Rectal examination may be performed in order to convince the patient that the possibility of a

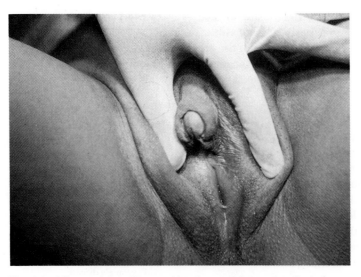

Fig. 8.1 Micropenis in a 25-year-old male pseudohermaphrodite before and after reconstructive surgery. 'Suicidal' preoperatively, he subsequently married and his wife underwent artificial insemination with donor sperm.

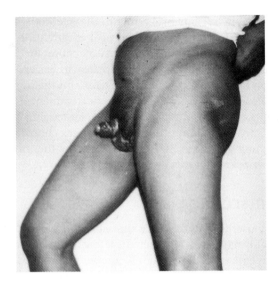

Fig. 8.2 Micropenis following reconstruction.

physical cause for his problem is being assiduously sought. Rectal examination is also desirable with regard to preventative medicine and unsuspected prostatic cancers are detected in approximately 1% of impotent men. The tone of the anal sphincter is noted during the rectal examination but it is of doubtful significance. The benefit of attempting to elicit the bulbocavernosus reflex (squeeze the glans penis and await the contraction of the anal sphincter) is also doubtful.

Examination of the cardiovascular and nervous systems

Taking the patient's blood pressure is always indicated as it is reassuring for the patient, important with regard to the aetiology of the erectile dysfunction, and good preventative medicine. Abdominal examination for an aortic aneurysm or abdominal bruits, together with examination of the legs for evidence of peripheral vascular disease, such as absent pulses and hair loss, is less rewarding.

A general neurological examination rarely detects any abnormality that was not suggested whilst taking the clinical history (see Ch. 6). The ankle reflexes should be checked and it is sometimes useful to check for vibration sensation and sensory loss. This is particularly of benefit in diabetics, in whom such signs of an autonomic

neuropathy suggest that this may be the cause for erectile failure.

BASIC INVESTIGATIONS

It is usually possible to have a good idea of the cause of the impotence after taking the history and conducting an examination. Many patients may be prepared to accept this, but others will require some confirmatory tests before they will readily accept appropriate management. It is essential to explain to the patient the possible diagnoses, future investigations and management options. At this stage, some patients may decide against further investigation, the main aim of which is to confirm the cause of the problem. There are four groups of causes and these should be discussed with the patient in the context of his own history and clinical examination. The clinician should also discuss the implications of further investigations for the treatment options that are available.

1. *Metabolic and hormonal*. These are fairly obvious from the history and may be diagnosed by simple laboratory investigations carried out on a blood sample.

2. *Neurological*. These causes are usually evident in the history or the examination.

3. *Vascular*. This is suggested by the nature of the impotence and the presence of other factors such as smoking, diabetes and cardiovascular disorders (Virag et al 1985).

4. *Psychological*. In some patients, the nature of the problem suggests a psychological aetiology but no clear factors emerge from the history to account for this. It is often desirable to exclude an organic basis at an early stage in order to concentrate on a possible hidden psychological causation.

During the subsequent discussion it is possible to prepare the patient for the next visit. If the patient's partner was not seen at the first visit she should be encouraged to attend on the next visit, as there is little point in pursuing some options if the partner does not wish to cooperate.

General investigations

These are arranged at the time of the first visit. It is always worthwhile to exclude diabetes, and to check liver function tests in those patients with a possible history of alcohol abuse. It is useful to determine the plasma testosterone level and a good case may be made for measuring the prostate specific antigen level, which is raised in carcinoma of the prostate, if any hormonal therapy is to be considered in the elderly male.

Diabetes

Impotence is common in diabetics and may be due to diabetic complications in addition to those aetiological factors which are possible in all men. Many younger diabetics have found that it is necessary to ingest sugar before anticipated periods of prolonged and strenuous sexual activity. Some hyperglycaemic patients presenting with impotence find that their potency improves when the diabetes is brought under control. Measurement of the glycosylated haemoglobin is useful in assessing the degree of diabetic control. In some diabetics, the impotence is irreversible due to an autonomic neuropathy or arteriopathy. In a study of a population of diabetics in a general practice together with age-matched controls, Dickinson (unpublished data) found a greater incidence of impotence amongst the diabetics ($p = 0.01$–0.001) and the mean age of the impotent diabetics was 6 years younger than impotent controls (Table 8.2).

Endocrine screening

Routine screening of serum testosterone is performed in most clinics but a significantly low value is only found in about 1% of patients who do not have clinical evidence of hypogonadism (Maatman & Montague 1986; Freidman et al 1986). The cost of screening all patients with such a low incidence of endocrine pathology has to be considered against the background of overlooking a potentially serious problem and the need of some patients for assurance that proper attention is being given to finding a physical cause for the problem. Such reassurance makes it easier for them to accept a psychological cause for the impotence and adopt less resistance to treatment. It is unnecessary to measure prolactin, luteinizing and follicle stimulating hormones or sex hormone binding globulin (SHBG) levels unless the initial testosterone level is low.

THE SECOND VISIT

It is useful to commence the second interview by enquiring to see whether there has been any improvement in the patient's erectile function. The results of the initial investigations are reviewed and the need for further investigation assessed. In practical terms, it may be difficult to be sure that there is no occult neurological causation or to distinguish between, or determine the relative importance of, vasculogenic and psychogenic factors. The result of an intracavernous injection of a vasoactive agent at this stage simplifies the diagnostic pathway (Fig. 8.3) and facilitates the choice of treatment.

Diagnostic injection of vasoactive agents

The observations that the injection of papaverine (Virag 1982) or alpha-adrenoreceptor blocking agents (Brindley 1983) into the corpora cavernosa was capable of provoking erection has revolutionized the investigation of impotence. The technique has been widely used as a diagnostic tool, although the test has not been standardized (Buvat et al 1986; Strachan & Pryor 1987; Zentgraf et al 1988). More recently the naturally occurring substance, prostaglandin E1 has been used (Stackl et al 1988). The use and side effects of vasodilators in treatment is discussed in Ch. 11.

Choice of drugs

Papaverine. Papaverine hydrochloride is an opium alkaloid that causes relaxation of smooth muscle. It has been used for many years in vascular surgery to treat peri-operative arterial spasm and it was for this reason that it was first used by Virag (1982).

Table 8.2 Incidence of impotence in diabetics in a general practice and in age-matched controls

| | POTENT | | IMPOTENT | |
	number	mean age (years)	number	mean age (years)
Diabetics	18	(61.0)	20	(67.6)
Non-diabetics	27	(61.0)	6	(74.0)

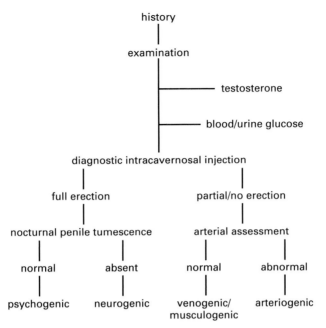

Fig. 8.3   Diagnostic pathway for the investigation of impotence.

The flaccid state of the penis is dependent on the contraction of the cavernous muscle through continuous stimulation by sympathetic nervous activity. This activity may be blocked by alpha-adrenoreceptor blocking agents. The intracavernous injection of papaverine relaxes the smooth muscle of the arterial wall and is associated with an increase in penile arterial flow (Juenemann et al 1986) and also causes relaxation of the smooth muscle of the corpora cavernosa with a decrease in the outflow of blood from the corpora (Virag et al 1984; Juenemann et al 1986).

As the vascular spaces within the corpora fill and the pressure rises towards arterial levels, the venous outflow is mechanically obstructed. The complications of papaverine are the induction of a prolonged erection which may even progress to a priapism (see below). There is also a significant incidence of penile fibrosis and this may occasionally occur after a single injection.

Papaverine has been stated to be hepatotoxic but the incidence of abnormal liver function tests during its usage is so small that most centres no longer monitor them in patients on a self-injection programme.

Alpha-adrenoreceptor blocking agents. These were investigated by Brindley (1983) and although phenoxybenzamine was at first preferred, it was subsequently abandoned because of a possible carcinogenic effect in beagle puppies. For this reason, phentolamine mesylate has been preferred and its use was popularized by Zorgniotti & Lefleur (1985). Phentolamine acts by blocking sympathetic nerve impulses to the cavernous and arterial smooth muscle. In practice, phentolamine (0.5 mg) is used in combination with papaverine (30 mg) and is said to have a synergistic effect. Phentolamine can produce hypotension, tachycardia and cardiac arrhythmias but these symptoms are unusual with the dosage used for erectile dysfunction.

Prostaglandin E1. Prostaglandin E1 is a natural substance found in many body tissues and is a potent vasodilator. Its sole medical use to date has been to bring about the closure of a patent ductus arteriosus. Intracavernous injection with PgE1 may be slightly more uncomfortable than with papaverine, but otherwise it appears to have few systemic side effects (Ishii et al 1988; Stackl et al 1988; Stackl et al 1990) and has no local side effects in animal studies (Aboseif et al 1989). Like papaverine, the response is dose dependent but unlike papaverine, there is a low risk of painful prolonged erections when higher doses are used (see Ch. 11).

At the present time prostaglandin E1 is expensive, difficult to store and requires dilution before use. Should it become packaged in a more convenient form, it would be the drug of choice for intracavernosal injection.

Combinations of drugs

The combination of papaverine and phentolamine has been widely used and some authors use a combination of prostaglandin (10 µg) and phentolamine (1 mg). Papaverine, phentolamine and prostaglandin is another combination and Virag (personal communication) has used a combination of six agents. There would seem to be little justification for using such polypharmacy.

Diagnostic intracavernous vasoactive drug injection — the papaverine test

This diagnostic procedure has greatly simplified the diagnosis of the aetiology of impotence. The response to the test not only depends upon the underlying arterial inflow but also the concentration of the drug used, the capacity of the cavernous smooth muscle to relax and the neurogenic control of the smooth muscle — be it denervated or overstimulated through anxiety. The choice of drug and its dosage is a matter of personal choice and it is desirable that the physician should become familiar with the drug of his or her choice. Papaverine in a dosage of 80 mg should elicit a full erection in most patients but the dosage may be reduced to 1 mg/year in young patients or when the cause is likely to be neurogenic.

The patient should always be asked to compare the drug induced erection with his normal erections, since the problem may be one of perception rather than one of deficiency. When the response is less than expected, e.g. in someone thought to have psychogenic impotence, the possibility of a false negative response should be considered. This may occur in 10% of patients (Buvat et al 1987) and is probably the result of anxiety, particularly in those patients who are very apprehensive of injections or find them painful. The addition of phentolamine may help to lessen the risk of a false negative response. When there is a conflict between the history and the result of the test, the test should be repeated with the addition of phentolamine or the patient investigated further with nocturnal penile tumescence monitoring.

A fully rigid erection excludes a significant vascular cause for the impotence. The main problem when using intracavernosal agents is the difficulty in interpreting a less than full response. Such a result could be due to an arteriogenic cause, veno-occlusive dysfunction, cavernous muscle pathology or a psychological inhibition. Buvat et al (1987) found that 44% of patients without significant vascular abnormalities and 33% with psychogenic impotence failed to respond fully to papaverine.

The vasoactive agent is injected through the posterolateral aspect of the penis — thereby avoiding the corpus spongiosum and the dorsal neurovascular bundle — into the corpus cavernosum using a syringe and a 25 gauge needle. The drug is massaged throughout the penis and an erection should occur within 5–10 minutes. It is unnecessary to place a elastic band around the base of the penis but it is desirable to allow the patient to relax in privacy. Manual stimulation may assist the response and this may also be enhanced by the provision of visual sexual stimuli — be it suitable magazines or videos.

The ideal duration of response for diagnostic purposes is less than 1 hour. Some physicians prefer to avoid the risk of a prolonged erection by injecting a small dose of the vasoactive agent in the first instance and then increasing the dose on subsequent occasions. It seems more logical when using the technique for diagnostic purposes to avoid the risk of failure by injecting a larger dose on the first occasion, particularly as the main objective is to separate psychological and vascular causes of impotence. However, if this is done, it is preferable for the patient to wait in the hospital or clinic until the erection subsides — particularly if they have a long distance to travel. Patients should always be warned to return to the clinic if there is a prolonged erection or if the erection becomes painful. The safe duration for an erection is uncertain and it is unlikely that any harm will result if the persistent erection does not become painful.

The instruction to the patient to return should the erection persist is governed by practical considerations. With a diagnostic injection, a time limit of 6 hours is convenient and it is desirable not to inject the patient in the late afternoon. After a therapeutic self-injection at home it may be more convenient to instruct the patient to report back to the clinic next morning. On rare occasions, the drug induced erection begins to subside when the patient is still in the clinic but subsequently recurs once the patient is on his way home, or is even at home several hours later. This erection may be prolonged and the mechanism for this is uncertain.

The response to intracavernous injections may be graded empirically (Table 8.3) and although there may be some difficulty in grading patients with a moderate tumescence, in clinical practice this is not usually a problem. Wespes et al (1987) preferred to assess the response by measuring the angle the erect penis makes to the body when the patient is standing. The 'angle of dangle' should be greater than 90° in the normal male. The assessment of response for therapeutic purposes is a little different (see Ch. 11).

The production of a full erection with intracavernous drugs excludes a significant vascular lesion (arterial or venous). Such patients may need further investigation to exclude a neurological lesion and the most reliable of these is the monitoring of sleep erections. An impaired response to a full dose of the test drug suggests a vasculogenic cause for the impotence, which may be arteriogenic or venogenic. It is only necessary to distinguish between these elements if surgical treatment by arterial reconstruction or venous ligation is being considered. The diagnosis of venous incompetence may be suggested by facial flushing when phentolamine has been used (Williams et al 1988) or if the erection is augmented by the patient standing.

Prolonged erections

The duration of a drug induced erection is very variable and prolonged erections with papaverine have occurred with a dose as low as 10 mg (Buvat

Table 8.3 Simple assessment of response to intracavernosal agents

Grade 0 — No change
Grade 1 — Moderate increase in size; slight rigidity
Grade 2 — Marked increase in size; firm submaximal rigidity
Grade 3 — Normal erection

(After Buvat et al 1987; Collins & Lewandowski 1987)

et al 1987). The majority of prolonged erections subside spontaneously, but in general terms it is undesirable for any erection to last more than 4–6 hours, particularly if it is associated with pain. The simplest treatment is to aspirate blood from the corpus (Padma Nathan et al 1986; Buvat et al 1987). If this fails, then metaraminol (Brindley 1984; Block et al 1987) or phenylephrine (Sidi & Chen 1987; Albrecht et al 1991) may be injected to reverse the erection. Virag et al (1984) proposed that all patients who have a full response to papaverine when used for diagnostic purposes should have the erection reversed before leaving the clinic. Failure to treat prolonged erection can lead to permanent impotence (Halstead et al 1986; Buvat et al 1987) due to the tissue anoxia which causes necrosis of the cavernous muscle and fibrosis.

Treatment of prolonged erection or priapism

Following the diagnostic injection of papaverine or alternative, patients are recommended to wait until the erection begins to subside. This may be facilitated by the patient walking up and down stairs. Some physicians have found that the use of nasal vasoconstrictor drugs may help and Alexander (1989) recommended the use of an exercise bicycle. Should these first aid measures not succeed, it is necessary to inject vasoconstrictor agents into the cavernous tissue. It is preferable to carry this out under controlled circumstances as the patient may become severely hypertensive. It is important to monitor the blood pressure during such treatment.

A 19 gauge butterfly needle is inserted into one corpus and 50 ml of blood aspirated. This may bring about detumescence and no additional treatment is required. Phenylephrine hydrochloride solution is the preferred vasoconstricting agent as it is much shorter acting than metaraminol, which is associated with more prolonged hypertension and has been linked with the rupture of cerebral berry and abdominal aortic aneurysms. A solution containing 1 ml (10 mg) of phenylephrine is diluted with 9 ml of normal saline and 2–3 ml of the mixture is injected into the corpus cavernosus. Further 2–3 ml injections of the solution may be given until detumescence occurs. The patient should be warned not to engage in any form of sexual activity for the rest of the day.

SUMMARY

It is usually possible to have a good idea of the cause for the impotence by the end of one or two visits, as is shown in Figure 8.3. Many patients do not require additional diagnostic tests; these are generally only necessary for those wishing to be considered for reconstructive procedures.

REFERENCES

Aboseif S R, Breza J, Bosch R J L H, Benard F, Stief C G, Stackl W, Lue T F, Tanagho E A (1989) Local and systemic effects of chronic intracavernous injection of papaverine, prostaglandin E1 and saline in primates. Journal of Urology 142: 403–408

Albrecht A D, Bar Moshe O, Vandendris M 1991 Treatment of pharmacological priapism with phenylephrine. Journal of Urology 146: 323–324

Alexander W D 1989 Detumescence by exercise bicycle. Lancet i: 735

Block T, Sturm W, Ernst G, Schmiedt E 1987 The intracavernous application of alpha-adrenergic drugs in the treatment of priapism. World Journal of Urology 5: 178–181

Brindley G S 1983 Cavernosal alpha-blockade: a new technique for investigating and treating erectile impotence. British Journal of Psychiatry 149: 332–337

Brindley G S 1984 New treatment for priapism. Lancet ii: 220

Buvat J, Lemaire A, Dehaene J C, Buvat-Herbaut M, Guieu J D 1986 Venous incompetence: critical study of the organic basis of high maintenance flow rates during artificial erection test. Journal of Urology 135: 926–928

Buvat J, Lemaire A, Marcolin G, Dehaene J L, Buvat-Herbaut M 1987 Intracavernous injection of papaverine (ICIP): assessment of its diagnostic and therapeutic value in 100 impotent patients. World Journal of Urology 5: 150–155

Collins J P, Lewandowski B J 1987 Experience with intracorporeal injection of papaverine and duplex ultrasound scanning for assessment of arteriogenic impotence. British Journal of Urology 59: 84–88

Freidman D E, Clare A W, Rees L H, Grossman A 1986 Should impotent males who have no clinical evidence of hypogonadism have routine endocrine screening? Lancet i: 1041

Halstead S H, Weigel J W, Nobel M J, Mebust W K 1986 Papaverine induced priapism: 2 case reports. Journal of Urology 136: 109–110

Ishii N, Watanabe H, Irisawa C, Kikuchi Y, Kawamura S, Suzuki K 1988 Studies on male sexual impotence, report of therapeutic trial with prostaglandin E1 for organic impotence. Japanese Journal of Urology 77: 954–962

Juenemann K P, Lue T F, Fournier G R, Tanagho E A 1986 Haemodynamics of papaverine and phentolamine induced penile erection. Journal of Urology 136: 158–161

Maatman T J, Montague D K 1986 Routine endocrine screening in impotence. Urology 27: 499–502

Padma Nathan H, Goldstein I, Krane R J 1986 Treatment of prolonged or priapistic erections following intracavernosal papaverine therapy. Seminars in Urology 4: 236–238

Sidi A A, Chen K K 1987 Clinical experience with vasoactive intracavernous pharmaco-therapy for treatment of impotence World Journal of Urology. 5: 156–159

Stackl W, Hasun R, Marberger M 1988 Intracavernous injection of prostaglandin E1 in impotent men Journal of Urology 140: 66–68

Stackl W, Hasun R, Marberger M 1990 The use of prostaglandin E1 for diagnosis and treatment of erectile dysfunction. World Journal of Urology 8: 84–86

Strachan J R, Pryor J P 1987 Diagnostic intracorporeal papaverine and erectile dysfunction. British Journal of Urology 59: 264–266

Virag R 1982 Intracavernous injection of papaverine for erectile failure. Lancet ii: 938

Virag R, Frydman D, Legman M, Virag H 1984 Intracavernous injection of papaverine as a diagnostic and therapeutic method in erectile failure. Angiology 35: 79–87

Virag R, Brouilly P, Frydman D 1985 Is impotence an arterial disorder? Lancet i: 181–184

Wespes E, Delcour C, Rondeux C, Struyven J, Schulman C C 1987 The erectile angle: objective criterion to evaluate the papaverine test in impotence. Journal of Urology 138: 1171–1173

Williams G, Mulcahy M J, Hartnell G, Kiely E 1988 Diagnosis and treatment of venous leakage: a curable cause of impotence. British Journal of Urology 61: 151–155

Zentgraf M, Baccouche M, Juenemann K P 1988 Diagnosis and therapy of erectile dysfunction using papaverine and phentolamine. Urology International 43: 65–75

Zorgniotti A W, Lefleur R S ,1985, Auto-injection of the corpus cavernosum with a vasoactive drug combination for vasculogenic impotence. Journal of Urology 133: 39–41

9. Special investigations

John P. Pryor   Ian K. Dickinson

DIAGNOSIS OF VASCULOGENIC IMPOTENCE

Vasculogenic impotence is likely when the associated factors of cigarette smoking, obesity, diabetes, hypertension or other cardiovascular disorders are present (Virag et al 1985a). Vasculogenic impotence is characterized by a history of incomplete or absent erection which is constant during all forms of sexual activity. Furthermore, the early morning erection, which is often ascribed by the patient to a full bladder, is also weak or absent. There are, in addition, two specific but uncommon syndromes associated with arteriogenic impotence. In the Leriche syndrome there is an obstructive lesion at the bifurcation of the aorta and the patient also complains of intermittent claudication (pain in the calf muscles when walking) (Leriche 1923). The gluteal steal syndrome is characterized by a decrease in erectile capacity during coitus as a result of an increase in blood going to the gluteal muscles during thrusting, and the blood is therefore stolen from the internal pudendal artery supplying the cavernous tissue (Michal et al 1978).

Assessment of arteriogenic impotence

The diagnosis of arteriogenic impotence may be suspected from the history and an impaired response to intracavernous drugs. Further investigation is only required in those patients who are being considered for reconstructive surgery, and at the present time colour Doppler duplex ultrasound scanning is the preferred technique.

Measurement of penile blood pressure

The measurement of penile blood pressure and comparison of this with the brachial blood pressure was an attempt to diagnose arteriogenic impotence. Its measurement, and indices derived from it, are only useful when the ratio between penile and brachial systolic blood pressures is less than 0.6 (Metz & Bengtsson 1981), as the false negative rate is high above this ratio. One major problem with all techniques that measure the penile blood pressure is that they rely upon the detection of a pulse, and there may be no means of determining whether this is in the dorsal penile or cavernous arteries. Furthermore, measurement of penile blood pressure in the resting state does not assess the potential for vessels to dilate during erection. This problem is overcome by using colour Doppler ultrasonography. Attempts to increase the value of penile blood pressure measurements by using stress in the form of exercise (Goldstein et al 1982) or hyperaemia (Bell et al 1983) have not been found successful.

Padma Nathan (1989) introduced measurement of the cavernous arterial occlusive pressure, performed at the time of cavernometry. When the intracavernous pressure is greater than the arterial pressure, it is no longer possible to hear the penile pulses. As the intracavernous pressure falls, it is possible to determine the point at which the arterial pressure becomes audible. The application of Doppler ultrasound (Velceck et al 1980; Forsberg et al 1982) to study penile blood flow refined the technique further, but was still unsatisfactory as it relied upon the identification of penile arteries which have a low flow in the flaccid state. When the test was performed after intracavernous injection of papaverine and phentolamine, Gall et al (1989) found a good correlation between the Doppler waveform analysis and the arteriographic

115

findings. The use of a Doppler technique, in association with high resolution ultrasound imaging of the vessels before and after the injection of papaverine (Collins & Lewandowski 1987; Lue et al 1985) has become the method of choice. Although a sophisticated technique, the equipment is now available in many radiology departments for the investigation of other vascular disorders.

Radioisotope studies of the penis (Shirai & Nakamura 1975; Fanous et al 1982; Nseyo et al 1984; Blacklay et al 1985; Townell et al 1985; Chaudhuri et al 1989; Lin et al 1989) provide non-invasive methods that are useful in those centres which use these techniques for the investigation of other vascular disorders. It is desirable to perform these tests before and after intracavernosal papaverine injection.

Colour Doppler ultrasound

Principles of colour Doppler ultrasound. High frequency sound waves, usually 2–10 MHz, are emitted from a crystal at the tip of the probe which is held at an angle of approximately 45° to the patient's skin. Coupling gel is placed on the probe to improve the skin contact and the ultrasound beam is directed towards the vessel under investigation. The movement of the red blood cells towards or away from the probe causes the frequency of the reflected ultrasound beam to increase or decrease. The difference between the frequency of the emitted and received ultrasound beam is known as the Doppler shift and is converted to an audible signal. It should be noted that blood cells flow faster in the centre of the blood vessel than closer to the walls (*axial flow*) and it is necessary to correct for this. The basic Doppler examination was by continuous auscultation alone, but in duplex ultrasound, a real time binode ultrasound transducer is combined with a pulsed Doppler within one probe. This permits excellent imaging of the tissues, and the vessels may be identified. It is possible to observe the Doppler waveforms in any blood vessel as well as to obtain a measurement for blood flow velocity with the aid of computer analysis. Such equipment is expensive but is now available in many radiology departments.

This technique has been popularized by Lue et al (1985; Lue 1990) and gives the most reliable assessment of penile blood flow. It is carried out on an outpatient basis and is relatively non-invasive. Its main limitation is the availability and cost of the equipment.

Results. Ultrasound scanning is capable of detecting fibrosis or calcification within the erectile tissue. The penile arteries may be identified and, although small in the flaccid state, they are easily visible following the intracavernous injection of a vasoactive agent. Measurements of any increase in the lumen size are unreliable as even after dilation the vessel may be less than 1 mm in diameter. The addition of colour enables the vessels to be identified with much greater ease and it is possible to measure the peak velocity of the blood, which in a normal man should be greater than 25–30 cm/sec (Figs 9.1 & 9.2). The blood velocity should be measured in each of the dorsal and cavernosal arteries before an erection occurs as the flow decreases when the intracorporeal pressure rises. Examination of the waveform provides further indication of the normality or otherwise of the penile circulation.

When the diastolic as well as the systolic blood flow is taken into consideration, it is possible to calculate the resistance index in order to evaluate

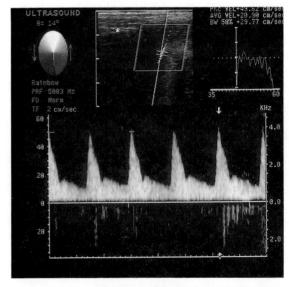

Fig. 9.1 Doppler ultrasound study in a man with normal flow in right dorsal penile artery (peak velocity 49.6 cm/sec).

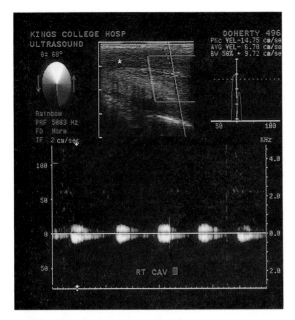

Fig. 9.2 Doppler ultrasound study of the right cavernosus artery of the same man as in Fig. 9.1, who had vasculogenic impotence (peak velocity 14.8 cm/sec).

the penile circulation and corporeal resistance (Juenemann et al 1990; Meuleman et al 1990).

$$\text{Resistance index} = \frac{\text{peak systolic velocity} - \text{diastolic flow velocity}}{\text{peak systolic flow velocity}}$$

It is emphasized that the maximum flow velocity should be measured at an early stage, and before erection occurs, because the flow diminishes as the intracorporeal pressure rises.

Magnetic resonance imaging (MRI)

Magnetic resonance imaging has been used to study the placental circulation (Schmid-Schönbein 1988; Panigel et al 1988). Sohn et al (1991) have used this technique to study the penile circulation. Its value is undetermined at the present time but it does offer the possibility to study the microcirculation within the corpora.

Arteriography

Most patients with arteriogenic impotence are not suitable for a reconstructive procedure and radiology is unnecessary. The radiology of impotence owes much to the studies of Genestie (1978) and Michal (Michal & Pospichal 1978; Michal et al 1980). Arteriography of the common iliac vessels and internal iliac vessels is straightforward but for the smaller vessels phalloarteriography (Figs 9.3 & 9.4) should always be carried out following the injection of a vasoactive agent. Some

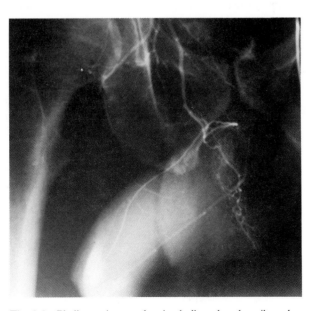

Fig. 9.3 Phalloarteriogram showing bulbar, dorsal penile and cavernosal arteries in a man with a high flow priapism.

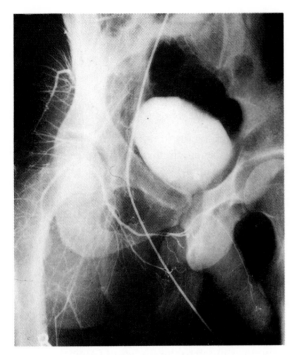

Fig. 9.4 Phalloarteriogram showing normal dorsal penile artery with occlusion of the cavernous artery (courtesy of Mr K Desai).

scribed at the turn of the century, but it was not until the last decade that the concept has received widespread support. At first, the diagnosis was established radiographically (Ebbehoj & Wagner 1979) but the trend has been to make the diagnosis by cavernometry and to reserve cavernosography for visualization of atypical leakage of blood from the corpora. The monitoring of the changes in intracorporeal pressure in response to the infusion of saline was first reported in 1979 (Virag 1981; Virag et al 1984) and studied in more detail by Wespes (Wespes et al 1984; Wespes & Schulman 1984, 1985). More recently, the test has been combined with the intracavernosal injection of vasoactive agents (Wespes et al 1986; Lue et al 1986; Bookstein et al 1987; Freidenberg et al 1987). The advantage of combining intracavernous pressure measurement with the papaverine test is that it attempts to separate arterial and venous causes for the impotence. The test is not without its drawbacks and care is needed to interpret the results (Newman & Reiss 1984; Buvat et al 1986; Porst et al 1987; Desai & Gingell 1988; Dickinson & Pryor 1989).

prefer to inject vasoactive drugs through the internal pudendal artery whilst carrying out the arteriography, whereas others utilize the intracavernosal injection of papaverine. Digital subtraction angiography (Nessi et al 1987) permits better imaging of the vessels and will be of increasing importance in the assessment of vasculogenic impotence prior to any reconstructive procedure.

Assessment of venous impotence

Dorsal vein ligation to cure impotence was de-

Cavernosometry

Cavernosometry is performed after injection of a vasoactive agent and, in an attempt to standardize the technique, dynamic cavernosometry is performed after giving 80 mg papaverine and recording intracorporeal pressure for 10 minutes before performing an artificial erection test (Dickinson & Pryor 1989). Five patterns of response were noted (Table 9.1). Some patients develop a full rigid erection within 10 minutes. These patients are considered to have no significant vascular abnor-

Table 9.1 Results of pharmacocavernometry in 126 patients (Dickinson & Pryor 1989)

Response	Number	Cavernous pressure 10 min after papaverine (mmHg)	Flow to create erection (ml/min)	Flow to maintain erection (ml/min)	Cavernous pressure after perfusion (mmHg)	Diagnosis
I	17	61	31	10	71	Normal
II	22	27	38	11	63	Normal
III	47	21	56	23	25	Arteriogenic impotence
IV	21	15	98	73	11	Venogenic impotence*
V	19	13.5	>120	not possible	13	Venogenic impotence*

*Arteriogenic impotence should be excluded by Doppler studies.

mality (see Ch. 8) and do not need to proceed further with the test.

A second group of patients do not respond to papaverine but continue to have an erection after the artificial erection test. The initial absence of response is though to be due to anxiety. These patients usually respond to papaverine at home and so, again, are thought to have no significant vascular lesion. The third group of patients do not respond to papaverine and do not continue to have an erection after the artificial erection test. The flow to maintain is less than 50 ml/min and therefore they have do not have veno-occlusive dysfunction. These patients are thought to have an arteriogenic impotence. The fourth group of patients, like the previous group, have no response to papaverine and do not continue to have an erection after the artificial erection test. The flow to maintain is greater than 50 ml/min and therefore they have veno-occlusive dysfunction. The final group do not respond to papaverine and do not get an erection during the artificial erection test. These patients have massive venous leakage.

In patients who develop and maintain erections, blood may be aspirated through the infusion line. This prevents a prolonged erection and only occasionally has it been necessary to inject phenylephrine (1–2 mg) into the corpus to ensure detumescence. It is unnecessary to perform cavernometry in all patients and better to reserve it for those patients with incomplete erections and where there is a normal arterial inflow.

Cavernosography

Cavernosography (Ebbehoj et al 1980; Herzberg et al 1981) carried out on the flaccid penis is only of benefit to show the extent of cavernous fibrosis or the persistence of shunts following surgery (Fig. 9.5). Cavernosography may also be performed with the penis erect and filling defects within the corpora or any abnormal bulges in the albuginea may be noted as well as any abnormal venous drainage channels. The test may be performed using a rapid blood-giving apparatus and it is only necessary to infuse both corpora in men with exstrophy (Woodhouse & Kellett 1984).

The main indication for cavernosography is to identify the site of 'venous leakage'. It used to be considered abnormal for the glans to fill during cavernosography but it is now recognized to occur in approximately one-third of patients. (Herzberg et al 1981; Delcour et al 1988). Some patients develop a spontaneous erection during cavernosography and at that time the venous outflow from the corpora is no longer visible. Venous leakage should be identified by observing the drainage of the penis at the time of full tumescence and a failure to obtain full tumescence with high flows is usually, though not invariably, pathological.

Much of our knowledge of the anatomy of the

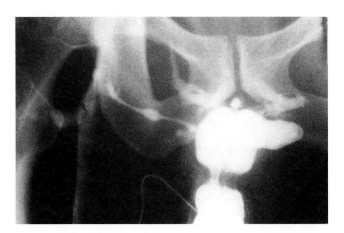

Fig. 9.5 Cavernosogram showing patent anastomosis of the long saphenous vein to the corpus cavernosum in a patient with veno-occlusive dysfunction following the shunt procedure for priapism.

venous drainage of the penis is due to the studies of Fitzpatrick (1975; Fitzpatrick et al 1975; Fitzpatrick 1982), although radiological studies of the veins have not been found helpful in planning treatment. The corpora drain by perforating veins into the corpus spongiosum, into the superficial and deep dorsal veins of the penis and through the crural veins into the pelvis. The role of cavernosography is of particular importance in the investigation of impotence following priapism. The impotence may be the result of penile fibrosis or due to the persistent patency of shunt operations to cure the priapism.

DIAGNOSIS OF NEUROGENIC IMPOTENCE

It is not possible to make a direct study of the neural pathways necessary for normal erection; indirect methods range from the monitoring of penile erections during sleep or in response to visual erotic stimuli, assessment of autonomic nerve function, or neurophysiological studies of the motor and sensory function of the somatic pelvic nerves. The monitoring of nocturnal penile tumescence (NPT) was for many years considered to be the 'gold standard' with regard to the diagnosis of organic impotence, but its importance has been reduced by the use of diagnostic papaverine. The disadvantages of nocturnal penile tumescence testing are clearly recognized and these, together with the simplicity of diagnostic papaverine, have contributed to its virtual demise. Nevertheless, the test remains an essential diagnostic procedure in some patients. It is, in addition, also useful to have an outpatient test for the diagnosis of an autonomic neuropathy.

Monitoring of nocturnal penile tumescence (NPT)

It is 50 years since the occurrence of erections during sleep was first observed in infants and subsequently found to be associated with the sleep pattern characterized by rapid eye movements. Fisher (Fisher et al 1975) and Karacan (Karacan & Moore 1982) realized the importance of these findings with regard to the diagnosis of organic impotence. Healthy 15-year-old males have approximately four episodes of nocturnal penile tumescence which last for a total of approximately 185 minutes in each night. The frequency of sleeping erections diminishes with increasing age and by the age of 70 years, there are on average two tumescent episodes each night lasting a total of 90 minutes (Karacan & Moore 1982).

Simple methods for monitoring nocturnal tumescence

Simple methods for monitoring sleeping erections have been described in an attempt to avoid the necessity of admitting the patient to hospital or a sleep laboratory overnight. The observations of the partner may be useful in assessing the presence and quality of sleeping erections. These techniques may provide useful information but their accuracy is questionable. The tests provide a means of monitoring the increase of penile girth during sleep and to a variable extent rely upon an increase in intracavernosal pressure. It is sometimes useful to initiate these tests at the time of the first consultation but it must be remembered that the results are subject to interference by the patient.

A relatively simple technique for monitoring penile tumescence is for the patient to place a ring of postage stamps around the penis and observe whether the perforations are broken during sleep (Barry et al 1980; Marshall et al 1982). A variety of similar techniques have been described (Jonas 1982; Morales et al 1983; Ek et al 1983; Bertini & Boileau 1986) and whilst they have the merit of simplicity, they do not overcome the need for formal monitoring of nocturnal penile tumescence in some patients.

Full monitoring of nocturnal penile tumescence

This usually requires the patient to be admitted to hospital for the monitoring of penile erections on three consecutive nights, but home monitoring equipment is now available. This is accomplished by placing two mercury filled strain gauges around the penis (one at the base and the other just below the glans). The electrical impedance of the strain gauges increases when the penis expands during erection, and this is recorded. It is no longer considered essential to monitor other changes that occur during rapid eye movement sleep.

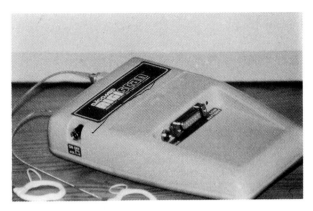

Fig. 9.6 Rigiscan machine for monitoring sleeping erections.

It is important to remember that the patient must sleep properly and this may not occur on the first night of admission to a strange environment (Wein et al 1981). It is also important to ensure that the patient is not taking any drugs or alcohol that may interfere with sleeping erections. It is unnecessary for the patient to remain in hospital once normal erections have been demonstrated.

The monitoring of nocturnal penile tumescence is no longer considered to be essential in order to confirm the diagnosis of organic impotence and attention has been focused on the defects in the test (Wasserman et al 1980; Marshall et al 1981;

Metz & Wagner 1981; Wein et al 1981; Pressman et al 1989). It is recognized that the sleeping erection may be accompanied by a full increase in the girth of the penis and yet the penis remains too soft to permit sexual intercourse. In an attempt to overcome such difficulties the erect penis may be examined and photographed by the patient, technician or nurse. The Rigiscan system (Dacomed Corporation, Minneapolis, USA) is a sophisticated computerized system which monitors rigidity as well as the increase in girth that occurs during sleeping erections (Figs 9.6, 9.7 & 9.8) (Bradley et al 1985). Other authors have developed other

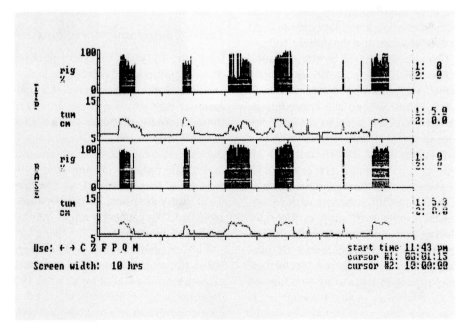

Fig. 9.7 Printout of Rigiscan trace of man with normal sleeping erections.

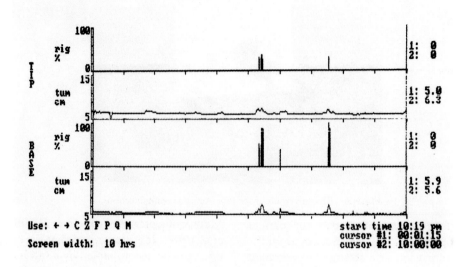

Fig. 9.8 Printout of Rigiscan trace of man with impaired sleeping erections.

methods for recording penile rigidity (Virag et al 1985b; Desai et al 1988b) and such techniques certainly increase the value of monitoring nocturnal penile tumescence.

A problem common to all attempts to monitor nocturnal tumescence is the fragility of the penile sensors, particularly when applied by the patient or doctors or nurses who are unaccustomed to their use. The cost of admitting the patient to hospital overnight has been reduced by the development of portable machines (e.g. the Tumistore machine, Lifetech Corporation, Houston, Texas, USA) or the use of hostel/hotel accommodation. An alternative approach has been to monitor the erectile response to erotic visual stimulation (Virag et al 1985b; Blacklay et al 1985), but not all patients respond to such stimuli (Earls et al 1983).

The main indication for monitoring nocturnal penile tumescence is in those patients with recognized neurological lesions in whom it is uncertain whether this is the cause of their erectile impotence, e.g. in multiple sclerosis or in men with lumbar disc lesions. The test may be performed in patients who appear to be unduly sensitive to papaverine or in whom an occult neuropathy is suspected, or in those patients who fail to respond to papaverine at all. NPT is sometimes useful to

convince patients with psychogenic impotence that normal erections occur during sleep. It is important to remember that a history of full nocturnal erections, either from the patient or his partner, is usually sufficient to avoid the need for this investigation (see Ch. 6, p. 88).

Tests of autonomic nerve function

It is not possible to perform direct testing of parasympathetic efferent fibres associated with erection. Some authors have examined the cardiovascular reflexes, but these are often negative in those impotent diabetics with a known neuropathy and absent ankle reflexes. Impotence may be the earliest symptom of an autonomic neuropathy in diabetic patients (Ewing et al 1980) and it has been said that pathological changes in diabetic neuropathy are nerve length dependent (Said et al 1983) and the earliest changes may be expected by examination of the feet.

The integrity of the body's longest unmyelinated fibres may be examined by testing thermal sensation in the feet (Fowler et al 1988). Thermal thresholds for both warming and cooling were measured in a group of 17 diabetic men and identified 14 patients with a neuropathy. Other symptoms of neuropathy were present in 8 of these patients, but the remainder had no other symptoms suggestive of a neuropathic origin for their impotence. It is of interest that 9 of the 15 men with a loss of perception for warming — conducted in unmyelinated fibres — had normal thresholds for cooling — conducted in small, myelinated fibres. This observation is in keeping with the hypothesis that impotence may be the earliest symptom of unmyelinated fibre neuropathy in diabetics. It is also of interest that the papaverine response was impaired in 9 of the 12 diabetics with evidence of a neuropathy. This suggests that the erectile dysfunction may be due to a combination of small fibre neuropathy and a microangiopathy.

Testing for reflex sweating of the feet may also be used as early evidence of an autonomic neuropathy, and a quantitative test for plantar sweating has recently been described and validated in a group of 24 impotent diabetic patients (Ryder et al 1988). These authors confirmed that testing the longest nerve fibres in the feet was the most sensitive method for detecting abnormalities of the autonomic nervous system.

Single potential analysis of cavernous electrical activity (SPACE)

Attempts to investigate neurogenic causes of impotence by direct measurement were unsuccessful until the report of Stief et al (1990). Wagner, Gerstenberg & Levin (1989) had drawn attention to the importance of electrical activity in the corporal muscle but had used needle electrodes to obtain the data. Stief et al also used needle electrodes but were able to show that in normal subjects the cavernous muscle acts synchronously and that erection was associated with smooth muscle relaxation. They have subsequently suggested that the muscular activity can be monitored by surface electrodes, however other groups have not been able to reproduce this work. It is clearly of great importance to have a direct means for monitoring the neuromuscular processes involved in erection/flaccidity.

Other neurophysiological tests

These tests are indirect assessments of neuro-

muscular function and have contributed to our understanding of impotence. They were of greater importance with regard to research than in the direct clinical management of patients. It is possible to monitor vibration sensitivity of penile skin (Newman 1970) but Fowler (personal communication) found difficulties in obtaining a consistent assessment of thermal thresholds of penile skin. Penile skin sensation may be tested by recording the production of cortical activity on the electroencephalogram (Lin & Bradley 1985) and these recordings give a measure of nerve conduction velocity. Desai recorded the sensory perception threshold (defined as the mean of 3 estimations) for the dorsal nerve of the penis and of the posterior urethra (Desai et al 1988a). Goldstein suggested that patients with a sensory deficit of the penis may have difficulty in sustaining a penile erection during coitus (Goldstein et al 1985).

Bulbocavernosus latency (Siroky et al 1979; Blaivas et al 1980; Barrett 1984; Blaivas 1984; Galloway et al 1985; Sarica & Karacan 1987; Desai et al 1988a; Parys et al 1988)

This test has been described as the urologist's knee jerk (Galloway et al 1985) and is based upon the bulbocavernosus reflex (S2–4) which is elicited by squeezing the glans penis and detecting a contraction of the anal sphincter. The latency time is measured by stimulating the penis with a current of variable frequency and duration and observing the time taken to record a reflex contraction of the bulbocavernosus muscle with the use of an electromyographic needle placed in the bulbocavernosus muscle. This is a test of the integrity of the sacral cord segment and its afferent and efferent fibres. It has been widely used to investigate urological disorders, including impotence.

A modification of the bulbocavernosus latency test involves the use of a concentric needle electrode to record individual units from the urethral sphincter, and the response time following the stimulation of penile skin is recorded (Fowler et al 1988).

Sacral evoked responses

Bradley (1972) described the urethro-anal response

(the posterior urethra is stimulated and the response monitored by the contraction of the anal sphincter). This is a similar test to the bulbocavernosus reflex and reflects the integrity of the slower conducting autonomic afferent fibres. Significantly delayed latency times have been found in a large population of men with impaired nocturnal penile tumescence (Sarica & Karacan 1987).

Pudendal motor evoked potentials

A method for the non-invasive electrical transcranial stimulation of the brain was described in 1980 and modified to allow magnetic stimulation of the brain. The latency time to the bulbocavernosus or anal sphincter has been recorded and compared to the time taken for those muscles to contract following stimulation of the sacral root (Opsomer et al 1986).

Bladder cystometry

The widespread availability of this test led to its use in the assessment of impotence. The test would appear to be too non-specific to have much diagnostic importance.

SUMMARY

It is usually possible to diagnose the cause of erectile dysfunction from the history and clinical examination of the patient. Further investigation may be necessary in order to convince the patient that there is not a significant organic component to his problem, or in order to evaluate the exact nature and significance of that component. The intracorporeal injection of papaverine has a major role to play in this assessment but the clinician must be aware of the pitfalls and complications of this test.

Further investigation is necessary in those centres embarking on surgical procedures to improve the quality of erectile function. Arterial reconstruction is confined to those men with major vessel disease or to a small group of young patients with congenital or traumatic arterial problems. These patients require a full assessment of the arterial system and it might be argued that so, too, do patients with venous incompetence. The diagnosis of veno-occlusive dysfunction, by cavernosometry, is easy but unfortunately the results of surgical correction are variable, with a 30% failure rate. Further refinements in diagnostic techniques are required.

Finally, and despite its drawbacks, there is still a necessity to perform nocturnal penile tumescence testing in some patients. The causes of erectile dysfunction are many and a clear understanding of the physiology of erection is essential in order to select and interpret wisely the many diagnostic techniques that are available.

REFERENCES

Barrett D M 1984 Electromyography: the practical approach. In: Barrett D M, Wein A J (eds) Controversies in neuro-urology. Churchill Livingstone, New York p. 85–92

Barry J M, Blank B, Boileau M 1980 Nocturnal penile tumescence monitoring with stamps. Urology 15: 171–172

Bell D, Lewis R, Kerstein M D 1983 Hyperemic stress test in diagnosis of vasculogenic impotence. Urology 23: 611–613

Bertini J, Boileau M A 1986 Evaluation of nocturnal penile tumescence with Potentest. Urology 27: 492–494

Blacklay P, Friedman D, Lumley J 1985 Penile skin blood flow measurement using photoplethysmography. In: Virag R, Virag-Lappas H (eds) Proceedings of the 1st world meeting on impotence. CERI, Paris p 129–132

Blaivas J G 1984 Electromyography: other uses. In: Barrett D M, Wein A J (eds) Controversies in neuro-urology. Churchill Livingstone, New York p 103–116

Blaivas J G, O'Donnell T F, Gottlieb P, Labib K B 1980 Comprehensive laboratory evaluation of impotent men. Journal of Urology 124: 201–204

Bookstein J J, Valji K, Parsons L, Kessler W 1987 Penile pharmacocavernosography and cavernosometry in the evaluation of impotence. Journal of Urology 137: 772–776

Bradley W E 1972 Urethral electromyelography. Journal of Urology 108: 563–564

Bradley W E, Timm G W, Gallagher J M, Johnson B K 1985 New method for continuous measurement of nocturnal penile tumescence and rigidity. Urology 26: 4–9

Buvat J, Lemaire A, Dehaene J C, Buvat-Herbaut M, Guieu J D 1986 Venous incompetence: critical study of the organic basis of high maintenance flow rates during artificial erection test. Journal of Urology 135: 926–928

Chaudhuri T K, Fink S, Burger R H, Netto I C V, Palmer J D K 1989. Physiological considerations in radionuclide imaging of the penis during impotence therapy. American Journal of Physiological Imaging 4: 75

Collins J P, Lewandowski B J 1987 Experience with intracorporeal injection of papaverine and duplex ultrasound scanning assessment of arteriogenic impotence. British Journal of Urology 59: 84–88

Delcour C, Wespes E, Vandenbosch G, Schulman C C, Struyven J 1988 Opacification of the glans penis during cavernosography. Journal of Urology 139: 732–733

Desai K M, Gingell J C 1988 Saline induced artificial erection without papaverine: a potential source of error in diagnosing cavernosal venous leakage. British Journal of Urology 62: 176–178

Desai K M, Dembrig K, Morgan H, Gingell J C, Prothero D 1988a Neurophysiological investigation of diabetic impotence. Are sacral responses of value? British Journal of Urology 61: 68–73

Desai K M, Floyd T J, Follett D H, Peake D R, Gingell J C 1988b Development of a penile rigidity indicator and new concepts in the quantification of rigidity. British Journal of Urology 61: 254–260

Dickinson I K, Pryor J P 1989 Pharmacocavernometry: a modified papaverine test. British Journal of Urology 63: 539–545

Earls C M, Morales A, Marshall W L 1983 Penile sufficiency: an operational definition. Journal of Urology 139: 536–538

Ebbehoj J, Wagner G 1979 Insufficient penile erection due to abnormal drainage of cavernous bodies. Urology 13: 507–510

Ebbehoj J, Uhrenholdt A, Wagner G 1980 Infusion cavernosography in human unstimulated and stimulated situations and its diagnostic value. In: Zorgniotti A W, Rossi G (eds) Vasculogenic impotence. Proceedings of the 1st international conference on corpus cavernosum revascularization. Thomas, Springfield, Illinois p 191–196

Ek A, Bradley W E , Krane R J 1983 Snap-gauge band: new concept in measuring penile rigidity. Urology 22: 63

Ewing D J, Campbell I W, Burt A A, Clarke B F 1980 The natural history of diabetic autonomic neuropathy. Quarterly Journal of Medicine 193: 95–108

Fanous H N, Jevtich M J, Chen D C P, Edson M 1982 Radioisotope penogram in diagnosis of vasculogenic impotence. Urology 20: 499–502

Fisher C, Schiavi R, Lear H, Edwards A, Davis D M, Witkin A P 1975 The assessment of nocturnal REM erection in differential diagnosis of sexual impotence. Journal of Sex and Marital Therapy 1: 277–289

Fitzpatrick T J 1975 The corpus cavernosum intercommunicating venous drainage system. Journal of Urology 113: 494–496

Fitzpatrick T J 1982 The penile intercommunicating venous valvular system. Journal of Urology 127: 1099–1100

Fitzpatrick T J, Cooper J F 1975 A cavernosogram study on the valvular competence of the human deep dorsal vein. Journal of Urology 113: 497–499

Forsberg L, Olsson A M, Neglen P 1982 Erectile function before and after aortoiliac reconstruction: a comparison between measurements of Doppler acceleration ratio, blood pressure and angiography. Journal of Urology 127: 379–382

Fowler C J, Ali Z, Kirby R S, Pryor J P 1988 The value of testing for unmyelinated fibre sensory neuropathy in diabetic impotence. British Journal of Urology 61: 63–67

Freidenberg D H, Berger R E, Chew D E, Ireton R, Ansell J S, Schwartz A N 1987 Quantification of corporeal venous outflow resistance in man by corporeal pressure flow evaluation. Journal of Urology 138: 533–538

Gall H, Baehren W, Scherb W, Stief C, Thon W 1989 Diagnostic accuracy of Doppler ultrasound technique of the penile arteries in correllation to selective arteriography. Cardiovascular and Interventional Radiology 11: 225–231

Galloway N T M , Chisolm G D, McInnes A 1985 Patterns and significance of the sacral evoked response (the urologist's knee jerk). British Journal of Urology 57: 145–147

Genestie J F, Romsieu A 1978 Radiologic exploration of impotence. Martinus Nijhoff Medical Division, The Hague

Goldstein I, Siroky M B, Nath R C, McMillan T N, Menzoian J O, Krane R J 1982 Vasculogenic impotence: role of the pelvic steal test. Journal of Urology 128: 300–306

Goldstein I, Tejada I S, Heeren T, Davidson M M, Sax D S, Krane R J 1985 Dorsal nerve impotence: a clinical study of the mechanism. Journal of Urology133: 187A

Herzberg Z, Kellett M J, Morgan R J, Pryor J P 1981 Method, indications and results of corpus cavernosography. British Journal of Urology 53: 641–644

Jonas U 1982 Erectionmeter: ein einfacher und sicherer test in der diagnostik der erektilen impotenz. Aktuel Urologie 13: 324–327

Juenemann K P, Siegsmund M, Rassweiler J, Alken P 1990 Calculation of the resistancy index for differential diagnosis of vascular and non-vascular impotence. International Journal of Impotence Research 2: 207

Karacan I, Moore C A 1982 Nocturnal penile tumescence: an objective diagnostic aid for erectile dysfunction. In: Bennett AH (ed) Management of male impotence. Williams & Wilkins, Baltimore p 62–72

Leriche R 1923 Des obliterations artérielles hautes, causes des insuffisances circulatoires des membres inférieurs. Bull Mem Soc Chir 49: 1404–1406

Lin J T, Bradley W E 1985 Penile neuropathy in insulin dependent diabetes mellitus. Journal of Urology 133: 213–215

Lin S N, Chang L S, Liu R S, Yeh S H, Yu P C, Kuo J S 1989 Diagnosis of vasculogenic impotence: combination of penile xenon-133 washout and papaverine tests. Urology 34: 28–32

Lue T F 1990 Impotence: a patient's goal-directed approach to treatment. World Journal of Urology 8: 67–74

Lue T F, Hricak H, Marich K W, Tanagho E A 1985 Evaluation of arteriogenic impotence with intracorporeal injection of papaverine and the Duplex ultrasound scanner. Seminars in Urology 3: 43–48

Lue T F, Hricak H, Schmidt R A, Tanagho E A 1986 Functional evaluation of penile veins by cavernosography in papaverine induced erection. Journal of Urology 135: 479–482

Marshall P, Morales A, Surridge D M 1981 Unreliability of nocturnal penile tumescence recording and MMPI profiles in assessment of impotence. Urology 17: 136–139

Marshall P, Earls C, Morales A, Surridge D 1982 Nocturnal penile tumescence recording with stamps: a validity study. Journal of Urology 128: 446–447

Metz P, Bengtsson J 1981 Penile blood pressure. Scandinavian Journal of Urology and Nephrology 15: 161–164

Metz P, Wagner G 1981 Penile circumference and erection. Urology 18: 268–270

Meuleman E J H, Bemelmans B L H, Van Asten W N J C, Doesburg W H, Skotnicki S H, Debruyne F M J 1990 Doppler color flow imaging (DCFI) in the evaluation of penile circulation. International Journal of Impotence Research 2: 216–217

Michal V, Pospichal J 1978 Phalloarteriography in the diagnosis of erectile impotence. World Journal of Surgery 2: 239–248

Michal V, Kramar R, Pospichal J 1978 External ileac 'steal syndrome'. Journal of Cardiovascular Surgery 12: 355–357

Michal V Pospíchal J Blazková J, 1980 Arteriography of the

internal pudendal arteries and passive erection. In: Zorgniotti A W, Rossi G (eds) Vasculogenic impotence. Proceedings of the 1st international conference on corpus cavernosum revascularization. Thomas, Springfield, Illinois p 169–179

Morales A, Marshall P G, Surridge D H, Fenemore J 1983 A new device for diagnostic screening of nocturnal penile tumescence. Journal of Urology 129: 288–290

Nessi R, Flaviis L de, Bellinzoni G, Fiori F, Salvini A 1987 Digital angiography of erectile failure. British Journal of Urology 59: 584–589

Newman H F 1970 Vibratory sensitivity of the penis. Fertility and Sterility 21: 791–793

Newman H F, Reiss H 1984 Artificial perfusion in impotence. Urology 24: 469–471

Nseyo U O, Wilbur H J, Lang S A, Flesh L, Bennett A 1984 Penile xenon (133Xe) washout: a rapid method of screening for vasculogenic impotence. Urology 23: 31–34

Opsomer R J, Guerit J M, Wese F X, van Cangh P J 1986 Pudendal cortical somatosensory evoked responses. Journal of Urology 135: 1216–1218

Padma Nathan H 1989 Evaluation of the corporal veno-occlusive mechanism: dynamic infusion cavernosometry and cavernosography. Seminars in Interventional Radiology 11: 225–231

Panigel M, Coulam C, Wolf G, Zeleznik A, Leone F, Podesta C 1988 Magnetic resonance imaging (MRI) of the placental circulation using gadolinium-DTPA as a paramagnetic marker in the rhesus monkey in vivo and the perfused human placenta in vitro. Trophoblast Research 3: 271–282

Parys B T, Evans C M, Parsons K F 1988 Bulbocavernous reflex latency in the investigation of diabetic impotence. British Journal of Urology 61: 59–62

Porst H, van Ahlen H, Vahlensieck W 1987 Relevance of dynamic cavernosography to the diagnosis of venous incompetence in erectile dysfunction. Journal of Urology 137: 1163–1167

Pressman M R, Fry J M, DiPhillipo M A, Durante R T 1989 Avoiding false positive findings in measuring nocturnal penile tumescence. Urology 5: 297–300

Ryder R E J, Marshall R, Johnson K, Ryder A P, Owens D R, Hayes T M 1988 Acetylcholine sweat spot test for autonomic denervation. Lancet i: 1303–1305

Said G, Slama G, Selva J 1983 Progressive centripetal degeneration of axons in small fibre diabetic polyneuropathy. Brain 106: 791–807

Sarica Y, Karacan I 1987 Bulbocavernous reflex to somatic and visceral nerve stimulation in normal subjects and in diabetics with erectile impotence. Journal of Urology 138: 55–58

Schmid-Schönbein H 1988 Conceptual proposition for a specific microcirculatory problem. Maternal blood flow in hemochorial multivillous placentae as percolation of 'porous medium'. Trophoblast Research 3: 17–38

Shirai M, Nakamura M 1975 Diagnostic discrimination between organic and functional impotence by radioisotope penogram with 99mTc. Tokoku Journal of Experimental Medicine 116: 9–15

Siroky M B, Sax D S, Krane R J 1979 Sacral signal tracing: the electrophysiology of the bulbocavernous reflex. Journal of Urology 122: 661–664

Sohn M H, Wein B, Bohndorf K, Handt S, Jakse G 1991 Dynamic magnetic resonance imaging (MRI) with paramagnetic contrast agents: a new concept for evaluation of erectile impotence. International Journal of Impotence Research 3: 37–48

Stief C G, Djamilian M, Schaebsdau F, Truss M C, Schlick R W, Abicht J H, Allhoff E P, Jonas U 1990 Single potential analysis of cavernous electric activity — a possible diagnosis of autonomic impotence? World Journal of Urology 8: 75–79

Townell N H, Siraj Q H, Hilson A J, Dick R, Morgan R J 1985 Isotope phallogram: a preliminary communication. Journal of the Royal Society of Medicine 78: 562–566

Velceck D, Sniderman K W, Vaughan E D, Sos T A, Muecke E C 1980 Penile blood flow index utilizing a Doppler pulse wave analysis to identify penile vascular insufficiency. Journal of Urology 123: 669–672

Virag R, 1981 Syndrome d'érection instable par insuffisance veineuse. Journal des Maladies Vasculaires 6: 121–124

Virag R 1984 Initial investigation of impotence. In: Virag R & Virag-Lappas H (eds) Proceedings of the 1st world meeting on impotence. CERI, Paris p 122–128

Virag R, Frydman D, Legman M, Virag H 1984 Intracavernous injection of papaverine as a diagnostic and therapeutic method in erectile failure. Angiology 35: 79–87

Virag R, Brouilly P, Frydman D 1985a Is impotence an arterial disorder? Lancet i: 181–184

Virag R, Virag H, Lajujie J 1985b A new device for measuring penile rigidity. Urology 25: 80–81

Wagner G, Gerstenberg T, Levin R J 1989 Electrical activity of corpus cavernosus during flaccidity and erection of the human penis. Journal of Urology 142: 723–727

Wasserman M D, Pollak C P, Spielman A J, Weitzman E D 1980 Theoretical and technical problems in the measurement of nocturnal penile tumescence for the differential diagnosis of impotence. Psychosomatic Medicine 42: 575–585

Wein A J, Fishkin R, Carpiniello L, Malloy T R 1981 Expansion without significant rigidity during nocturnal penile tumescence testing: a potential source of misinterpretation. Journal of Urology 126: 343–344

Wespes E, Schulman C C 1984 Parameters of erection. British Journal of Urology 56: 416–417

Wespes E, Schulman C C 1985 Venous leakage: surgical treatment of a curable cause of impotence. Journal of Urology 133: 796–798

Wespes E, Delcour C, Strugven J, Schulman C C 1984 Cavernometry and cavernosography. European Urology 10: 229–232

Wespes E, Delcour C, Stragven J, Schulman C C 1986 Pharmacocavernometry–cavernography in impotence. British Journal of Urology 58: 429–433

Woodhouse C R J, Kellett M J 1984. Anatomy of the penis and its deformities in exstrophy and epispadias. Journal of Urology 132: 1122–1124

Treatment of erectile dysfunction

10. Psychological approaches to treatment

Martin Cole

HISTORICAL OVERVIEW

Before the arrival of the new sex therapies in the 1960s, most patients with sexual problems, if they were provided with more than 'medication and general advice', were offered treatment largely based upon psychoanalytical theory. Though some behavioural therapy was just beginning to emerge (Wolpe 1958), it was then assumed that most sexual disorders were symptoms of deeply repressed and unresolved, unconscious conflicts acquired in childhood and that the recognition and resolution of these conflicts, through treatment based upon psychodynamic theory, could lead to normal sexual functioning.

Inevitably, treatment programmes of this nature were denied to all except the wealthy and those with time to spare, but even with the high motivation that one would expect in such a patient sample, the treatment outcomes were rarely successful (Cooper 1978; Ellis 1980; Allgeier & Allgeier 1984).

The 1960s and 70s heralded the arrival of Masters & Johnson (1966, 1970), Helen Kaplan (1974, 1979) and a therapeutic renaissance from which were born the 'new sex therapies'. Imperfect as they may appear in some respects nowadays, at that time they were welcomed almost unconditionally and uncritically, largely because of the relatively simplistic way in which they portrayed sexual dysfunction. They introduced, for the first time, ideas and methods based upon an empiricism initiated some 20 years earlier by Kinsey (1948, 1953). For example, Masters & Johnson (1966) recognized four stages in the sexual response cycle: excitement, plateau, orgasm and resolution — an interpretation later to be reformulated by Kaplan (1974) into her triphasic model of desire/drive, arousal and orgasm — a model generally accepted today.

From this theoretical base, the new sex therapies evolved a directive, interventionist approach to treatment, relying heavily upon behavioural and psychoeducational methods. However, there remained the contribution of the less tangible humanistic psychotherapies (and in Helen Kaplan's case psychodynamic methods) all aimed at encouraging self-knowledge, attitudinal change, permission-giving and self-acceptance. This complex mix of the psychodynamic, behavioural and humanistic persists to this day in sex therapy.

More recently, this therapeutic triumvirate has been joined by cognitive and cognitive-behavioural methods and their future place is assured in sex therapy (Hawton 1989). It was, however, Ellis (1975, 1976, 1980) who was largely responsible for introducing these cognitive methods into sex therapy, laying emphasis as he did upon the role that disturbed thinking plays in maintaining sexual problems. He stressed that it is the individual's negative evaluations of his problem that causes distress as much as the problem itself, and that by challenging these beliefs substantial progress could be made in dealing with most sexual difficulties, including erectile problems.

Most recently has come the realization that a significant proportion of men presenting with erectile dysfunction have an organic aetiology (e.g. Melman et al 1984). Such an awareness does not diminish the role of the psychological therapies — indeed it will have the opposite effect and add to their status. If proper diagnoses are now made, the effectiveness of the psychological therapies should improve, since time and energy will not be wasted treating those patients with predominantly organic aetiologies purely with psychological therapies.

THE CAUSES OF ERECTILE DYSFUNCTION

Introduction

Most sex disorders have a multifactorial basis and erectile dysfunction is no exception. The many factors involved can be divided into those which have an organic or physical basis, and those which are the result of learning or experience; these latter are said to have a psychological basis. Organic factors are those where an innate or largely innate aspect of anatomy, physiology or behaviour is responsible for the erectile disorder, or where, as a result of disease, the individual's physical response has been adversely affected. Psychological factors refer to the multitude of causes best described as *experiential* which include all life experiences, e.g. early childhood conditioning, physical and psychological traumata, and the impact of relationships and their interaction with 'innate/preprogrammed/temperamental' patterns of response to experiences.

Whilst it is relatively easy to assign a cause to one or other of these categories (though difficulties do arise, to be discussed later) it is by no means as easy to define impotence as being either organogenic or psychogenic, since it is difficult to imagine any physical or organic factor which does not impinge upon the mental state of the patient. For example, impotence in diabetic men cannot correctly be described as organogenic since the patient's evaluation of the harmful effects of the disease, once diagnosed, may even exceed its physiological effect. A constructive view is probably to regard the contribution of organic and psychological factors as belonging to two orthogonal (independent) dimensions (LoPiccolo & Stock 1986). Both sets of factors can then vary independently of each other, either or both being strong or weak. However, even this is simplistic as interactions between the dimensions occur.

Notwithstanding this obvious and complex interaction between physical and psychological factors, it is important to recognize the distinction between organic and psychological causes, if only to focus the clinician's mind on the need for an early and accurate diagnosis of the presenting problem. It is only when such a diagnosis is reached that the deployment of whatever therapeutic resources are available can be accomplished with the greatest efficiency. The first part of this chapter will consider the multitude of psychological factors which may be implicated in the development of erectile dysfunction. The psychological basis for *normal* function is described in Chapter 2. The second part of this chapter describes the more commonly employed treatment options.

Kaplan (1974, 1979) divided the psychological causes of sex disorders into *remote* and *immediate*. Her 'remote' causes included those factors which had their effect early in the formative years of development, such as a repressive traditional and sexually repressive upbringing, early trauma — a rape or sexual abuse, or maladaptive relationships with parents in childhood; indeed, she included any early aversive experiences and longstanding neurotic conflicts under this heading. Her 'immediate' causes, on the other hand, included ignorance, inappropriate attitudes to sex, a poor relationship, excessive anxiety about sexual feelings and, in particular , performance fears.

Hawton (1985) neatly divided the psychological causes of sexual dysfunction into *predisposing factors*, *precipitating factors* and *maintaining factors* (see Table 6.1) His predisposing factors, which roughly correspond to Kaplan's remote causes, refer to those early experiences which predispose, but do not pre-determine, a later sexual disorder. His precipitants are events such as the discovery of infidelity, depression and anxiety or the presence of a dysfunction in one's partner. Finally, his maintaining factors are those which he argues are the only ones amenable to modification, e.g. performance anxiety, poor communication between partners and a fear of intimacy.

The multifactorial nature of erectile dysfunction — a checklist

The aetiological factors implicated in erectile loss, and listed below, have been classified into four categories. The *organic* category is the most easily defined and includes those factors where either neurophysiological processes, disease or psychopathology are responsible for the erectile difficulties. Though they are of no direct concern to us in this chapter, they are presented here to complete the picture. The *interactive* category includes those causes which cannot be easily ascribed to either the organic or experiential categories, and clearly comprise elements of both.

Those factors listed under *experiential* and *relationship* headings identify causes which would in current parlance be regarded as 'psychological'. In other words, they refer to events which, either acting in the distant or recent past or in the 'here and now', have resulted in high levels of maladaptive learning sufficient to have made a substantial contribution to the erectile problem.

It is tempting to regard these so-called psychological factors as being qualitatively different from those which have a much more clearly defined physical or organic basis. It is as if learning and experience are believed to operate in some way independent of the hereditary or biological make-up of the developing individual. Of course this is not true. Each genetically unique individual will respond to a set of environmental circumstances in a correspondingly unique manner. Thus, some men will be particularly resistant to stress (or more specifically sex-stress) and will be able to survive many more environmental insults than another more genetically precarious individual, who might become an early casualty (see Fig. 10.1).

Since the aetiology of erectile impotence is so obviously multifactorial, it is a good idea if the clinician prepares a checklist (if only in his mind)

of the more salient factors that he believes to be implicated in the presenting condition. This list can obviously be revised in the light of further investigations. Such an approach imposes an important discipline upon the diagnostic process and if the patient can also become involved in this detective work his awareness and understanding of the nature of his problem can become part of the therapeutic process. Some patients and many clinicians may need a little encouragement before they can warm to this idea and it is, unfortunately, time consuming. Moreover, many clinicians are very reluctant to disclose too much information to the patient. This is understandable if the diagnosis is unclear, though every effort should be made to be open and honest with the patient.

To assist the clinician in the preparation of a checklist, the more important causal factors implicated in the aetiology of erectile disorders are summarized below. They form the basis of a retrospective survey of the author's patients with erectile problems, presented later (see p. 142).

ORGANIC (physical)

1. *Disease*: a clinically defined condition which is known to affect erectile function, e.g. multiple sclerosis, diabetes, epilepsy, cardiovascular disorders.
2. *Iatrogenic (drugs)*: current medication which is thought to be responsible for the erectile dysfunction (see Ch. 6).

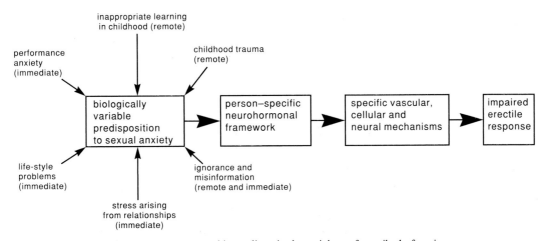

Fig. 10.1 The role of sex-stress, remote and immediate, in the aetiology of erectile dysfunction.

3. *Psychosis*: history of, or a currently presenting, clinically diagnosed psychosis which is also thought to be relevant to the presenting erectile dysfunction (see Ch. 6).

4. *Neurohormonal dysfunction*: a well-defined neurohormonal dysfunction, e.g. low testosterone or hyperprolactinaemia, which has been diagnosed by investigations and which may also result in erectile loss; or a condition diagnosed (or inferred) as a result of anatomical abnormalities, e.g. hypogonadism, undescended testes, intersexual state, e.g. Klinefelter syndrome (see Ch. 3).

5. *Substance abuse*: sustained ingestion of a drug (including alcohol but excluding prescribed medications) which can be incriminated as a cause of erectile dysfunction.

6. *Vasculogenic or neurogenic disorder*: a clinically defined condition where, as a result of investigation, either the vascular or nerve supply to the penis has been implicated in the erectile dysfunction.

7. *Personality disorder (or borderline psychosis)*: a clinically evident personality disorder which would be expected to affect sexual response and behaviour.

8. *Mental or physical handicap*: erectile dysfunction causally or specifically related to a mental or physical handicap, e.g. cerebral palsy.

9. *Physical trauma*: injury affecting erectile capacity, e.g. spinal injury.

10. *Iatrogenic (other)*: erectile dysfunction caused by medical intervention, e.g. surgery, dialysis, prostatectomy.

INTERACTIVE (organogenic and experiential)

11. *Low sex drive*: in men under 50, a total outlet of less than one orgasm a week, together with a general subjective lack of interest in sex as an erotic experience; in men over 50, a correspondingly lower drive.

12. *Personality type*: where a clearly defined constellation of personality traits signals a lack of interest or performance deficits in sexual response, e.g.:

    a. a rigid, anxious, obsessional, low-affect male with traditional antisexual values.
    b. an emotional, high-affect male who, as a result of well established and powerful defences, has repressed his feeling states.
    c. an inadequate, unassertive, underconfident male who feels deeply rejected and may have developed masochistic behaviours.

13. *Homosexual needs*: clear evidence of homosexual or bisexual needs, either overt or in fantasy, which could interfere with heterosexual erectile response.

14. *Age*: advancing years will have a synergistic effect upon the other aetiological factors listed, so that, all other things being equal, the erectile capacity of the ageing adult becomes more precarious. (No arbitrary age can be identified, but those men over 50 are more vulnerable.)

15. *Paraphilias*: overt, unusual sexual behaviours which are obsessive and play a significant role in the individual's sex life (or make up a significant part of his sexual fantasies).

16. *Depression*: a clinically diagnosed depressive illness which can be related in time to the erectile dysfunction.

17. *Dyspareunia*: pain in intercourse (actual or anticipated, i.e. phobic) resulting from phimosis, Peyronie's disease or a sexually transmitted disease.

18. *Severe anxiety states*: generalized, or specific, e.g. agoraphobia or panic attacks.

19. *Poor self-image*: specific physical problems believed by the individual to have eroded his ego-strength and thereby contributed to his erectile problem, e.g. acne, eczema, psoriasis, bad teeth, physical handicap, disfigurement.

20. *Gender identity conflicts*: evidence of transsexual or transvestite needs and behaviours which have interfered with heterosexual erectile response.

EXPERIENTIAL (excluding relationship problems)

21. *Restricted upbringing*: this refers specifically to a 'Victorian', 'puritanical', repressive,

antisexual upbringing which has resulted in the denial of sexual feelings in the adult and strong feelings of guilt.

22. *Religious pressures*: as above, but related specifically to religious pressures.

23. *Disturbed family relationships*: a wide range of scenarios where there may be a loss of a parent figure resulting in separation anxiety, over-attachment, unresolved oedipal problems or where parent figures may be disturbed themselves and have created an early traumatic environment for the young child.

24. *Lifestyle problems*: a loss of erection which can be specifically related to a well-defined lifestyle problem, e.g. fatigue resulting from work, unsocial hours, stress from money worries, children's behaviour.

25. *Psychological trauma*: specific event(s) in adolescent or adult life, the consequences of which have a profound psychological effect on the individual's sexual responses, e.g. adult rape, observing infidelity of partner; including traumatic learning where a significant, single, negative event has a far-reaching effect on sexual performance.

26. *Child abuse*: reported sexual or physical abuse which appears clearly related to the presenting erectile dysfunction.

PROBLEMS WITH RELATIONSHIPS

27. *Performance anxiety*: a loss of erection specifically resulting from anxiety generated by a history or expectation of perceived failure and particularly the need to obtain an erection to please one's partner.

28. *Rejection (loss of partner)*: loss resulting from death, divorce or separation (widower syndrome).

29. *Rejection by partner*: erectile dysfunction thought to be caused by overt or covert rejection within the relationship or by refusal of partner to have sex.

30. *Heterophobia*: the presence in the adult of anxiety, specifically relating to heterosexual courtship and sex play, which is sufficiently powerful to have prevented the formation of relationships or, where intercourse has been

attempted, erectile inadequacy is experienced as a result of this anxiety.

31. *Specific sexual incompatibility*: where the behaviour of a sexually demanding female partner leads to performance anxiety in the male or, conversely, where a deeply inhibited female partner cannot respond sexually.

32. *Fears of intimacy*: sexual anxiety in a man generated by a close relationship (may not be separate from 33).

33. *Loss of attraction (habituation)*: man no longer regards his partner to be sexually attractive or sexually significant (see Ch. 2) (may not be separate from 32).

34. *Dysfunction in partner*: the presence of a *specific* sexual problem in his partner (e.g. vaginismus, sexual aversion) which leads to erectile dysfunction in a man.

35. *Poor communication*: erectile problems resulting from the inability of a couple to communicate effectively; the relationship is thus bedevilled by anger and resentment.

Psychological factors implicated in erectile dysfunction

Attention has already been drawn to the difficulties involved in distinguishing between the 'organic' and the 'psychological' causes of erectile impotence. To help overcome these difficulties, a third category of causes, the 'interactive', is proposed, where both organic and psychological factors interacting together are implicated. In this section, factors which are *interactive* and *experiential*, together with those which are *relationship-based*, are considered in more detail. The role of the organic factors has been dealt with in previous chapters. References in the text to 'my patient sample' refer to the analysis of the prevalence of these factors in the survey, the results of which are presented on page 142.

Low sex drive

It is common knowledge that sex is very important for some people and of little significance to others. Sex, for some, dictates their lives from puberty until death. They have orgasms most days of their lives either through masturbation or intercourse, they have a rich fantasy life and derive an enormous amount of erotic pleasure from sex one way or another. At the other end of the distribution curve there are men who can adopt a 'take it or leave it' attitude to sex — they start their sex lives late and stop early, indeed there may be long intervals in their lives, perhaps up to six months or more, where they do not have an orgasm or any interest in sex. This may be because of stress, the lack of a partner or simply because they are not interested. Even when they do masturbate, often they do it for 'relief' rather than for any positive need to enjoy the erotic experience of fantasy and orgasm. For this group, even when they are happily married, the frequency of intercourse is low, perhaps only once every three to four weeks at the most.

Walen & Roth (1987), along with other authors, identify sexual underarousal as being an important feature in many sex disorders, though they view this low arousal from a purely cognitive standpoint. However, since the low sex drive category is so well represented in patients who have presented with erectile problems (see p. 142), clearly more attention should be directed to examining the role that drive plays in the aetiology of sexual dysfunction in general and erectile disorders in particular.

Low sex drive is a condition aetiologically distinct from inhibited sexual desire (Kaplan 1979). These two conditions are not always distinguishable in women though in men they are not so easily confused. A man with a low sex drive is globally disinterested in sex, whereas disorders of desire in men are usually situational and partner-dependent, his drive being unaffected in self-masturbation or in coitus with other partners. Inhibited sexual desire is an important cause of erectile dysfunction and has been dealt with separately under the categories of 'fear of intimacy' and 'loss of attraction' (see p. 139).

Personality type (not personality disorder)

It does appear from clinical impressions that there are certain constellations of behaviours (personality types) which are more likely to show a propensity to develop erectile problems than others. Those crudely identified earlier (see p. 132) appear more frequently than one might expect by chance. It is important to try to identify those who are more likely to develop problems, if only because the treatment programmes available may not be equally suited to each type. One might assume, for example, that individuals with low affect would respond more readily to the cognitive therapies, whilst those with high affect would be more likely to benefit from the behavioural approach; or that introverts would gain more from sensate focus than would extroverts with their short attention span.

Homosexual needs

It is not uncommon to find men who, as a consequence of feeling inadequate heterosexually, believe themselves to be homosexual or at least to have 'homosexual tendencies'. Indeed, some hold on to those beliefs without any other strong evidence that they are gay. With skilled counselling these fears can often be put in perspective or laid to rest and heterosexual skills encouraged.

However, these men contrast with others, many of whom may also have erectile problems, where their homosexual needs are more clearly expressed either covertly in fantasy or overtly in homosexual or bisexual behaviour.

If, for whatever reason, neurohormonal or experiential, gay needs form a significant part of the sexual repertoire of a patient, these needs can be expected to impair his capacity to become aroused heterosexually. However, there is probably little point in trying to change or eliminate these homosexual needs: it may be more profitable to try to help the patient understand and accept his homosexual behaviour and, if necessary, modify his life-style accordingly.

Age

It is to be expected that advancing age will play a part in increasing the vulnerability of a man to erectile disorders. Age, unfortunately, is inexorable and inescapable: however, attitudes to age are not. In my patient sample, as in many other studies, age appeared to play an important part in predisposing to erectile problems. It was surprising to discover the extent to which some men experienced problems adjusting to the fact that as they get older they cannot expect to maintain the level of drive, frequency and performance that they may have enjoyed previously.

The clinician has a difficult task and it is crucial that he takes a balanced view. He should avoid defeatist comments like, 'What do you expect at your age?', instead, he should take care to explain that false and unrealistic expectations of sexual performance in later life may actually lead to anxiety related sexual problems. He needs to emphasize that whilst physiological changes do result in the slowing down of sexual responses, there is no intrinsic reason why sex should ever stop. Two points do need stressing, however. First, that for a man to be able to enjoy sex in later life he needs a motivated partner to whom he is still attracted — very often sex stops in a relationship simply because the partner says, 'No more' or he no longer finds her attractive. Second, it should be emphasized that individual men differ dramatically in their sexual needs. Some are quite happy to stop in their fifties and never give sex another thought; others would be devastated by that prospect and see sex as an ongoing and important part of their lives, well into their sixties, seventies or later. If there is a large age difference between the man and his younger partner, this may also create sexual problems by creating performance anxiety in him as a result of his need to please his more sexually demanding partner.

The paraphilias (unusual sex)

Many patients with erectile problems said they enjoy incorporating unusual sex (fetishistic and sadomasochistic behaviours in particular) into their masturbatory fantasies: a few reported that they practised these behaviours overtly. The desire for unusual sex, either in fantasy or reality, provides an insight into the roots of an individual's sexual needs and it is not unreasonable to assume that if these needs are at variance with those demanded by a conventional relationship, then his capacity to become aroused may be impaired. Without speculating on the causes of these paraphilias (see Ch. 2), there is little evidence to suggest that therapeutic intervention can do much to eliminate them permanently from an individual's sexual repertoire.

Thus one is left with the need to concentrate upon helping the patient understand and accept what he may regard as an unacceptable part of himself; indeed by so doing, one may reduce anxiety which, in turn, will reduce his dependence upon the paraphilia. It may also be necessary to suggest that he change his lifestyle in a way that might help him reconcile his sexual needs with those of his relationship and family. Those who prefer a more interventionist behavioural approach to treatment should consult Walen & Roth (1987) and Bancroft (1989).

Depression

It is well known that depression, acting centrally, may suppress the sex drive which, in turn, may affect erectile response, although it is somewhat surprising that a heightened sex drive may also accompany depression (Mathew & Weinman 1982). Conventional sex therapy is of little use whilst the depression persists and, clearly, therapy should be directed initially towards dealing with the depressive illness. Unfortunately, antidepressant medication, often the chosen form of therapy, may also reduce the sex drive, though there is usually a rapid return to normal response once the medication is withdrawn and the depression has lifted. Alternatively, or in combination, if the opportunity and skills are available, 'cognitive' methods can be used to treat the depression equally effectively but without sexual side effects (Hawton et al 1989; Gelder 1990).

The patient may not be aware of the connection between his depression (indeed, he may not even know that he is clinically depressed) and his sexual problem. However, once it has been explained to him that his erectile difficulties are likely to be linked to his depression, and that these difficulties are temporary, one major source of anxiety will have been removed. If he is also being prescribed antidepressant medication the possible effects of this on his sexual response should be explained.

Dyspareunia

Reports of dyspareunia were unexpectedly frequency in my sample of patients with sexual problems. Phimosis, a tight foreskin, and a fear of paraphimosis, the foreskin tightly encircling and strangulating the penis below the glands, are problems best solved by circumcision, supported by counselling and psychotherapy. More rarely, one meets patients who present with anxieties of phobic proportions, their fears being triggered by actual or imagined attempts to retract the foreskin even when there is no evidence that the foreskin is tight (a male equivalent of vaginismus!).

Severe anxiety states

Even with the exclusion of the heterophobe and those with personality disorders, patients very occasionally present with high levels of anxiety unrelated to sexual function or performance. Naturally, these anxiety states may indirectly inhibit sexual responses and attention should be directed towards dealing with the causes of the anxiety before any sex therapy is contemplated. Anxiolytic medication may suppress the sex drive (Riley & Riley 1986) and the patient should be told about this.

Poor self-image

Those patients who present with a poor self-image and low self-esteem exhibit a variety of thinking and feeling states. The causes of these are complex and may involve personality type, early experiences, psychiatric illness and 'learned helplessness'. These feelings of inadequacy may be without foundation and patients may attempt to rationalize them by attributing them to an imagined physical deficiency. A favourite one is penis size. Many underconfident men present complaining about the size of their penis as a means of justifying their sexual anxiety, yet I can recall only one or two who had a penis that was significantly smaller than average. Most had a normal sized penis and some had even quite large ones.

Low self-esteem and poor self-image may also result from physical conditions, e.g. acne, eczema or psoriasis, which, when severe, can have a profound effect on sufferers. If such conditions are present in childhood the effects can be even more damaging. If ego-strength is particularly low, the poor self-image so generated can prevent or delay normal development and the acquisition of normal social and courtship skills. Low self-esteem is

well addressed through the use of cognitive therapy (see p. 155).

Gender identity conflicts

A man may be confused about his sexual identity and gender role and perhaps also uncertain about whether he is heterosexual, homosexual or bisexual. In these circumstances, he may also find it difficult to establish relationships which provide him with adequate sexual arousal, with the result that he may develop erectile problems. The application of the classic treatment paradigm: know and understand yourself, accept yourself, change yourself, is clearly one method of approach, though much time and patience is needed if realistic help is to be given. Complex therapy of this kind is very often best done by pursuing an optimal strategy calling upon one's intuitive skills to help achieve the best possible solution to what is often a very complex and perhaps unresolvable problem. In situations such as this, I am reminded of Reinhold Niebuhr's prayer: 'God grant me the serenity to accept things I cannot change, the courage to change things I can and the wisdom to know the difference'.

Restricted upbringing

A strict, antisexual, so-called Victorian upbringing was not uncommon a generation or more ago, and the casualties of this kind of oppression are still presenting with their sexual problems. The cumulative effect of these early experiences, which led to the denial of sexual feelings, labelling them as sinful or dirty, are long-lasting. The banning of nudity in the home, punishment for any behaviours regarded by the parents as even remotely sexual, the censorship of TV or, more ominously, the absence of any display of affection in the home and the avoidance of any discussion about sex, all play their part in interfering with the normal development of the child. The effects are even more dramatic if he has no siblings and has to carry this load on his own.

Religious pressures

It appears from my patient sample that religious pressures have played a small but significant role in reinforcing negative attitudes to sex. A restrictive upbringing, where the child is inculcated with the belief that all sex is shameful and sexual feelings should be denied, need not necessarily be administered through religious doctrine (nor, may it be stressed, are all religions oppressive). However, when religion does become the vehicle for this kind of antisexual oppression, it can be particularly devastating in its effect. Sometimes the clinician is faced with the difficult task of getting the patient to confront the need to change his views about sex, even though this change may lead him into conflict with his religious beliefs. One might find, however, that some patients would rather change their sexual expectations and it may be that counselling to reconcile the conflict in that direction is required. Such changes cannot be achieved overnight and careful counselling is often required if the patient is to be liberated from the constraints of his upbringing.

Disturbed family relationships

Most therapists and clinicians, and sex therapists are no exception, recognize a crude distinction between those patients whose problems appear to stem from a so-called 'psychodynamic' aetiology and those whose condition seems to be better explained 'behaviourally'. Those men who present with erectile dysfunction and appear to have a 'psychodynamic' aetiology are often those who provide histories where the early family relationships were profoundly disturbed in one way or another. Problems such as over- or under-attachment, oedipal conflicts and exaggerated separation anxiety are common in this group of patients, although it is not clear whether such 'problems' are any less common in the general population.

Treatment of these patients is not easy and in spite of its so-called psychodynamic aetiology, psychoeducation, behavioural and cognitive methods (see p. 155) are the methods most likely to succeed, given sufficient patient motivation to accept this approach. Indeed, in some cases, analytical psychotherapy may do more harm than good by encouraging the patient to focus too closely upon those early traumatic experiences when instead he should be encouraged to face the 'here and now' in a more pragmatic manner.

Lifestyle problems

Problems of this kind are fortunately usually of relatively short duration. However, in times of stress where worries about family, money or work impinge upon the psychological health of a man, then clearly his sexual response may be affected. One of the consequences of stress is the lowering of sex drive, with the result that sex may stop altogether until circumstances improve. However, some men might still find themselves under pressure to please their partner despite their lack of sexual desire and fail because they are sexually anxious or depressed.

Unemployment is likely to have an adverse affect on sexual behaviour as indeed may a change of job or retirement. I can recall a number of patients who had either lost status as a result of job changes or found it difficult to adjust to being at home most of the day after retirement and who then developed erectile problems.

Adolescent or adult psychological traumata

These appear rarely in my patient sample but when present may result in traumatic learning, the effects of which can be long-lasting. Rape, the discovery of a partner in bed with her lover, humiliation by a girl in an early sexual encounter are instances which can have devastating effects on performance. The clinician, however, should always be on the lookout for false assumptions. Patients often incorrectly exaggerate the role that a particular experience may have played in the causation of their erectile problem. If this appears to be the case, the patient's attention should be directed towards what are the more likely explanations for his problem.

Child abuse

Child abuse has not been widely reported in this male patient sample. Nevertheless, when it does occur, it may predispose the individual to sexual problems in adulthood. Since so much depends upon the nature and extent of the abuse and the degree to which the young boy was traumatized at the time, it is dangerous to generalize. The evidence available would suggest that young girls are more likely to suffer from harmful sequelae following abuse than boys, but that may be simply because girls are more often the target for abuse. Wilkins (1990) draws attention to the fact that women also frequently abuse young boys, indeed, in one study, women were found to be responsible for nearly one quarter of the abuse of boys. Naturally, the patient should be encouraged to talk about the experience, if he wishes, but consistent with a cognitive-behavioural approach he should not be encouraged to dwell upon the experience obsessionally.

Performance anxiety

Problems with erection, once they appear, may or may not persist. Many men report temporary loss of erection due to stress, fatigue or anxiety experienced at the beginning of, say, a new relationship — however, most of these difficulties disappear without recourse to treatment. Some erectile problems are, however, more persistent and unquestionably performance anxiety is one of the most important factors responsible for initiating and maintaining this erectile loss. A man may have a very strong need to please his partner sexually and if his capacity to get an erection is impaired in any way, expectations of failure, whether based upon real or imagined circumstances, will produce in him high levels of anxiety which will in turn add to his chances of failure. This cycle of anxiety and failure then becomes self-fulfilling as the patient enters the vicious circle of 'fear of fear'.

Performance anxiety can be covert and experienced cognitively or overt and result in the more usual subjective visceral feelings of anxiety (I recall one patient who said that he was so nervous about his impending sexual failure that his partner was prompted to enquire whether there was a burglar in the house!). Performance anxiety can result from imagined events or actual past experiences and it can survive the passage of time long after the original triggering experiences have been forgotten.

Masters & Johnson were correct in attaching the importance they did to the role played by performance anxiety, if only because it is eminently treatable. Frequently, however, it is only one of many aetiological factors involved in the causation of erectile problems and, naturally, it is important

that the complex multifactorial nature of any one patient's condition is understood before treatment is begun.

Not all forms of anxiety associated with sexual behaviour are as damaging to sexual response as performance anxiety. Barlow and others have shown that some forms of anxiety may actually enhance sexual arousal (Barlow 1986). Anxieties of this kind, which are often part and parcel of the agony and ecstasy of some sexual experiences, are best described as *expectation anxieties* and are quite distinct from performance anxiety in their effect (see p. 143). Furthermore, it seems likely that men differ in their response to anxiety. Men with erectile dysfunction respond adversely to anxiety whereas men without commonly show increased arousal (see Ch. 2).

Rejection — loss of partner

The loss of a valued and loved partner, however it happens, can have a dramatic effect upon a man's sexual responses. Whether it is death, divorce or separation the grief experienced can sometimes take years to dissipate, particularly in the older man. Kolodny et al (1979) called this loss of sexual function, following bereavement, 'the widowers' syndrome' and it figures prominently in most patient samples presenting with erectile difficulties. Indeed, this shutdown in sexual response is often so complete that many patients believe that there may be a physical cause for their lack of interest in sex. One would naturally expect a period of grief, depression and a temporary shutdown of sexual response following a loss of this kind, though men do vary considerably in the time they take to recover. Some start their sex lives again almost immediately, others may need to wait perhaps for as much as two or three years.

This interval depends upon a number of factors: first, the extent to which the loss is felt. This will obviously vary from relationship to relationship; secondly, the age of the survivor — if he is young, his recovery will be more rapid than if he is in his fifties or older; thirdly, the extent of his previous extra-marital or extra-relationship experience; and fourthly, the degree to which he can judge correctly when he is ready to embark upon a new sexual encounter, whether it is part of a new serious relationship or not. The reappearance of regular night or morning erections may be a good signal, indicating that the neurohormonal mechanisms responsible for sexual arousal are beginning to function normally again.

Unfortunately, some men underestimate the time it takes to come to terms with their loss, attempt a sexual relationship prematurely, fail and trigger a sequence of crippling performance fears which may take some time to sort out. Moreover, a strong need to please his new partner may magnify even slight inadequacies in his performance and result in such high levels of anxiety that total erectile failure is almost inevitable.

Rejection by partner

Also figuring prominently in the list of causes of erectile dysfunction is rejection of a different kind. This is where a 'secret divorce' has taken place and, whilst the couple may remain together and even share a bed, the patient's partner refuses sex or, if she agrees, becomes a totally uninvolved partner. Whether this rejection is overt or covert the message he receives is loud and clear — 'I am not interested in you'; 'I don't fancy you'; 'Get on with it if you must but don't expect me to enjoy it'. A sexually precarious man will naturally be badly affected by the lack of response from his partner and may develop erectile loss as a consequence. Treatment is not easy, often the only option is either to put up with it or get out of the relationship.

Sometimes women will reject their partner at menopause believing that this event marks the end of their sex lives. Simple counselling may be adequate to solve this problem.

Heterophobia

Heterophobia means fear of the opposite sex (Cole 1986, 1988b). Most heterosexuals will experience some degree of anxiety in opposite sex transactions, whether they are at a social or sexual level. However, it is only when this anxiety reaches unacceptable levels that blocks in courtship, sex play and intercourse emerge. Heterophobia is prominent in my patient sample as a cause of erectile dysfunction because of the large number of part-

nerless individuals included. Sexual anxiety, however, is a universal experience and few men can claim not to have experienced its often unwelcome attentions some time in their lives.

The lack of social and sexual skills, so often a feature of the heterophobe, cannot always be explained in terms of the blocking effects of anxiety. In some men, there appears to be a total lack of awareness of what they should do to acquire a partner, engage in sex play and proceed to intercourse, a deficiency which does not appear to be simply the result of maladaptive learning or overt anxiety, and it may be that a neurophysiological explanation will be found. The therapeutic strategies best suited to the treatment of the heterophobe are detailed in Chapter 15.

Specific sexual incompatibility

The successful integration of sexual and loving needs into a relationship is clearly important if that relationship is to survive and flourish. However, couples may fall 'in love,' yet with sex playing little or no part in the transaction. As long as the couple are compatible and their priorities do not change too much with the passage of time, clearly this presents no problem, since loving relationships between couples can and do exist in the absence of sex. However, not infrequently, the 'immature' parameters, upon which the initial attraction was based, change over the years and sex may then become increasingly more important for one or other of the partners. Either way, this may disrupt the relationship: if she becomes sexually demanding, he may develop performance anxieties; similarly if his sexual needs are not satisfied because of her lack of interest (for whatever reason), he may feel rejected — both scenarios can lead to erectile loss.

Fear of intimacy (inhibited sexual desire)

One does not have to be an adherent of Freud to recognize that fears of intimacy may play an important part in the genesis of many sex disorders. Powerful feelings which, for want of a better word, can be described as incestuous may lead to blocks in sexual desire, arousal and hence erectile capacity. Very often, blocks in the erectile responses caused by fears of intimacy are partner-specific and as a result the prognosis of the condition is often poor (De Amicis et al 1985). Sexual problems caused in this way often disrupt a relationship and, unfortunately, the cycle is often repeated in subsequent relationships. The couple should be helped to understand the true nature of their 'problem': to see it objectively and in perspective so that they can each (and collectively) take responsibility for whatever decisions about their future, if any, are necessary.

Loss of attraction (inhibited sexual desire)

Sex therapists (and many others) have been reluctant to identify loss of attraction for one's partner as an important cause of sexual problems. One reason for this is undoubtedly because it is difficult, if not impossible, to 'treat'. There is also the fear that recognition of 'loss of attraction' as a major cause of sex dysfunction may challenge the implicit values of our society, namely that this doesn't happen, or rather that it shouldn't happen. Be that as it may, loss of attraction is a potent force endangering sex lives and disrupting relationships, with the result that blocks in sexual arousal may then lead to erectile loss (see also Ch. 2). This is often partner-specific and will have a poor prognosis, if only because the affected partner will discover that his sexual responses are unaffected in other relationships. Loss of attraction (*habituation*) as a cause of erectile loss may not be distinguishable from the previous category, 'fear of intimacy', except that in the latter the cause can be more readily identified whereas in the former it cannot.

Dysfunction in partner

A specific sexual dysfunction in his partner will obviously affect the quality of a man's sex life. It is well known that the partners of women with severe vaginismus may develop erectile problems and that inhibited sexual desire in the partner may also have the same effect. Remedies may not be easy but given high motivation in both, conventional sex therapy can help.

Case vignette: Rejecting partner/dysfunctional partner. Alan and his wife, Doreen, had been

separated for three months when they decided to make another attempt to rescue their marriage. Alan, an electronics engineer, is 28 and Doreen, who works in a building society, is 26. They have been married for five years. Alan is a fairly quiet, reserved man and somewhat obsessional; Doreen is more extrovert and assertive. Alan had developed erectile inadequacy a year ago and now they were together again they hoped that 'his' problem could be treated. Neither had had intercourse with anyone else before they met five years ago, Alan because of his shyness and Doreen because she had been brought up very strictly. She wanted to wait until they were married before beginning their sex lives, but they did attempt intercourse once or twice: however Alan failed to get an erection so they decided to wait.

Even after they were married, things did not go well. Doreen had been brought up to believe that the man should take the initiative. She was unhappy about touching Alan's penis and found it very difficult to relax when they began foreplay. Eventually, the quality of Alan's erection improved and they did achieve intercourse but Doreen did not enjoy it very much, never reached a climax and derived very little pleasure from love-making. As the years passed, the frequency of intercourse dropped to once a month or even less and Doreen's evident distaste for sex upset Alan so much so that he resorted to self-masturbation, having no difficulty with his erection. However, he felt emotionally and sexually rejected and as the months passed he found that his earlier erectile problems returned when they attempted intercourse, and eventually their sex lives stopped.

Although Alan was clearly sexually precarious, the main cause of his erectile problem was Doreen's inability to respond sexually to him because of her guilt and anxiety about sex. This lack of response in her signalled a total lack of love and a rejection which Alan could not handle.

After a considerable amount of counselling, Doreen did learn to relax and begin to accept her own sexual feelings as being good and desirable. This acceptance helped her to respond to Alan, his capacity to erect returned and intercourse, though not frequent, became rewarding to them both.

Poor communication

On its own, poor communication is probably not a very important cause of erectile inadequacy. However, where problems already exist, or where the relationship is sexually precarious, the ability to communicate openly and honestly is likely to be of considerable benefit. Couples are often deterred from talking honestly to each other about their sexual feelings because of the embarrassment caused by the intimacy so generated: this is particularly evident in relationships of some years' duration or where both have 'well-defended' personalities. An additional problem is that couples may not wish to hurt each other and end up by not talking to each other at all. The role of the clinician or counsellor is to act as a facilitator and help catalyse meaningful communication within the relationship. Once this has been achieved, it may be possible to establish better patterns of communication in the future.

Having said this, it should not be overlooked that many relationships may have become highly ritualized and stylized in their behaviours and that the open and honest sharing of feelings can be harmful and disruptive. Couples have, over the years, learnt to communicate through various codes and rituals and if these are to be challenged, the clinician or counsellor must proceed cautiously or he may do more harm than good by disturbing well tested patterns of behaviour.

A case vignette. The details of the history of this couple are presented here to illustrate the multifactoral aetiology typically found in patients with an erectile problem.

Peter and Sylvia had both been happily married before, but both had lost their partners through bereavement: they married each other a year ago. Peter is 65 and Sylvia 61. Neither had experienced any sexual problems in their marriages, though sex had never been particularly important for either of them. Peter's medical history is important. Angina and high blood pressure were diagnosed about 15 years ago and he was prescribed the β blocker, oxprenolol, at that time and has been taking it ever since. By this time, his sex life with his first wife had become somewhat episodic, since his wife was ill, and regular sex ceased with her about 10 years ago. Five years later she died of cancer after a long illness. As a result, Peter was completely celibate for about 4 years, masturbating only infrequently.

Shortly after his wife died, Peter met a woman with whom he attempted intercourse: this was a complete failure and he recalled how guilty he felt about the whole experience. Two years later, he met Sylvia. Peter, now retired, was an accountant. He has a highly obsessional, rigid personality, holds very traditional values and is a perfectionist in all he undertakes. He is meticulously dressed and Sylvia volunteered the observation that his attention to detail and obsessive tidiness at home can be very annoying. Peter can get a moderate erection in self-masturbation and reports reasonably good morning erections.

Neither Peter nor Sylvia attempted intercourse before they got married (Peter's traditional values saw to that) and Peter claims that he was somewhat surprised when he discovered that he was unable to make love to his new wife. He was naturally very upset by this discovery since his idea of sexual fulfilment is entirely centred on pleasing his partner, even though Sylvia insists that his erectile inadequacy doesn't really matter to her. At the time of presentation, he had not achieved intercourse with Sylvia, losing his partial erection just before penetration.

A number of separate factors have contributed to Peter and Sylvia's problem; they are listed below, though not in order of importance. Any one of these factors alone probably would not in itself have had any effect upon the patient's sexual response. However, the additive effect of them all was sufficient to tip the scales, producing erectile dysfunction. Whilst no attempt has been made to weight the contribution of these factors, there is little doubt that performance anxiety has played and continues to play a major role in maintaining the problem. Though clearly both organic and psychological factors have contributed to the manifestation of their problem, it was thought that the couple would respond adequately to psychological methods of treatment. The part thought to be played by these physical factors was explained to the couple and then a modified Masters & Johnson approach was undertaken.

The more significant factors presumed to be implicated in the aetiology of this presenting problem are:

1. Age
2. Medication
3. Cardiovascular problems
4. Personality type
5. Loss of wife and 'widowers' syndrome'
6. Medium to low sex drive
7. Performance anxiety.

Peter's capacity to achieve a good erection was never fully restored and intercourse was achieved only very occasionally. Of more importance was the fact that they both felt better about 'the problem', were able to put it in perspective, realizing that their relationship was rewarding in so many other respects.

A SURVEY OF PATIENTS

To provide some idea of the relative contribution of the aetiological factors previously discussed, a retrospective analysis was undertaken on those patients who had consulted the author between 1971 and 1989. From a total available sample of over 2000 patients, their records revealed that approximately 36% had presented with a clearly defined erectile dysfunction. From this latter sample, 384 patients were selected for the final analysis on the basis that their notes provided sufficient information to provide a fairly accurate assessment of the aetiology of their erectile problem. The mean age of this final sample was 40.9 years (SD = ± 10.4 years). At the time of presentation, 35% had a stable relationship and 65% were without any relationship. A total of 718 observations (factors) were extracted from the notes of 384 patients, giving a mean of 1.9 observations per patient.

The factors chosen initially were those thought likely to be of importance in the aetiology of erectile disorders from information gained from personal clinical impressions, together with the help of previous relevant publications, e.g. Masters & Johnson (1970), Kaplan (1974), Hawton (1985) and Bancroft (1989). An original list of 41 factors provided a starting point for the exercise, but subsequently this was reduced to 35 (see p. 143). Those factors which were later thought not to play any, or only a very small part, and were therefore excluded were, e.g. pregnancy in partner, specific neurotic conditions (e.g. obsessional or phobic behaviours) and ignorance and misinformation.

No attempt was made to ensure that the final list of factors were independent of each other or even mutually exclusive. Such a task would have been beyond the scope of this preliminary investigation, though a full multivariate factor analysis of the aetiolology of erectile disorders is long overdue. Instead, the purpose of this exercise was simply to highlight, in a relatively unsophisticated way, the relative contribution of those factors thought to be playing some role in the causation of erectile disorders. 65% of the sample analysed were without a meaningful relationship at the time of presentation. This fact will obviously introduce some bias into the results, perhaps by exaggerating the role of the interactive at the expense of the experiential factors. The incidence of problems associated with relationships is relatively unaffected because many of those without relationships at the time of presentation suffered from erectile disorders as a direct consequence of the loss of the relationship.

Subject to the inevitable approximations involved in the collection of retrospective data (see Fig. 10.2) a number of general observations can be made:

i. Strictly organic factors do not figure very predominantly in this survey (17.7%) largely because opportunities were not available, in the early years particularly, to pursue full diagnostic investigations. There is little doubt, therefore, that many instances of neurohormonal dysfunction and vasculogenic or neurogenic impotence have been missed or classified under other headings (low sex drive, for example).

ii. 'Diseases' of various types have played an important part in the aetiology of erectile disorders (8.0%), particularly in advancing years.

iii. Those factors included in the 'interactive' sections share both genetic and learnt aetiologies. Together they contribute over 35% of the total causes identified. A few are clearly amenable to some form of therapeutic intervention (severe anxiety states, poor self-image, dyspareunia, depression); others less so.

iv. Of particular interest is the significant contribution that low sex drive and personality type appear to have played. Together, they have contributed over 16% of the total effects observed; indeed, of all the observations made these two factors are the most frequently recorded.

v. The part played by the so-called 'experiential' factors, whilst of undoubted importance (13.4%), is less so than might have been expected. However, early childhood experiences have proved to be of undoubted relevance, as have the iatrogenic effects of drugs.

vi. It is no surprise that problems associated with relationships have been found to be of considerable significance (31.7%) in the aetiology of erectile problems. Naturally, performance anxiety is crucially important, as is rejection by one's partner in whatever form. Anxiety specifically related to heterosocial and

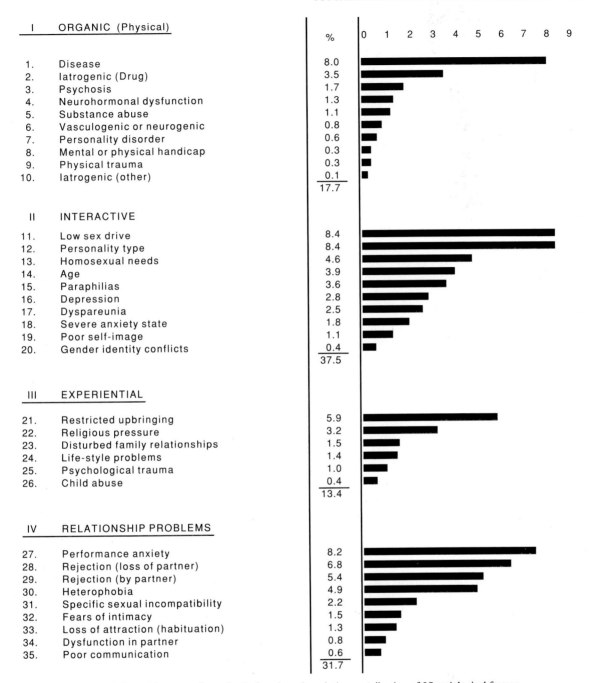

Fig. 10.2   The multifactorial nature of erectile dysfunction: the relative contribution of 35 aetiological factors.

heterosexual behaviours (heterophobia) also plays an important role.

The role of anxiety in sexual dysfunction

Psychoanalysis, learning theory and the new sex therapies all have in common the assumption that 'anxiety' is instrumental in causing many sex disorders and erectile loss in particular (Masters & Johnson 1970; Kaplan 1982). This assumption is not unreasonable. Most men will, from personal experience, be able to recall circumstances where

consciously experienced feelings of either generalized or performance anxiety will have resulted in
a temporary loss of their erection, a loss which
disappears on a later occasion when the stress is
removed. Experience of this kind led to the widely
held belief that up to 95% of erectile problems are
psychogenic, e.g. Hastings (1963), McCary (1967),
Johnson (1968), Masters & Johnson (1970).

Given this almost universal belief in the negative effects of anxiety on sexual performance, it
was not surprising that methods of anxiety reduction figured prominently in the armamentarium
of most sex therapists, whatever school they represented: the analytic (Fenichel 1945); the behavioural (Wolpe 1958); the eclectic (Masters &
Johnson 1970; Kaplan 1974) and the cognitive
(Ellis 1962, 1975). Moreover, it should not be
forgotten that methods of anxiety reduction were
also regarded as being respectable and tested (they
were already widely used in the treatment of other
problems in the 1960s) and relatively easy to ad-
minister. Masters & Johnson (1970) summarized
the current feelings at that time when they stressed
that in a relaxed individual the sexual reflexes will
operate normally. Other workers, e.g. Patterson
& O'Gorman (1986, 1989, 1990), also invoke
anxiety as a significant determinant in sex dysfunction, and clearly anxiety does play a major
role in blocking sexual responses.

However, the situation becomes more confused
when adequate recognition is given to the important role that organic (physical) causes are playing
in the aetiology of sex disorders and, more importantly, the discovery that far from inhibiting sexual
response, anxiety may actually increase sexual
arousal in some men (and women) (see Ch. 2).

In the early 1940s, Ramsay (1943) reported
non-erotic erections in boys where fear or excitement, near accidents or being chased by
the police acted as the stimulus. Later, Sarrel &
Masters (1982) also reported erections in men
who had been molested by women armed with
knives and commented that even in these circumstances, these men had been able to achieve intercourse. Norton & Jehu (1984), in their review
of the role of anxiety in sex dysfunctions, also
provided support for the view that consciously
experienced anxiety is so common a feature of
good sex that it would not be sensible to believe

that sexual anxiety was always a liability. Further
evidence that anxiety can potentiate sex arousal
came from Stoller's (1976) observation that those
men who enjoy 'unusual sex' (the voyeurs, pae-
dophiles and exhibitionists, for example) are
often aroused as much by the fear of the forbidden
and the risk of being caught as by the practice
itself.

Laboratory experiments also provide support
for the view that anxiety plays an important part in
sexual arousal. Hoon et al (1977) and Wolchick et
al (1980) report how an initial exposure of men
and women to an anxiety-provoking film led to an
increase in sex arousal when the subjects were
later exposed to an erotic film. An increase in
arousal was not found when a matched control
had instead viewed a 'neutral' film before the
erotic film.

These findings may appear to contradict the
previously stated assumption that anxiety is a
cause of erectile dysfunction. However, it should
be remembered that experiments on the effects of
anxiety on arousal are carried out on normal, non-
dysfunctional men. Thus, Barlow (1986) was able
to show that subjects who have a sex dysfunction
are more likely to be inhibited by anxiety than
those who function well, who, in contrast, may
be aroused by an anxiety provoking experience.
Moreover, he and others were also able to distinguish between generalized and performance anxiety in their contribution to sex-stress, the latter
playing a more important inhibitory role (Barlow,
Sakheim & Beck 1983; Beck et al 1984). From
a therapeutic point of view, this evidence is of
considerable importance, if only because it
draws attention to the fact that the global and
indiscriminate use of anxiety-reduction methods
cannot always be relied upon (Cole 1985).
Clearly, it is very important to be able to distinguish between those patients who will best
respond to the anxiety reduction methods of
sex therapy and those who may require other
forms of intervention, e.g. flooding, a largely
cognitively based approach or the help of
pharmacotherapy.

Patients, however, do not always fall clearly into
functional and dysfunctional categories. For example, patients may present for help with situational erectile problems, where they can respond

effectively in some circumstances but not others. An understanding of the role that anxiety may be playing in these differing circumstances may not only help the clinician to provide the patient with more insight into the causes of his unpredictable erectile response, but also lead to changes in the patient's behaviour, enabling him to respond more effectively in a wider spectrum of circumstances.

Of course, it is not always possible to intervene successfully. This makes it imperative that the apparently contradictory role of anxiety in the expression of erectile response be more fully understood.

The role of anger in sexual dysfunction

The relationship between anger and sexual arousal is as complex and contradictory as that observed in the response to anxiety (see Ch. 2). In some individuals, anger increases sexual arousal whereas in others anger inhibits the sexual response. Clinicians need to recognize this fact if only to disabuse themselves of the popular view that sexual responses can only take place when the patient is calm and relaxed.

The role of cognitions in sexual dysfunction

Expectations of sex performance can be, and often are, a self-fulfilling prophecy — indeed, this is the basis of what is normally understood as performance anxiety. For example, Briddell et al (1978) showed that sexually functional subjects rarely had any doubts about their ability to achieve a good sex response. Moreover, Laws & Rubin (1969) and Henson & Rubin (1971) found that sexually effective subjects could, if they wished, deliberately suppress their erections by self-distraction whilst watching an erotic film, or alternatively produce an erection to order by engaging in sexual fantasies. This kind of cognitive interference was, of course, recognized by Masters & Johnson (1970) and Kaplan (1974) when they described these competing cognitions as 'spectatoring', 'performance demand characteristic' and 'failure self-statements'.

Masters & Johnson, however, tended to focus on the negative effects of cognitions and disre-garded their positive role when they proposed that erections cannot be 'willed', they only 'happen' (Masters & Johnson 1966). This is clearly not true.

On the basis of his research, Barlow (1986) suggested a new working model for psychogenic sex dysfunction. In brief, he proposed that negative or distracting thoughts (cognitive interference) interact with autonomic arousal (the physiological components of anxiety and sexual response) to block sexual performance. He argues that if the physiological arousal mechanisms are not synchronized or compatible with the psychological responses, but instead compete with them, then sexual response may be blocked. If this hypothesis proves to be correct, it would explain why anxieties can be seen to be acting both as a potentiator or as an inhibitor of sexual arousal, depending upon the associated cognitions (i.e. if anxiety is read as being rewarding, its presence will arouse; if it is coded as being punishing, it will inhibit). Barlow suggests that these competing task irrelevant thoughts, spectatoring, failure self-beliefs, indeed any distracting cognitions in those who are dysfunctional, stem from early experience, though why some men become dysfunctional and others, with the same learning history, do not, is unclear.

The role of the relationship

The interface between marital and sex therapy is ill-defined and though each discipline has evolved its own style and methodologies (Crowe 1978; Dryden 1985; Bancroft 1989) their areas of interest will often overlap. The clinician, when dealing with erectile problems, for example, will be unable to escape the reality of the complex interplay between relationship factors and sexual response, and some of these factors have been referred to earlier (see p. 138).

It is not easy to make any constructive generalizations about the role played by the relationship in precipitating erectile inadequacy for the simple reason that the relationship scenarios that exist are so varied and complex. At one extreme, one meets a patient who can only respond to his partner sexually in a loving, secure and intimate relationship and where his prime concern is to please and satisfy her. This feeling of his is not a posture — he genuinely only becomes aroused and obtains pleasure from love-making if she also enjoys the experience; his primary source of pleasure is in her response — his arousal may only be of secondary importance.

In contrast to those men who only see the expression of sex as part of a whole-person relationship, there are others whose sexual constructs are quite different. They find the intimacy of close relationships sexually threatening, they habituate quickly and may find they only become fully aroused in new relationships. They have no difficulty in focusing on their own sexual needs and though they will be pleased if their partners are responsive, this response is not essential to their enjoyment. Naturally, if these two types of patient present for help with an erectile problem it should be apparent that the approach to treatment will be quite different in each case.

A distinction can be made between those aetiological factors which stem largely from the needs of the individual (*intrinsic problems*) and those which are clearly contingent upon the relationship (*situational or contingent problems*). Such a distinction is important because intrinsic problems may not respond so readily to couple therapy (requiring instead more attention from individual therapy) any more than contingent problems will respond easily to individual therapy. Intrinsic problems are those where blocks to arousal result primarily from the patient's own autonomous needs and which are not a product of the relationship. For example, erectile difficulties arising from homosexual needs, a profound fear of intimacy or a low sex drive would fall into this category. Good examples of situational or contingent problems, on the other hand, would most forms of performance anxiety, rejection by one's partner or any form of sexual incompatibility.

Patients will not normally have presented for help unless either, sex is very important to one or other (or both) or, as sometimes happens, they sadly only seek assistance because their relationship has reached the point of irretrievable breakdown — perhaps as a kind of token gesture to atone or appease their consciences.

Conflicts within a relationship can, of course, exist for many years but if these conflicts are kept within acceptable limits the sex may remain tolerably good. When, however, these conflicts become overt, often one of the first casualties is the couple's sex life. Of course, the reverse is equally if not more common: poor sex may damage a relationship that is otherwise tolerably good and the strain of enforced abstinence or perfunctory sex can be powerfully disruptive (Sanders 1983). It is very difficult to assess the strength of this disruptive effect because different couples attach such widely disparate values to sex. For example, Smith (1990) found in a cross-section of adult US males and females that one in five had not had sex in the previous year and even amongst the currently married, one in ten were abstinent in the preceding year. Sex may therefore be disruptive, or cohesive, or appear to play no part at all in the relationship, depending upon the couple.

Sometimes neither marital nor sex therapy is able to restore the couple's sex life to an acceptable level. Every clinician must be prepared, therefore, to meet failure and attention needs to be paid to this eventuality by providing suitable support and counselling. The couple should be encouraged to put their problem in perspective and not to magnify the negative consequences of their difficulties. Alternative strategies of love-making can be suggested and, of course, other medical approaches to the treatment of erectile problems considered (see Chs 9–12).

At a counselling level, however, one useful approach is to try to help the couple see the relationship in the context of the 'pay off' paradigm. Relationships only survive because of the cohesive effects of a large number of rewards which provide a 'pay off' to each partner. If these 'pay offs' drop below a certain ill-defined and intangible threshold (or more rewarding 'pay offs' are discovered elsewhere), disruptive forces will exceed the cohesive forces and the relationship may end. Each couple will attach quite different values to these 'pay offs'. Some will regard sex as being very important, others will not when instead perhaps money, the children, companionship, emotional dependence or even the need for a nice house which would otherwise be lost, will figure prominently. Regardless of how each couple measures the quality of their relationship, there is inevitably a multitude of reasons for maintaining a relationship. The loss of sex will only be one factor out of many and the couple or aggrieved partner may be helped to see the possibility that the credits for staying (even without good sex) may still exceed the debits should the relationship end. Sometimes the disruptive role of poor or absent sex is potentiated by the high and often false expectations that the aggrieved partner may have about sex in general and their own sexual needs in particular. Counselling may help him (or her) to put these expectations into a more objective perspective.

Sometimes it is clear that the man's inability or refusal to have intercourse with his partner arises simply from the difficulties he experiences in reconciling 'sex' and 'love'. His need for an intimate, cooperative and stable relationship is in stark contrast to an equally strong need in him for sexual variety. This conflict will increase with the passage of time as 'incestuous' feelings in the relationship gain strength (see Ch. 2). Such a conflict often leads to problems of frequency dissatisfaction and lack of arousal which may in turn become manifest in erectile problems. Disorders in sexual desire arising from this kind of dynamic are notoriously difficult to treat, and whether the relationship survives or not often depends upon whether therapy can help put the sexual problem in perspective. Sex and love do not have to be packaged together for a relationship to survive, indeed sex does not necessarily lead to affection nor its absence alienation. Many unconsummated marriages survive and flourish and arguably a relatively asexual relationship is just as likely to survive as one where both partners are sexually active (Cole 1985). Ultimately, however, the resolution of problems of this kind depend upon the needs and personalities of the individuals involved and unless these can be reconciled (or tolerated) sex can and will play a powerfully disruptive role in relationships.

Finally, it should not be overlooked that many men do not currently have, or may never have had, a sexual relationship. Nevertheless they may still have an erectile problem — proven or suspected. Indeed, those who find the formation and maintenance of a stable relationship difficult are likely to have more than their fair share of sexual and emotional problems. They will therefore be correspondingly more difficult to treat for many reasons, not least of which is that they will require the help of a cooperative partner (Cole 1986, 1988b). The treatment of this group of patients is discused fully in Chapter 13.

Assessment and diagnosis — an algorithm

A full and correct assessment and diagnosis of patients with erectile problems is crucial (see Chs 6–8) and though it may be tempting to dispense with some investigations because a psychogenic aetiology appears so obvious, this temptation should be resisted if the resources are available.

Conversely, it is even more tempting to assume a medical aetiology and dispense with psychological treatments. This is particularly easy when patients present with a clear history of disease or the iatrogenic effects of medication or surgery. Whatever the presumed direct consequences of these physical events are, it must *always be assumed that some performance anxiety may be present*. This should be investigated and, if possible, treated, however unlikely a successful outcome appears initially (Gregoire 1990).

The accompanying algorithm (Fig. 10.3) is provided to help the clinician arrive at a correct diagnosis and assist in the search for the most appropriate psychological treatment programme.

TREATMENT

The therapeutic contract

At the first meeting, the therapist or clinician should allow time for the patient to discuss what he believes he needs from the consultation, and for the clinician, to the best of his ability, in turn to tell the patient what he can and cannot offer. It is important, therefore, to arrive at some form of mutual understanding. This is known as a therapeutic contract and helps to avoid later misunderstandings or false expectations. In addition, practical matters such as the frequency and length of appointments (ideally at weekly intervals and roughly an hour's duration) and the likely length of the treatment programme (5–15 weeks) and the cost (if any), can be discussed and, if necessary, negotiated.

If possible, it is also desirable to discuss with the

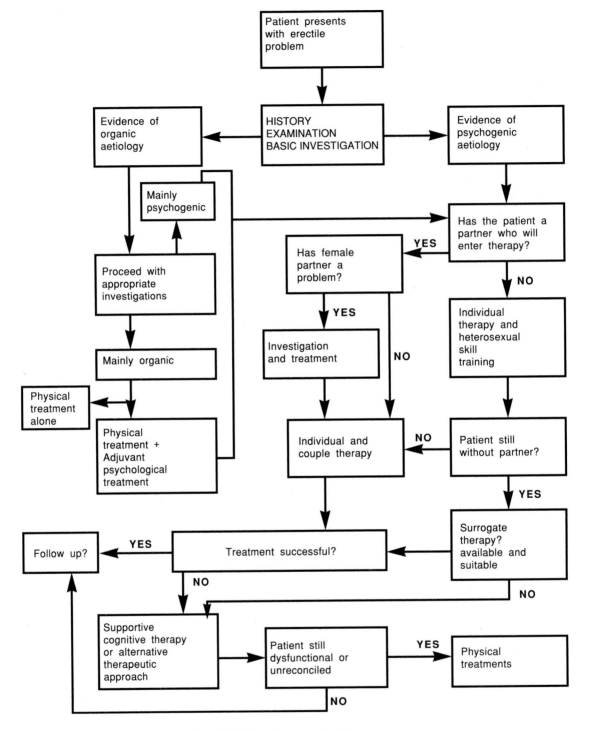

Fig. 10.3 Psychological treatments of erectile dysfunction — an algorithm.

patient details of the methods of assessment that he (the clinician) is likely to call upon; how he will arrive at his diagnosis and the alternative forms of treatment open to him. Though in practice these may be limited to a modified Masters & Johnson programme, with greater or lesser emphasis placed upon the humanistic and cognitive therapies, it is helpful to try to inform the patient about the nature of these therapies. It is also important to remember that the effectiveness of any form of therapy is strongly linked to the clinician's counselling skills. He needs to be able to offer acceptance, empathy, genuineness and good communication — skills that, unfortunately, are not always widely found amongst the medical profession. Indeed, it is argued by some (Truax & Carkhuff 1967; Rogers 1980) that the successful involvement of these skills in therapy is often more important then the choice of a specific therapeutic programme. Whether this is true or not in the case of sex therapy, whose methods tend to be brief and directive, remains to be established.

A critically important part of any therapeutic interaction with the patient (including physical treatments) is the provision of information about the nature of the problem and the choice of appropriate available treatments. It is usually best to supplement verbal information with handouts or recommended books. A list of particularly useful books for this purpose is given in Appendix 10.1.

Individual versus couple therapy

In the 1970s and 80s it was conventional wisdom to adhere to Masters & Johnson's doctrine of 'the relationship is the patient', and few in the mainstream of sex therapy have challenged what appears at first sight to be a fairly sensible way of dealing with sexual problems. Such an approach is known as *couple* or *conjoint therapy* and is based upon the idea that the focus of treatment should be directed towards the complex transactions which take place in the presenting relationship (Dicks 1967; Masters & Johnson 1970; Duddle 1975; Kaplan 1979; Hawton 1985; Bancroft 1989). Although such an approach would clearly not be possible if the patient presents without a partner, the tradition of treating the relationship has become so entrenched in sex and marital therapy that when patients do come along on their own with a problem, as they frequently do, they are sometimes told that psychological therapies will not be available unless they come with a partner.

An alternative therapeutic strategy is one where the clinician instead places greater emphasis and focuses his attention on the *individuals* in the relationship, seeing them separately, at least in the initial stages of treatment. Treating the couple from the start may present the practitioner with far too complex a scenario, and it is often very difficult to begin to deal with the complex task of therapeutic negotiations when neither individual has fully considered what they want for themselves. By focusing on the individual at this early stage, a much clearer picture can be obtained by everyone concerned, about expectations, needs, priorities, hopes and fears. Such an approach may also help the individuals involved to take responsiblity for their own feelings instead of projecting (blaming) them on to their partner.

Few clinicians would argue that individual therapy should replace couple therapy entirely, or conversely, few devotees of couple therapy would deny the importance of seeing individuals on their own from time to time. What is required is a shift of emphasis towards the recognition that the individual may need to be helped to sort out his or her own problems and to take responsibility for them before they can begin to enter into the complex requirements of couple therapy.

A number of theoretical issues are raised by this polemic of individual versus couple therapy. These issues will become increasingly important as the stable, monogamous, nuclear family continues to be replaced by those seeking alternative social and sexual lifestyles, and as a consequence, more and more people present for therapy as partnerless individuals. One of the questions that needs to be addressed urgently is how far is it legitimate to regard the 'relationship' as an entity in its own right and then target it in the treatment programme? Indeed, those who are strongly motivated towards treating the relationship may sometimes be tempted to ascribe to the 'relationship' an objectivity which many believe is not justified. Ellis put this point of view succinctly when he wrote 'in most instances disturbed marriages (or premarital relationships) were a product of disturbed spouses and if people were truly to be helped to live happily with each other they would first have to be shown how they could live peacefully with themselves' (Ellis 1962, p. 3).

The psychodynamic therapies

Most of the new sex therapies, which are characterized by a brief, direct interventionist approach addressing the 'here and now', rely heavily on the behavioural and psychoeducational elements of therapy, which have been joined more recently by cognitive behavioural methods (see p. 155). The psychodynamic (psychoanalytic) contribution to sex therapy which until the 1960s played an important part, has more recently not been able to withstand the assault of the more empirically based therapies.

The psychoanalytic interpretation of erectile disorders is that they are the product of the guilt and fear generated by unconscious castration anxieties, which in turn arise from unresolved oedipal conflicts. Normal sexual functioning can only be restored, according to psychoanalytic theory, if these unconscious conflicts can be resolved.

Partly as a result of the work of Kaplan (1974), the psychodynamic approach still appears to play a small but significant role in modern sex therapy (Cooper 1986, 1988). Kaplan, in proposing that the initial focus of attack should be behavioural, to be followed, only if no progress was made, by a more psychodynamically oriented programme, was able to achieve a seemingly remarkable marriage between the psychodynamic and behavioural schools. So well did she succeed that a 'quasi-eclectic, modified Masters & Johnson × Kaplan hybrid programme' appeared to to be the chosen method of sex therapists, at least in the UK (Cole 1985). Further evidence of this kind of almost paradoxical eclecticism is illustrated by Crown & d'Ardenne when they stated that 'we embed our behavioural approaches firmly in the psychodynamic attitude' (Crown & d'Ardenne 1982, p. 72).

There is little doubt that some erectile problems are in part a consequence of deep-seated emotional disturbances and may present as symptoms of underlying conflicts acquired in childhood (Kaplan 1974). However, there is little or no evidence to support the view that attention directed towards the discovery and resolution of these conflicts by the application of analytical type therapies

will lead to normal sexual functioning. Indeed, if anything, it could be argued that since psychodynamic methods assume that humans are, in the main, driven by internal forces beyond their immediate control, to focus upon these conflicts too closely could actually make matters worse. To be fair, O'Connor & Stern (1972) report a 77% improvement and a 36% cure in a sample of 96 patients with sexual problems who were treated analytically: though how far this study would stand up to modern methods of statistical evaluation is open to doubt.

The behavioural therapies

Strictly behavioural methods have in the past been used to treat men with erectile problems, e.g. relaxation and desensitization, operant conditioning, flooding, aversive conditioning and training in assertive behaviour (Friedman & Lipsedge 1971; Kockott et al 1975; Reckless & Geiger 1978; Ellis 1980). However, because most of these approaches have disregarded the importance of the interpersonal element in sexual arousal, they have not proved their worth and as a result have not been widely adopted. Indeed, much of the strength of the Masters & Johnson therapies springs from the unique way in which they were able to integrate this behavioural approach with the psychoeducational and interpersonal elements required of sex therapy. This they achieved, for example, in sensate focus (see p. 152), where relaxation and systematic desensitization are elegantly combined with interpersonal communication. Some of these behaviour therapies, systematic desensitization and assertion training in particular, have a clearer role in the treatment of partnerless individuals (see Ch. 15).

The Masters & Johnson therapies

Masters & Johnson's ideas and approach to the treatment of sexual problems still have a profound influence upon mainstream sex therapy throughout the world. It is not easy to encapsulate in a few words the reasons for their success because much of their approach was somewhat doctrinaire, providing as it did a unique type of therapy which was both eclectic yet also singularly theirs.

Masters & Johnson focused primarily on the

couple (the relationship is the patient); they always used two therapists, one male one female (cotherapy), and relied largely on the use of a rapid residential treatment programme lasting about two weeks, which was then followed by homework (home assignments). Not surprisingly, their course of treatment was expensive and their patient sample highly selected. They placed great emphasis upon encouraging a positive and accepting view of sex (permission giving) by providing factual information and attempting to dispel the many sexual myths which had become part of folklore. In contrast to their predecessors, Masters & Johnson did not believe that the kind of sexual problems they met with at St. Louis were normally caused by any preexisting psychopathology, but that high levels of anxiety were in the main responsible for the problems they encountered.

Undoubtedly the most significant aspect of their work, which contributed to the popularity and acceptance of their methods, was the way in which they prepared a series of treatment packages designed specifically for each problem. These mini-programmes were not only readily understood by the patients but also by their therapists and clinicians!

The two essential elements in their approach were an initial *ban on intercourse*, during which time the couple practised *sensate focus*. Sensate focus is an exercise in mutual pleasuring where the couple caress and touch each other and learn how to enjoy the experience without the need for it to end in penetrative sex or orgasm.

The modified Masters & Johnson approach

One of the most important features of the new sex therapies is the innovation, popularized by Masters & Johnson, of giving the couple (or individual) 'homework'. If therapy is based largely upon a cognitive-behavioural framework, where new skills have to be learnt or perceptions and evaluations changed, this requires practice, hence the necessity for home assignments. A once weekly or fortnightly consultation with the clinician would be inadequate on its own.

The programme is normally divided into three stages: *non-genital sensate focus, genital sensate focus* and *vaginal containment*.

Although the details of the programme are quite simple to explain and to follow, it is a good idea for the clinician to have a supply of typed instructions describing sensate focus to give to the patient to take away and which will act as an aide-mémoire to supplement his verbal instructions. Suitably brief accounts appear in Bancroft (1989), Cole & Dryden (1989) and Lloyd & Brown (1989).

It is impossible to dictate how long should be spent on each stage, so much depends upon individual circumstances and particularly the rate of progress the couple are making. Having said that, it is desirable that a minimum of 4–6 homework sessions should be spent on each stage if possible. Throughout the programme, the couple need to be guided by a professional. For example, the clinician should see the couple before they decide to move from one stage to the next, and this decision should be made by all three. Any indecision or uncertainty on the couple's part, brought about by a lack of supervision, will obviously be counterproductive.

It is important that the couple to do their very best to foster a sense of closeness and understanding during these early stages of the programme. If they can communicate their fears and wishes about what they really enjoy in bed, the likelihood of a successful outcome will be increased. However, this is not as easy as it sounds. Many couples find it difficult to talk to one another about their sexual feelings, partly because with the passage of time, blocks evolve in relationships which make this kind of sexual intimacy very difficult to achieve. For many years, they may have only communicated with each other in a very limited manner using non-verbal cues so that their sex life had become highly ritualized and stylized. Couples may have been making false assumptions about each other's sexual needs and preferences; instead they must try to foster more direct and honest methods of communicating with each other: 'No, I don't get an orgasm very often, but it doesn't matter', 'I enjoy sex much more when we do it slowly'. Had there been no problem, it may not have mattered and it would not have been necessary to attempt to disturb this pattern of behaviour. However, in couples presenting for treatment, these behaviours need to be changed if possible, and help provided to enable them to face their mutual fears of intimacy.

If the treatment is to be successful, it is crucial that the couple make available private time. Half an hour two or three times a week is all that is necessary, though it is essential that the time set aside should be free from any risk of interruption as far as possible. Tradesmen, telephones and children's needs, for example, are definitely contraindicated. A warm room, a low light and perhaps some music, if desired, all help. They should try to choose a time when they are not tired or stressed, e.g. avoid an occasion just before a dinner party or at 1.30 a.m. on a weekday. Alcohol at this stage is probably not a good idea.

During the first two stages of the treatment programme, there is ban on intercourse. The reasons for this ban should be explained to them. The idea is quite simple. To reduce performance anxiety, a careful balance between relaxation and arousal must be achieved. In the vulnerable partner, anxiety (cognitive or visceral) switches into the system very quickly and may irreversibly block further arousal. In order to prevent this happening, fear of any sort, but particularly the fear of failing, must to be kept to a minimum. It is almost as if arousal needs to creep in by the back door unannounced, and this is best achieved naturally when the patient is not bothered by any thoughts of having to please his partner. An initial ban on genital stimulation (and more significantly the ban on intercourse) will not only reduce performance needs but also may have a paradoxical effect and lead to an early erection.

Incidentally, if the couple have previously used condoms, an effort should be made to get them to find an alternative method of fertility control before sensate focus is undertaken. Sometimes methods of contraception are not discussed and I have known couples who by default have attempted vaginal containment using a condom experiencing failure as a result.

One of the most important functions of sensate focus is to prevent performance anxieties developing as a result of 'spectatoring'. If the patient persists in monitoring both his own and his partner's sexual responses — 'Is she enjoying this?', 'Will she have an orgasm?', 'Will I lose my erection?' — these anxieties will block his arousal and inhibit his erection.

The treatment programme

An integral part of most programmes of sex therapy which adopt a modified Masters & Johnson 'approach' involves the homework assignment known as sensate focus (Masters & Johnson 1970), so-called because it comprises a series of exercises where the couple practise focusing on feelings and sensations. The basic idea behind sensate focus is to help the couple experience each other's intimate physical company in a relaxed situation so that they can begin to enjoy their sexual and emotional feelings.

1. Non-genital sensate focus

This, the introductory stage, aims to provide the couple with an opportunity to establish closeness and physical intimacy but on the strict understanding that no genital stimulation is allowed. (There is also a total ban on intercourse until stage 3, which applies both inside and outside sessions). Some sex therapists also ban breast stimulation at this point, but this is optional. Touching, caressing, massage and communication are the important features of non-genital sensate focus, perhaps providing the first opportunity for a long time for the man with an erectile problem to be able to relax with his partner knowing that he doesn't have to perform and escalate the sex play into consummatory sex.

One of the fundamental ideas behind sensate focus is to encourage the couple to switch off the thinking (distracting thoughts about performance, the relationship, of inadequacy and so on) and switch on the immediate feelings experienced during the touching exercise. It will be much easier to achieve this goal if the couple *take it in turns* to touch, caress and fondle their partner. This alternate pleasuring will also enable them to be free from the distracting need to simultaneously please their partner and themselves. In this first stage of sensate focus the couple have both agreed to avoid genital stimulation (and, of course, intercourse) at the request of the therapist.

Once again it needs to be stressed that sensate focus means focusing on sensations: touch is often a neglected form of communication between people even when they make love, and whether this love-making is a sprint or a marathon, intercourse can be so performance oriented that individual moments are often not savoured to the extent that they might be.

The sequence of touching involved in sensate focus can be very gentle or quite firm and the whole body can be explored (except the penis and scrotum and vulva at this point) in whatever way that gives the greatest pleasure. Sometimes if words are difficult to find the best way to indicate to one's partner that a particular form of stimulation is good is simply to guide their hand. It is a good idea to recommend that couples try some perfumed body cream, baby oil or talc as a lubricant to help the massage process.

One way to start sensate focus is to begin to massage your partner while they are lying on their stomach. The stroking and caressing can start on the back and arms and then slowly move down to the buttocks and lower legs, finishing perhaps on the inside of the thighs which most people find particularly sensitive and sexy. When they turn over they can begin again on their arms, legs, breasts and abdomen. Pleasuring can end by kissing and cuddling.

After two or three sessions of this very relaxed approach some, but by no means all, men will find that the penis will begin to erect. They may not get a full erection yet and they should not expect to. For the older man, say over the age of 50, erections may take longer to appear and a first erection may not be possible until stage 2, where direct stimulation to the penis is allowed. It should always be remembered that as the purpose of sensate focus is not to provide the man with an erection, but to change his focus of attention from performance to pleasure, then clearly it does not matter when he begins to get aroused and erect. He should be warned against any temptation to 'use' his penis for sexual intercourse, just because it has appeared for the first time for a long time!

The patient needs to be told that he must be selfish and that, at this point in treatment, he must try to disregard his partner's needs entirely and focus on his own. After all, the greatest compliment he can pay her is to become sexually aroused himself, something he will not achieve if he remains preoccupied with trying to please her.

It is a good idea to divide non-genital sensate focus into two stages — in the first, each partner is told to consider only their own pleasure and that they should ignore pleasuring their partner; they need to learn to take pleasure; arousal occurs as a result of getting pleasure. In the second stage, the partners respond to both their own and partner's needs.

2. Genital sensate focus

Stage 1 should lead gradually and naturally into stage 2, where mutual stimulation of the penis and scrotum and vulva is allowed. Any sudden escalation of arousal should be avoided since it is crucial that the whole sensate focus programme should proceed smoothly and slowly, extending the repertoire of sex play at a speed determined by each couple's needs.

Whole body touching should be enjoyed as before but now this touching can extend to the genitals. Relaxation is still however the keynote of this stage, the aim being for the patient simply to focus upon and enjoy the luxury of the simple eroticism of the sensations he is experiencing, disregarding the size or firmness of his erection. Even an unerect or partially erect penis can signal exquisitely sexy feelings to the brain and it is these feelings which need to be focused upon.

Once erection has become a regular feature of sensate focus, it is a good idea for the man to deliberately allow himself to lose his erection: on regaining it he can then prove to himself that such a loss is not an irreversible disaster and is to be expected in normal love-making from time to time. If during this stage of sensate focus either partner reaches orgasm, this should be enjoyed. It may not happen at this point and of course no deliberate attempt to masturbate to orgasm should be undertaken, unless orgasm occurs very easily and naturally. Towards the final stages of genital sensate focus, the couple can begin simultaneous pleasuring until they are ready for penetration or vaginal containment.

3. Vaginal containment

This is the final stage just before intercourse begins, where the man, using one of several strategies described below, penetrates the vagina with his penis, enjoying the experience of vaginal containment for its own sake.

For many couples this is a crucial step in therapy. Many men can obtain and hold good erections in self- and partner-masturbation but lose their erection either just at the point of penetration or shortly afterwards. The moment at which the penis enters the vagina can be of great emotional and symbolic significance to some men and if these men are also sexually precarious, it is at this point that they may lose their erection — indeed, this is so common that this type of erectile loss has been described as penetration anxiety.

This stage of vaginal containment, however it is approached, can be divided into two stages: (i) without movement, so that he can simply enjoy the experience of penetration; and (ii) with movement where one or both can begin a more active role.

In order to ensure that his anxieties do not become raised unnecessarily at this point, one of two apparently contradictory strategies should be tried. One is for his partner to take control and for her to introduce his penis into the vagina. The best way to achieve this is for the man to lie on his back with his erect penis held vertical and for her to lower herself gently upon him, guiding his penis into the vagina with her hand. To ensure that this is easily achieved, oil or KY jelly should be applied liberally to the penis and vulva should there be any hint of vaginal dryness. An alternative strategy is for his partner to be totally passive, to lie on her side with her back to him and with her legs drawn up to her breasts exposing the vulva and vagina (the lateral position). Whilst he is also lying on his side, he can then place his erect penis at the entrance to the vagina and slowly penetrate — as long as she remains passive, his performance anxiety will be kept to a minimum. This approach works well if his partner is slim.

Whichever method is adopted, it is very important that at this stage there is no attempt at thrusting on his part or active movements on her part. Only a minimum amount of movement is required by one or other of them to maintain the erection. Naturally as the man's confidence improves either he or she can become more active. Penetration and vaginal containment can be practised two or three times at each session, remembering that the prime object is for the man to focus upon the pleasant feelings of vaginal containment rather than achieving an orgasm or pleasing his partner.

Sometimes progress is slow and a good erectile response difficult to achieve. When this happens, it may be helpful to try an alternative approach. The man (with his partner's help) should feed his unerect or semi-erect penis into the vagina as far as possible using whatever coital position feels most comfortable for them. Some patients in this relaxed and immobile position will find that the contained penis will then begin to erect more fully. Some men may regard this exercise as somewhat humiliating, almost an admission of defeat, however the method works often enough for it to be given a try.

Many couples find difficulties with sensate focus. Some complain of being bored, frequently they report it is too clinical and not infrequently, they break the ban on intercourse prematurely. Intervention by the clinician or therapist is important if these problems are to be addressed and resolved (Hawton 1989). The couple need all the encouragement they can get to make them persevere. If they are unclear about either the reasons for pursuing a course of action, or are confused about what they should do, clear explanations are required.

However, such interventions are not always successful and sensate focus has to be dispensed with otherwise the patients will drop-out, if they have not already done so. Alternative treatment strategies must then be tried. For example, marital therapy may provide a constructive alternative or, conversely, individual counselling may help establish why these blocks, which are sabotaging the sensate focus, are so powerful. Whatever the outcome, it is important that the clinician does not give up in the mistaken belief that if sensate focus doesn't work nothing will (see Fig. 10.3, p. 148). For example, the couple can be helped to accept that their relationship is still to be valued even if genital sex no longer plays an important part. And, even if the relationship ends, one or both can be helped to see that this may not be the catastrophe they imagine it to be. Whatever therapeutic approaches are chosen, the cognitive methods described below can be of considerable value.

Case vignette: Lifestyle changes. Rod and Pam, in their early fifties, have been married for 20 years.

They have no children and when Rod was offered early retirement, he decided to accept and try to get a part-time job to supplement his pension. This proved difficult and he found himself at home most of the day with Pam who was also unable to find work at the time. They had a good marriage and a reasonable sex life and Pam was looking forward to having Rod at home, since he had worked long hours at his job and their sex life had been somewhat intermittent because of this.

Though this change of lifestyle suited Pam, Rod was not quite so happy. He felt he had lost some of his independence and Pam's sexual approaches during the day (they had never made love in the daytime before, except on holiday) put him under pressure. Moreover, because of the time they had together, Pam wanted sex more often, so instead of having intercourse once a fortnight Pam wanted it once or twice a week. Rod was quite unable to respond to this pressure and found that he was losing his erection, ejaculating quickly and within two months of retiring couldn't get an erection at all.

They presented as a couple. Rod was investigated to eliminate any organic basis to his problem and although Rod was convinced there was a physical cause, none was found. Eventually, he came to accept that the loss of his erection (and his sex drive) had resulted from the sudden change in his lifestyle. His loss of status, earnings and his independence, together with the additional pressure that Pam was putting on him to make love more frequently, had created performance anxieties generated by his need to respond to and please his wife.

It was suggested he should make strenuous efforts to get another job or even do some voluntary work to enable him to have an independent life. They were counselled together and helped to see how they could work out a mutually acceptable frequency of intercourse. They were instructed to start with an initial ban on intercourse together with some sensate focus exercises until Rod began to feel aroused once more. This counselling also helped them to realize that physical intimacy need not always lead to penetrative sex. The result was the restoration of a good sex life and at follow-up six months later, this improvement had been maintained.

Cognitive approaches

Sexual functioning is shaped by three main sets of factors: biological events, environmental conditions and persistent negative processes, such as anger, anxiety and depression. The cognitive therapist believes that these destructive, negative processes are often sustained simply by the persistence of maladaptive and disturbed thoughts, attitudes and beliefs and that for treatment of any kind to be effective these irrational beliefs need to be challenged and then discarded (Kowalski 1985; Walen & Perlmutter 1988; Cole & Dryden 1991).

Rational emotive therapy

Albert Ellis, one of the pioneers of cognitive psychotherapy and well-known for his Rational Emotive Therapy (RET), provided a very simple model to show how cognitions influence feelings and behaviours with his $A \rightarrow B \rightarrow C \rightarrow D$ paradigm. Using this approach in the treatment of erectile dysfunction, A (the *activating* experience or event) would represent the opportunity to have sex and C (the emotional or behavioural *consequence*) might be performance anxiety and loss of erection. In Ellis' view, A does not cause C but instead is brought about by B, the individual's *belief* system, or more specifically, his evaluation of A. Using this model, Ellis sets out to instruct the patient to focus on B and dispute his irrational beliefs, replacing them with rational ones.

Thus when a man presents with a psychogenic erectile problem his irrational belief about A might be, 'If I don't get an erection, as I *must*, this will prove that I am inadequate as a man', 'It will be a disaster if I cannot please her', 'If I fail with her I will always fail from now on', 'My sex life is at an end,', and so on. However, he is told to argue with himself and to *dispute* (D) these *irrational beliefs* and negative evaluations (iB's) replacing them with new *rational beliefs* (rB's) such as, 'I would like to get an erection, it will be a pity if I don't and I will be disappointed, but it certainly won't be a disaster', 'My partner may be put out but this does not prove that I am inadequate', and so on. If he argues with himself in this way, substituting his irrational beliefs with new rational beliefs, he may still be disappointed but he won't be so anxious. Moreover, this reduction in anxiety may well enable him to get an erection. Ellis' ideas are not new but, incorporated into his ABCD framework, they provide a very convenient working model which is usually readily understood by most patients without too much difficulty. A simple account of RET is to be found in Dryden & Gordon (1990).

Munjack et al (1984) report that there was a significant improvement in men with erectile dysfunction using RET over a control group which was assigned to a waiting list, and though this improvement was not fully maintained at follow-up, significant progress was achieved over pretreatment levels of performance. Everaerd & Dekker (1985) also showed that RET led to an improvement in both sexual functioning and satisfaction with the relationship.

Psychoeducation

Misinformation, disinformation, prejudice and sheer ignorance are part and parcel of the subject of sex. It is therefore essential that from the outset patients are provided with an opportunity to obtain a basic and factually sound source of information about sex, since this often goes a long way towards liberating them from many of their anxieties. Every clinician should have available copies of a list of books which he has examined and can personally recommend to his patients. This booklist should be comprehensive and be suitable for a wide range of reading abilities (see Appendix 10.1, p. 164). Communication in the field of sex education is further complicated by the presence of a large number of so-called sexual myths (Zilbergeld 1980). These have become part of a sexual folklore and can be particularly disabling to a vulnerable or sexually precarious man. These myths need to be identified and then challenged. For example:

1. Men don't always want sex nor are they always ready for it — they are not sex machines. Indeed, it is not essential that all physical contact should lead to sex, nor should sex necessarily mean penetrative intercourse. For example, Bass (1986), using RET, focuses on trying to de-emphasize erection as a prerequisite of sexual satisfaction.
2. Men remain sexually responsive throughout their lives and though advancing age may slow down their responses, there is no particular

cut-off point at which a man's capacity to respond sexually disappears altogether. As men age, they require more direct and prolonged physical stimulation to the penis. It is important that they communicate this need to their partner verbally or non-verbally instead of hoping that their partner will discover this fact by telepathy or intuition. Some women find it very difficult to touch their partner's penis. Counselling will be needed to assist these shy women overcome their inhibitions.

3. It is often thought that by not masturbating a man can save himself and ensure a stronger and more long-lasting erection when the opportunity for intercourse arises. If anything, the reverse if true, possibly due to the drop in testosterone levels which is associated with decreased frequency of orgasm.
4. Quantity is not quality. It is not the duration of intercourse (nor the size of his penis) that matters, but the quality of the total experience. A man's attention should be drawn to the more subtle physical and emotional rewards afforded by extending precoital sex play. Most men, once they have penetrated, last only three or four minutes (Cole 1988a) and indeed women often complain that men go on too long.
5. A large number of women, perhaps as many as 1 in 2, do not achieve an orgasm in intercourse without some manual assistance (Sanders 1983; Kaplan 1989). This is a fact of life and it does not reflect badly on either him or her. Communication between them later can help solve any difficulty that may arise, though he must be reminded that both he and she can have good sex without her being orgasmic.

Other specific cognitive methods can be used in sex therapy to challenge the patient's view of things, replacing negative, damaging evaluations with a more rational and positive stance. The ideas outlined below have been developed by many authors and the list provided represents a distillate of some of their views. Those clinicians who are particularly interested in these cognitive methods are referred to Ellis (1975), Beck et al (1979), Walen (1980), Walen & Roth (1987), Walen & Perlmutter (1988), Hawton (1989).

Bishay (1988) used cognitive restructuring to treat patients who were particularly resistant to the more traditional methods of sex therapy. Although he used these methods to treat patients with vaginismus, avoidance of intercourse and delayed ejaculation, there is no reason why these methods cannot be adapted for use in the treatment of erectile disorders. For example, a patient unable to achieve an erection sufficiently hard to penetrate the vagina would be told to repeat to himself, several times a day, that there is no reason why he should not be able to obtain an erection strong enough to achieve intercourse. He should emphatically argue with himself and remind himself over and over again that since he can get an erection in self-masturbation there is no reason whatsoever why he should not be able to get an equally firm erection in the presence of his partner and retain it so that penetration and intercourse become possible. Rathus (1978) likewise used covert assertions in his treatment of a 25-year-old nurse with anorgasmia. She was told to rehearse and repeat orally statements like, 'I am attractive', 'I can enjoy sex as much as a man'. Once again this approach could be adapted to the treatment of erectile dysfunction.

Patients who present with erectile impotence, whatever their circumstances, are often devastated by their problem: they become obsessed with their inadequacy and their minds become crowded with negative and self-destructive thoughts. These thoughts can and must be challenged. Listed below are some of the ways by which these negative thoughts are maintained in a self-propagating and self-fulfilling style. Awareness of what is happening helps the patient to argue with himself and reassert some degree of rationality into his confused mental state.

Magnification: exaggerating, out of all proportion, the distressing consequences of an event.

Minimization: diminishing the benefit of an event.

Mustabation (need statements) (not masturbation!): insisting on an event taking place and not compromising — and being deeply upset when this goal is not achieved.

Personalization: taking things too personally.

Awfulizing: fostering an attitude of mind which is preoccupied with how AWFUL things are.

Selective abstraction: taking an event out of context, i.e. only seeing the bad things and ignoring the good.

The patient should be reminded continuously *that it is not the unfortunate experience (his erectile problem) which causes him the most distress, but rather the view that he takes about this problem.* Rethinking his attitudes, arguing with himself and substituting a positive view of things will have two beneficial effects: in the first place, the problem will not seem so bad if he can regard it in a more reasonable light — 'There is nothing good nor bad but thinking makes it so' — and, more importantly, the reduction in anxiety which will accompany a more rational view of things will itself help to resolve the problems he is experiencing with his erection.

There is no easy way to predict the relative effectiveness of the cognitive versus the behavioural therapies, though the way in which they catalyse change is quite different. One might therefore expect different individuals to respond differently to these two types of therapy. Adequate research in this area is long overdue (see p. 158).

The role of fantasy

Though the relationship between sexual fantasy and erectile response is complex, there is a positive correlation between the extent of sexual fantasy and sexual activity (Zimmer et al 1983). However, it appears that much of this fantasy is self-generating (it may be hormone dependent) and as such is not easily taught. Clinicians often find it difficult to motivate patients to engage in sexual fantasies to order, and this will naturally limit the value of fantasy training in particular and the use of fantasy in general to potentiate arousal.

Sexual fantasy may also have a negative role to play in that there is some evidence that those who enjoy their sexual fantasies most, often have poor sexual relationships with their partners (Bancroft 1989) and it is possible that the need for fantasy leads to the poverty of the sexual relationship rather than the reverse.

The use of erotic films or videos in therapy may therefore only have a limited role to play in fostering arousal, though there is no harm in suggesting that the couple experiment. Moreover, if they can give themselves permission to enjoy erotica it may not only arouse them and refresh their fantasies, but the experience may also be of value in their psychoeducation.

Alternative therapeutic strategies

The majority of professionals involved in helping men with erectile problems will have had either a formal medical training, qualified as a clinical psychologist, gained a qualification in human sexuality or maybe moved into sex and marital therapy from one of the other professions, e.g. nursing, family planning or social work.

Whatever their background, most practitioners will have settled for a fairly narrow therapeutic approach based largely upon the nature of their training and their personal inclinations and skills. Occasionally professionals change direction during their careers; most however do not. It is therefore important that from time to time, practitioners of whatever persuasion are reminded of the vast armamentarium of therapeutic strategies at their disposal. More often than not, these alternative approaches may prove to be inappropriate or unacceptable, but occasionally they may offer ideas which can be incorporated into the eclectic approach most of us should seek to practice. Moreover, being aware of these alternative approaches may help the professional to make a more informed decision if and when he decides to refer patients to colleagues in other disciplines. A simple list of the more important approaches is given below. Some of these are not discussed here, as a description of anything but the most important contributions to the treatment of erectile dysfunction is outside the scope of this chapter.

Psychodynamic therapies   Farrell (1981)
Behaviour therapy   Hawton et al (1989)
Cognitive therapy   Dryden & Golden (1986)
Psychoeducation   Zilbergeld (1980)
Group therapy   Kayata & Syzdlo (1988)
Hypnotherapy   Heap (1988)
Balint   Tunnadine (1983)
Rational emotive therapy   Dryden & Gordon (1990)
Transactional analysis   Stewart (1989)
Person centred therapy   Mearns & Thorne (1988)
Family therapy   Skynner & Cleese (1987)
Gestalt therapy   Korb et al (1989)
Personal construct therapy   Bannister & Fransella (1980)
Surrogate therapy   Cole (1988b)

A good general reference is Dryden (1990).

THE OUTCOME OF TREATMENT

In spite of the growth and popularity of sex therapy, its lasting effectiveness is still open to doubt (De Amicis et al 1985). This uncertainty is largely due to the almost insurmountable difficulties experienced in attempting to accurately assess treatment outcomes (Bancroft 1981; Bancroft et al 1986). Three difficulties in particular need to be overcome. First, it is important to be able to arrive at a clear and objective definition of the problem under examination; secondly, valid, and preferably standardized, methods of measuring the nature and severity of the patient's condition must be available (see Ch. 7); and thirdly, and in practice most difficult of all, a representative sample of adequate size must be obtained. Clearly, the smaller the expected effects of treatment, the larger the sample required to demonstrate these effects. Indeed, the majority of negative results in sex therapy outcome research have arisen simply because the sample size has been inadequate to detect anything but enormous clinical effects (Bancroft et al 1986).

Matters are made more complicated by the enormous heterogeneity of the population under study. A multitude of uncontrolled (and uncontrollable) variables, which may have effects on treatment and outcome, are associated with the diversity of sexual and marital relationship under treatment. The effects of these variables, (e.g. motivation, duration of dysfunction, premorbid sexual functioning, personality factors) can clearly have a profound effect on outcome, possibly masking the effects of any intervention. There are also the equally unpredictable effects arising from the clinician's personality and its impact upon the course of treatment. Last, but by no means least, are the difficulties met when attempts are made to establish which changes in the patients sexual responses, observed at the end of treatment and again in a later follow-up, do actually result from the treatment in question. There is the possibility that they would have occurred anyway. The only solution to this problem lies in using appropriate control groups — this has not been done in the majority of outcome studies. These difficulties are discussed fully by Reynolds (1977), Warner & Bancroft (1986) and Bancroft (1989),

Thus, because of the difficulties outlined, much of the published work on therapeutic outcomes must be considered highly suspect (Cole 1985).

A summary of the outcome of treatment for erectile disorders is given in Table 10.1. Although most of the reports refer to behaviourally oriented programmes, there still remains a wide variation in outcome. A first glance at the summary of results may give the impression that Masters & Johnson treatment programmes are reasonably effective. However, if the criticisms of outcome studies referred to earlier are taken into account, clearly some of these results must be regarded with considerable caution.

For example, De Amicis et al (1985) followed up 38 couples who had received sex therapy for various sex dysfunctions, including men with erectile difficulties. Their results were somewhat equivocal. Patients did appear to show an immediate response to therapy but these early changes were not generally maintained at the three year follow-up. Men with erectile problems showed a significant improvement in their ability to maintain an erection during intercourse but in those men who were unable to achieve an erection before intercourse, difficulties remained. The authors point out that some of these failures could be attributed to the fact that at the time of treatment it was not always possible to distinguish between organic and psychogenic impotence.

Some outcome studies may have influenced clinical practice. For example, a number of studies have not been able to demonstrate that the use of two therapists (cotherapy) produces consistently better results than a single therapist, or that there is any difference between intensive and widely spaced treatment programmes (Arentewicz & Schmidt 1983; Carney et al 1978; Crowe et al 1981; Mathews et al 1983; Heiman & Lopiccolo 1983; Heiman et al 1985). However, Warner & Bancroft (1986) wonder whether such negative findings should influence the nature of treatment

programmes. Of course, the preferred use of a single therapist may have been dictated not so much by these research findings but by logistic issues and its apparent cost-effectiveness.

It is not surprising that reviewers have not been universally over-enthusiastic about the benefits of sex therapy. For example, Wright et al (1977), in a comprehensive review of the treatment outcomes up to 1976, concluded that many claims for the overall effectiveness of the new sex therapies could not be justified. Hawton (1983) was equally cautious when referring to 'more or less consistent although undramatic evidence for the superiority of the Masters & Johnson approach over other methods of treatment or no treatment'. He added, 'there are considerable doubts about the long-term effects of sex therapy, especially because couples are lost to follow-up'. Watson & Brockman (1982) were also unsure of the overall usefulness of sex therapy for many patients since they found that therapy was often only a final attempt to avert an inevitable marital breakdown.

Hawton & Catalan (1986) looked at those factors most likely to lead to a satisfactory outcome following sex therapy. They discovered that the quality of the relationship, the couples' motivation for therapy and their commitment to the homework assignments indicated a good prognosis. It was not a surprise to find that outcome was also related to the extent to which each partner found the other sexually attractive, and that the presence of a psychiatric disorder in either led to a poor prognosis (Hawton 1982). Clearly, the role played by these prognostic factors must be taken into account in any adequately controlled outcome studies (Bancroft et al 1986).

Inevitably the reader is left with a somewhat confusing picture. This, however, is not surprising bearing in mind the problems encountered in sex therapy and its evaluation. One thing is clear: nothing approaching the successes claimed by Masters & Johnson have been achieved since they published their results, and until the results of further properly controlled outcome studies are available, no one can be certain of the effectiveness or otherwise of their methods. Unfortunately, even now there still remains a temptation on the part of some sex therapists to overestimate the simplicity and success of their methods. A notable

Table 10.1   Erectile dysfunction (ED) — outcome of treatment.

Author	Sample	Treatment programme	Outcome after treatment	Outcome at follow-up
Masters & Johnson (1970)	US couples 1° ED (n = 32) 2° ED (n = 213)	Masters & Johnson	Cured: 1° ED 60% 2° ED 74%	*At five years* Cured: 1° ED 60% 2° ED 63%
Duddle (1975)	ED (n = 15)	Masters & Johnson	65% 'consummated' 4% failed 29% not known	No data
Kockott et al (1975)	3 groups of 8 males (n = 24) 1° & 2° ED	Comparison of systematic desensitization, 'medication & advice' and waiting list	SD 25% 'cured' M&A 25% 'cured' WL no cure Additionally, one patient in the SD and M&A groups improved	No data
Ansari (1976)	Men with sex problems ED	Comparison of: modified Masters & Johnson, chemotherapy and no treatment	No difference between two treatments and controls	No data
Levine & Agle (1978)	US couples with 2° ED, age 25–29 Wide cross section (n = 16 couples)	Masters & Johnson and Kaplan programme	'Potent' 38% 'Improved' 25% 'No change' 37%	Only 1 patient maintained full erection after 1 year
Mears (1978)		The Balint approach: 'brief interpretative psychotherapy'	Successful outcome: 30%	No data
Crown & d'Ardenne (1982)	1° and 2° ED (n = 10)	Modified Masters & Johnson	Positive change 20% Some improvement 10% No change 50% Drop out 20%	No data
Hawton (1982)	(n = 26)	Masters & Johnson	Problem resolved or largely resolved 81% Largely unresolved 4% No change 15% Worse 0%	*3 month follow-up:* 69% 8% 0% Not known 23%
Arentewicz & Schmidt (1983)	(n = 57)	Modified Masters & Johnson	Cured 49% Improved 30% Slightly improved 4% No change 4% Dropped out 13%	*After one year* (n = 29) *compared*: The same 48% Better 14% Worse 24% Separated 14%
De Amicis et al (1985)	US couples (n = 15)	Modified Masters & Johnson	'Significant improvement in ability to maintain erection during intercourse.' 'No change in ability to obtain erection before intercourse.'	No data
Hawton et al (1986)	UK couples (n = 18)	Modified Masters & Johnson	'Gains made during therapy were reasonably well sustained at the long term follow-up.'	No data
Hawton & Catalan (1986)	UK couples (n = 34)	Modified Masters & Johnson	Problem resolved 41% Largely resolved 26% Largely unresolved 15% No change 15% Worse 3%	No data

example of this is Helen Kaplan who claims that over 90% of premature ejaculators can be cured within an average of 14 weeks of treatment (Kaplan 1989, p. 2). How does she manage to reconcile this with outcome studies of, for example, Hawton et al (1986) whose results were 'disappointing', or those of De Amicis (1985), where the improvements were not maintained at three year follow-up? If current methods of sex therapy are not working this fact needs to be faced and action taken.

It is not easy to summarize: perhaps all that can be said at present is that on the available evidence an unknown proportion of men will respond to the psychological approaches to treatment outlined in this chapter. Whether these benefits will be maintained and for how long is uncertain.

Given the current lack of good research data it is quite justifiable to resort to clinical experience and many clinicians are aware of individual patients who have responded well to psychological treatment (and remain well in follow-up). Whether these changes result from the specific application of therapy is, of course, another matter.

Finally, attention must be focused on the many benefits which follow from helping the patient, and his partner, to see their problem in a different perspective, i.e. outside the immediate context of the target problem (the erectile inadequacy). These include improvements in mood, mental satisfaction and self-esteem.

SUMMARY

A large proportion of men with erectile dysfunction, perhaps up to one half, owe their condition largely to the 'psychological' factors discussed in this chapter and many of them will respond to the treatment strategies presented.

Although it is now known that many medical conditions have a multifactorial causation, it is difficult to think of a condition which has a more diverse and complex array of aetiological factors than erectile inadequacy. Such a situation presents the clinician with a unique diagnostic and therapeutic challenge. If he gets it wrong he will waste valuable resources and may mislead his patients into either false hopes or false despair. If he gets it right it is both intellectually and emotionally rewarding.

Clinicians tend to be fairly conservative in their choice of a therapeutic method (Cooper 1986). They tend to avoid the complexities of a truly eclectic approach and choose a particular treatment strategy often because it is the only one they know about and understand, or because it fits in with their preconceived notions of human nature. A notable example is the emphasis placed on therapeutic interventions with couples in monogamous, heterosexual relationships. However, the degree to which individuals are experimenting in relationships through multiple sex partners, cohabitees and serial monogamy, or electing to live alone, presents the clinician with a new challenge which can no longer be ignored. One consequence of these changes is that the standard treatment programmes of Masters & Johnson and Helen Kaplan do not always provide the answers and sometimes the clinician may be forced to think laterally and dig more deeply into the well of his therapeutic armamentarium. For example, he may have to dispose of the sacred cow of always focusing treatment on the relationship and instead on occasion switch his emphasis towards some form of individual therapy. Allied to this is the need to recognize the possibility that where conventional sex therapy has failed, some of the 'alternative' treatment strategies referred to may help some men with their problems by targeting less on the presenting symptoms and more on the whole person. Naturally, the clinician himself may not want to become involved personally, but he should be prepared to refer his patient to appropriate colleagues.

As our understanding of the multifactorial character of erectile disorders increases, and we can more fully comprehend the nature of the complex interplay between organic and psychological aetiologies, so the effectiveness of the treatments on offer will improve. For example, as our knowledge of the neurophysiology of sexual behaviour becomes more complete it seems likely that organogenic diagnoses will continue to grow at the expense of the psychogenic, allowing greater scope for pharmacotherapy.

However, even the most dramatic advances in our understanding of sexual physiology will not alter the fact that most sex involves another person and it is the often intangible, indeed imponderable, elements of the relationship which also require close scrutiny. As Lief (1980) pointed out 'the sexual process in a couple's interaction involves the transfer of information from one partner's neurohormonal system to the other's in ways which are completely mysterious to us at present'. This mystery needs to be explored if real progress is to be made in helping those with sexual problems.

REFERENCES

Allgeier E R, Allgeier A R 1984 Sexual interactions. Heath, Lexington

Ansari J M A 1976 Impotence: prognosis (a controlled study). British Journal of Psychiatry 128: 194–198

Arentewicz G, Schmidt G 1983 The treatment of sexual disorders. Basic Books, New York

Bancroft J 1981 Some methodological aspects of treatment outcome research. Proceedings of the VII World Congress of Sexology, Israel

Bancroft J 1989 Human sexuality and its problems. Churchill Livingstone, London

Bancroft J, Dickerson M, Fairburn C G, Gray J, Greenwood J, Stevenson N, Warner P 1986 Sex therapy outcome research: a reappraisal of methodology. 1. A treatment study of male sexual dysfunction. Psychological Medicine 16: 851–863

Bannister D, Fransella F 1980 Inquiring man, 2nd edn. Penguin, Harmondsworth

Barlow D H 1986 Causes of sexual dysfunction: the role of anxiety and cognitive interference. Journal of Consulting and Clinical Psychology 54: 140–148

Barlow D H, Sakheim D K, Beck J G 1983 Anxiety increases sexual arousal. Journal of Abnormal Psychology 92(1): 49–54

Bass B A 1986 The elegant solution to the problem of impotence. Journal of Rational-Emotive Therapy 4: 113–118

Beck J G, Rush A J, Emery G, Shaw B F 1979 Cognitive theory of depression. Guilford Press, New York

Beck J G, Barlow D H, Sakheim D K, Abrahamson D J 1984 Sexual responding during anxiety: clinical versus non-clinical patterns. Paper presented at the 18th Annual Conference of the Association for the Advancement of Behavior Therapy, Philadelphia

Bishay N R 1988 Cognitive therapy in psychosexual dysfunctions: a preliminary report. Sexual and Marital Therapy 3(1): 83–90

Briddell D W, Rimm C D, Caddy G R, Krawitz G, Sholis D, Wunderlin R J 1978 The effects of alcohol and cognitive set on sexual arousal to deviant stimuli. Journal of Abnormal Psychology 87: 418–430

Carney A, Bancroft J, Mathews A 1978 Combination of hormonal and psychological treatment for female sexual unresponsiveness. British Journal of Psychiatry 132: 339–346

Cole M J 1985 Sex therapy — a critical appraisal. British Journal of Psychiatry 147: 337–351

Cole M J 1986 Socio-sexual characteristics of men with sexual problems. Sexual and Marital Therapy 1(1): 89–108

Cole M J 1988a Normal and dysfunctional sexual behaviour: frequencies and incidences. In: Cole M, Dryden W (eds) Sex therapy in Britain. Open University Press, Milton Keynes

Cole M J 1988b Sex therapy for individuals. In: Cole M, Dryden W (eds) Sex therapy in Britain. Open University Press, Milton Keynes

Cole M, Dryden W 1989 Sex problems: your questions answered. Macdonald Optima, London

Cole M, Dryden W 1991 Sexual problems. In: Dryden W (ed) Clinical problems: a cognitive-behavioural approach. Routledge, London

Cooper A J 1978 Treatment of male potency: the present status. In: LoPiccolo J, LoPiccolo L (eds) Handbook of sex therapy. Plenum Press, New York

Cooper G F 1986 Survey of sex therapists in Britain. Training and Consultancy Service, Birmingham, UK

Cooper G F 1988 The psychological methods of sex therapy. In: Cole M, Dryden W (eds) Sex therapy in Britain. Open University Press, Milton Keynes

Crowe M J 1978 Conjoint marital therapy: a controlled outcome study. Psychological Medicine 8: 623–636

Crowe M J, Gillan P, Golombok S 1981 Form and content in the conjoint treatment of sexual dysfunction: a controlled study. Behaviour Research and Therapy 19: 47–54

Crown S, d'Ardenne P 1982 Symposium on sexual dysfunctions: controversies, methods and results. British Journal of Psychiatry 140: 70–77

De Amicis L A, Goldberg D C, LoPiccolo J, Friedman J, Davies L 1985 Clinical follow-up of couples treated for sexual dysfunction. Archives of Sexual Behavior 14: 467–489

Dicks H U 1967 Marital tensions. Routledge and Kegan, London

Dryden W (ed) 1985 Marital therapy in Britain, Vols 1 and 2. Harper and Row, London

Dryden W (ed) 1990 Individual therapy: a handbook. Open University Press, Milton Keynes

Dryden W, Golden W (eds) 1986 Cognitive behavioural approaches to psychotherapy. Harper and Row, London

Dryden W, Gordon J 1990 What is rational emotive therapy? Gale Centre Publications, Loughton

Duddle C M 1975 The treatment of marital psycho-sexual problems. British Journal of Psychiatry 127: 169–170

Ellis A 1962 Reason and emotion in psychotherapy. Lyle Stuart, Secaucus, NJ

Ellis A 1975 The rational-emotive approach to sex therapy. The Counseling Psychologist 5: 14–22

Ellis A 1976 Sex and the liberated man. Lyle Stuart, New York

Ellis A 1980 Treatment of erectile dysfunction. In: Leiblum S R, Pervin L A (eds) Principles and practice of sex therapy. Tavistock Publications, London

Everaerd W, Dekker J 1985 Treatment of male sexual dysfunction: sex therapy compared with systematic desensitization and rational-emotive therapy. Behaviour Research and Therapy 23(1): 13–25

Farrell B A 1981 The study of psychoanalysis. Oxford University Press, Oxford

Fenichel O 1945 The psychoanalytic theory of neurosis. Norton, New York

Friedman D E, Lipsedge M S 1971 Treatment of phobic anxiety and psychogenic impotence by systematic desensitization employing methohexitone. British Journal of Psychiatry 118: 89

Gelder M G 1990 Psychological treatment for depressive disorders. British Medical Journal 300: 1087–1088

Gregoire A 1990 Physical or psychological: an unhealthy splitting in theory and practice. Sexual and Marital Therapy 5(2): 103–104

Hastings D W 1963 Impotence and frigidity. Churchill, London

Hawton K 1982 The behavioural treatment of sexual dysfunction. British Journal of Psychiatry 140: 94–101

Hawton K 1983 Recent research in the treatment of sexual dysfunctions. Paper presented to the meeting of the Association of Sexual and Marital Therapists (unpublished). Manchester, UK

Hawton K 1985 Sex therapy: a practical guide. Oxford University Press, Oxford

Hawton K 1989 Sexual dysfunctions. In: Hawton K, Salkovskis P M, Kirk J, Clark D M (eds) Cognitive behaviour therapy for psychiatric problems: a practical guide. Oxford University Press, Oxford

Hawton K, Catalan J, Martin P, Fagg J 1986 Long-term outcome of sex therapy. Behaviour Research and Therapy 24: 665–675

Hawton K, Catalan J 1986 Prognostic factors in sex therapy. Behaviour Research and Therapy 24: 377–385

Hawton K, Salkovskis P M, Kirk J, Clark D M (eds) 1989 Cognitive behaviour therapy for psychiatric problems: a practical guide. Oxford University Press, Oxford

Heap M 1988 Hypnosis: current clinical experimental and forensic practices. Croom Helm, London

Heiman J R, LoPiccolo J 1983 Clinical outcome of sex therapy. Archives of General Psychiatry 40: 443–449

Heiman J R, LoPiccolo J, Hogan D, Roberts C 1985 Effectiveness of single therapists versus co-therapy teams in sex therapy. Journal of Consulting and Clinical Psychology 53: 287–294

Henson D E, Rubin H B 1971 Voluntary control of eroticism. Journal of Applied Behaviour Analysis 4: 37–44

Hoon P, Wincze J, Hoon E 1977 A test of reciprocal inhibition: are anxiety and sexual arousal in women mutually inhibitory? Journal of Abnormal Psychology 86: 65–74

Johnson J 1968 Disorders of sexual potency in the male. Pergamon Press, Oxford

Kaplan H S 1974 The new sex therapy. Brunner/Mazel, New York

Kaplan H S 1979 Disorders of sexual desire. Baillière–Tindall, London

Kaplan H S 1982 The treatment of sexual phobias: the combined use of anti-panic medication and sex therapy. Journal of Sexual and Marital Therapy 8: 3–28

Kaplan H S 1989 PE: How to overcome premature ejaculation. Brunner/Mazel, New York

Kayata L, Szydlo D 1988 Sex therapy in groups. In: Cole M, Dryden W (eds) Sex therapy in Britain. Open University Press, Milton Keynes

Kinsey A C, Pomeroy W B, Martin C E, Gebhard P H 1948 Sexual behavior in the human male. W B Saunders, Philadelphia

Kinsey A C, Pomeroy W B, Martin C E, Gebhard P H 1953 Sexual behavior in the human female. W B Saunders, Philadelphia

Kockott G, Dittmar F, Nusselt L 1975 Systematic desensitization of erectile impotence: a controlled study. Archives of Sexual Behavior 4: 493–500

Kolodny R C, Masters W H, Johnson V E 1979 Textbook of sexual medicine. Little, Brown, Boston

Korb M P, Gorrell J, Van de Riet V 1989 Gestalt therapy practice and theory, 2nd edn. Pergamon, New York

Kowalski R 1985 Cognitive therapy for sexual problems. British Journal of Sexual Medicine 12: 64–66, 90–93, 131–135

Laws D, Rubin H 1969 Instructional control of autonomic sexual response. Journal of Applied Behavior Analysis 2: 93–100

Lief H I 1980 Forward In: Leiblum S R, Pervin L A (eds) Principles and practice of sex therapy. Tavistock Publications, London

Levine S B, Agle D 1978 The effectiveness of sex therapy for chronic secondary psychological impotence. Journal of Sex and Marital Therapy 4: 235–258

Lloyd P M, Brown P T 1989 Sensate focus in the treatment of sexual difficulties. British Journal of Sexual Medicine, May 195–198

LoPiccolo J, Stock W 1986 Treatment of sexual dysfunction. Journal of Consulting and Clinical Psychology 54: 158–167

McCary J L 1967 Human sexuality. Van Nostrand, Princeton

Masters W H, Johnson V E 1966 Human sexual response. Little, Brown, Boston

Masters W H, Johnson V E 1970 Human sexual inadequacy. Churchill, London

Mathew R J, Weinman M L 1982 Sexual dysfunctions in depression. Archives of Sexual Behaviour 11(4): 323–328

Mathews A, Whitehead A, Kellett J 1983 Psychological and hormonal factors in the treatment of female sexual dysfunction. Psychological Medicine 13: 83–92

Mearns D, Thorne B 1988 Person centred counselling in action. Sage, London

Mears E 1978 Sexual problem clinics: an assessment of the work of 26 doctors trained by the Institute of Psychosexual Medicine. Public Health 92: 218–233

Melman A, Kaplan D, Redfield J 1984 Evaluation of the first 70 patients in the center for male sexual dysfunction of the Beth Israel Medical Center. Journal of Urology 131: 53–55

Munjack D J, Schlaks A, Sanchez V C, Usigli R, Zulueta A, Leonard M 1984 Rational emotive therapy in the treatment of erectile failure: an initial study. Journal of Sex and Marital Therapy 10: 170–175

Norton G R, Jehu D 1984 The role of anxiety in sexual dysfunction: a review. Archives of Sexual Behavior 13: 165–183

O'Connor J F, Stern L O 1972 Results of treatment in functional sexual disorders. New York State Journal of Medicine 72: 1927–1934

Patterson D G, O'Gorman E C 1986 A questionnaire measure of sexual anxiety. British Journal of Psychiatry 149: 63–67

Patterson D G, O'Gorman E C 1989 Sexual anxiety in sexual dysfunction. British Journal of Psychiatry 155: 374–375

Patterson D G, O'Gorman E C 1990 Sexual anxiety in homosexuals. Sexual and Marital Therapy 5: 49–53

Ramsay G 1943 The sexual development of boys. American Journal of Psychology 56: 217

Rathus S A 1978 Use of covert assertion in cognitive restructuring of sexual attitudes. Behavior Therapy 9: 678

Reckless J, Geiger N 1978 Impotence as a practical problem. In: LoPiccolo J, LoPiccolo L (eds) Handbook of sex therapy. Plenum, New York

Reynolds B S 1977 Psychological treatment models and

outcome results for erectile dysfunction: a critical review. Psychological Bulletin 84: 1218–1238

Riley A J, Riley E J 1986 The effect of single dose diazepam on female sexual response induced by masturbation. Sexual and Marital Therapy 1: 49–53

Rogers C R 1980 A way of being. Houghton Mifflin, Boston

Sanders D 1983 How to avoid divorce. Woman, March 12: 27–30

Sarrel D M, Masters W H 1982 Sexual molestation of men by women. Archives of Sexual Behavior 11: 117–131

Skynner R, Cleese J 1987 Families and how to survive them. Methuen, London

Smith T W 1990 Adult sexual behavior in 1989: number of partners, frequency and risk. General Social Survey Topic Report No. 18. Paper presented to the American Association for the Advancement of Science, New Orleans

Stewart I 1989 Transactional analysis counselling in action. Sage, London

Stoller R 1976 Sexual excitement. Archives of General Psychiatry 33: 899–909

Truax C B, Carkhuff R R 1967 Towards effective counseling and psychotherapy. Aldine, Chicago

Tunnadine P 1983 The making of love. Jonathan Cape, London

Walen S R 1980 Cognitive factors in sexual behavior. Journal of Sex and Marital Therapy 6: 87–101

Walen S R, Roth D 1987 A cognitive approach. In: Gerr J H, O'Donohue W (eds) Theories of human sexuality. Plenum, New York

Walen S R, Perlmutter R 1988 Cognitive–behavioral treatment of adult sexual dysfunctions from a family perspective. In: Epstein N, Schlensinger S, Dryden W (eds) Cognitive-behavioral approaches to family therapy. Brunner/Mazel, New York

Warner P, Bancroft J 1986 Sex therapy outcome research: a reappraisal of methodology. 2. Methodological considerations — the importance of prognostic variability. Psychological Medicine 16: 855–863

Watson J P, Brockman B 1982 A follow-up of couples attending a psychosexual problems clinic. British Journal of Clinical Psychology 21: 143–144

Wilkins R 1990 Women who sexually abuse children. British Medical Journal 300: 1153–1154

Wolchick S A, Beggs V E, Wincze J P, Sakheim D K, Barlow D H, Mavissakalian M 1980 The effects of a subjective monitoring task in the measurement of genital response to erotic stimulation. Archives of Sexual Behavior 9: 533–545

Wolpe J 1958 Psychotherapy by reciprocal inhibition. Stanford University Press, Stanford

Wright J, Perreault R, Mathieu M 1977 The treatment of sexual dysfunction: a review. Archives of General Psychiatry 34: 881–890

Zilbergeld B 1980 Men and sex. Fontana/Collins, Glasgow

Zimmer D, Borchardt E, Fischle C 1983 Sexual fantasies of sexually distressed and non-distressed men and women: an empirical comparison. Journal of Sexual and Marital Therapy 9: 38–50

APPENDIX 10.1

RECOMMENDED BOOKS FOR PATIENTS

Men

It's Up to You by Warwick Williams. Thorsons, 1989 (Specifically about erectile dysfunction.)

Men and Sex by Bernard Zilbergeld. Fontana, 1980 (Male sexuality generally.)

Women

Women's Experience of Sex by Sheila Kitzinger. Penguin, 1985

Women and Sex by Anne Hooper. Sheldon, 1986

General

Sexual Happiness: a practical approach by Maurice Yaffe & Elizabeth Fenwick. Dorling Kindersley, 1986

The Book of Love by David Delvin. New English Library, 1974

Treat Yourself to Sex by Paul Brown & Caroline Faulder. Penguin, 1979

Sex Problems: Your Questions Answered by Martin Cole and Windy Dryden. Macdonald Optima, 1989

These books differ greatly in style and approach. It is strongly recommended that the clinician look at them before recommending them to patients.

11. Pharmacological treatments for impotence

Alain Gregoire

The use of intracavernosal injections of vasoactive drugs (IIVD) probably constitutes the most dramatic therapeutic advance in the treatment of sexual problems since the description of sex therapy by Masters & Johnson (Masters & Johnson 1970). The consequences of this development to both patient and clinician have been far reaching. It provides an alternative for patients who previously might have gone untreated because they did not want, or were not suitable for, both implants and sex therapy. For clinicians, IIVD has provided a greater understanding of the mechanisms of impotence, a diagnostic tool and a simpler, cheaper treatment alternative (see also Chs 5 & 8). The arrival of IIVD has produced an enormous increase in medical interest in erectile dysfunction, usually, although not always, with positive effects on patient care.

Indiscriminate use of physical methods of achieving erections is inevitably detrimental to some patients, whose problems are not simply the inability to achieve stiffness of the penis. This medicalization and apparently increased treatability of the problem has awakened the interest of the media, perhaps contributing to the widespread rise in demand for treatment from men with erectile problems. Nevertheless, this form of treatment is far from ideal, and more 'patient friendly' pharmacological approaches are being actively investigated. These oral and topical preparations, largely still in the development stage, will also be discussed.

INTRACAVERNOSAL INJECTIONS OF VASOACTIVE DRUGS

The use of IIVD to induce erections for therapeu-

tic purposes was first described by Virag in 1982. Brindley, working independently on the effects of phenoxybenzamine, an alpha-blocker, published results of the first major series of patients treated using IIVD (Brindley 1983, 1986). The effectiveness of vasoative drugs in producing erections when injected into the corpora cavernosa of normal and impotent men has been confirmed in both uncontrolled and double-blind placebo-controlled studies (Brindley 1983; Kieley et al 1987a).

The mode of action of these drugs, and the diagnostic significance of their effects, have been described in previous chapters. The present discussion will concentrate on the therapeutic use of IIVD, which differs from the diagnostic use in a number of ways. The physician using IIVD diagnostically is simply applying a procedure to obtain an answer to a question. There is no need to explain the finer details of the procedure to the patient and the role of the patient is largely a passive one.

From the very beginning, therapeutic use of IIVD is different. The patient is actively involved in selecting this mode of treatment, using the physician as an advisor. The physician's aim is to lead the patient towards not only correct and effective use of the treatment, but eventual improvement in his sexual relationships through its effects.

Indications for IIVD

Long term use

Much of the initial work on IIVD concentrated on the treatment of men with largely organic impotence. In such cases, there are few data to guide the clinician on which treatment options would be most suitable. The most important deciding factor, bar the small number of contraindications to IIVD (see below) becomes the patient's choice of which treatment he finds most attractive (or least unattractive!). The partner's views are obviously also a key determinant. Presenting all treatment options in an objective manner, with their advantages and disadvantages, is likely to lead to higher satisfaction rates once a choice has been made.

In patients whose impotence is largely or entirely due to organic disease, it is generally assumed that use of the injections will need to continue until the patient decides to stop, side effects become unacceptable or the treatment becomes ineffective.

In recent years, the use of therapeutic IIVD has gradually extended to include men with psychogenic impotence. The case for such a use is far less clear cut and the practice is not based on careful evaluation of results, but rather on an attempt to meet the ever growing demand for a simple and, in many cases, simplistic remedy which faces clinicians in this field. Furthermore, as urologists have been adopting an increasingly active role in this field, it is inevitable that many patients with largely psychogenic impotence will consult them and receive the treatments they offer.

IIVD is extremely effective in producing erections in this group of patients, as local penile function, on which the erectile response to intracavernosal vasodilators depends, is generally undamaged. This may add to the attractiveness of using the treatment with these patients.

Limited use

There are theoretical grounds for believing that psychological benefit may be obtained from the use of IIVD as a short term measure. It has been suggested that the restoration of adequate, reliable erections, allowing satisfactory intercourse, would lead to a reduction in sexual anxiety and would allow patients to learn to concentrate on their experiences, rather than their performance. Other more general effects, such as improved self-esteem and self-image and greater partner satisfaction, could also result. All these factors, which are important in psychological therapies, could produce

an improvement in erections in these men. Indeed, there are suggestions in the literature that a proportion of patients experience an improvement in their spontaneous erections after short courses of IIVD. The proportion of patients reported as responding in this way varies from less than 10% (Brindley 1986; Williams et al 1987) to 66% (Virag et al 1984). This wide range of results is not surprising as these studies do not specify their client population or their definitions of impotence and use different methods of assessing aetiology and measuring improvement.

It is not possible from the data available to draw conclusions about exactly which patients are more likely to show this improvement. Virag (1982) and Lue (1988) both conclude from their findings that patients with vascular and psychogenic dysfunction are those most likely to respond. Williams et al (1987) found that patients who showed improved erections were 'predominantly psychogenic', although three were also diabetic. Brindley (1986) noted that all 7 patients whose potency returned to some degree had only 'partial impotence' before treatment. No patients in his 'completely impotent' group showed improvement. Taken together these findings confirm that it is the psychological contribution to these patients' dysfunction which is treatment responsive, rather than any organic pathology reacting to a persisting (and unknown) pharmacological effect.

The significance of this improvement for clinical practice is at present difficult to interpret. It depends on whether the improvement is a lasting one, which patients are most likely to benefit, the incidence of side effects, and the effectiveness of this treatment compared to current psychological interventions. These questions, to which there are only partial answers, will be addressed in turn.

Follow-up data. Very little follow-up data on patients showing improved potency are available, although it seems from uncontrolled studies that a proportion of responders maintain the improvement for at least one year (Williams et al 1987; Virag et al 1984). However, results from a controlled study conducted by the author (Gregoire 1991a) demonstrate that on a number of measures, the significant improvement in sexual functioning experienced during IIVD was poorly sustained after treatment stopped.

Prognostic factors. Virag (1984) suggests that the best responders are those with high levels of performance anxiety, but there are no studies examining possible prognostic factors, such as degree and duration of impotence, presence of co-existing sexual dysfunction, quality of relationship and personality (e.g. suggestibility in those with high neuroticism scores). Conversely, some factors predicting a successful outcome have been established for sex therapy (Hawton & Catalan 1986). These include motivation for treatment, duration of the problem and premorbid sexual adjustment. It could be argued that patients with favourable prognostic factors for sex therapy should be given this treatment and only those patients with unfavourable conditions should be offered limited IIVD. However, it could also be argued that as the benefits of limited IIVD are psychologically mediated, the same factors may predict a favourable outcome to either treatment. If this were the case, the only factor which would differentiate between the two treatments for any given patient could be his level of motivation to take part in one or other treatment. We thus return to what is essentially selection of treatment according to the patient's choice. It is important to reiterate that in such situations the impartial advice and information provided by the clinician is essential in facilitating patient choice.

Unwanted effects. Reports of limited use of IIVD suggest a very low rate of side effects, although only very small numbers of patients are involved. However, support for this conclusion arises from the evidence regarding rates of side effects with long term use, notably incidence of fibrosis. This has been shown to rise in direct proportion to the number of injections administered (see p. 173).

Comparative effectiveness. In a study conducted by the author, men with psychogenic impotence were randomly allocated to either limited use of intracavernosal injections (defined as a course of six home injections of papaverine, each leading onto sexual intercourse) or modified Masters & Johnson type sex therapy (Gregoire 1991a). A consecutive series of men fulfilling the same entry criteria, but who only received an assessment and an appointment for treatment 3 months later, were used as a waiting list control group.

Erectile function and change with time was measured using the Golombok & Rust Inventory of Sexual Satisfaction (see Ch. 7), a clinical assessment and three 4 point scales measuring frequency, duration and severity, which were completed by the subject. By the end of treatment significant improvements in erectile function had occurred in both treatment groups compared to controls. This significant improvement was maintained in the sex therapy group at 3 months follow-up, but not in the group who had received limited intracavernosal injections. Interestingly, a significant improvement in premature ejaculation scores on the GRISS occurred in the limited IIVD group at the end of treatment and this was maintained at 3 months follow-up.

Even if it appears to be inferior to sex therapy in the long term, there are compelling reasons for adding limited use of IIVD to our range of possible secondary treatments for predominantly psychogenic impotence. Many men either do not respond to or are unwilling to undergo sex therapy for a variety of reasons, and in some cases the partner is unwilling or unavailable to take part in sex therapy. Although it is often desirable to tackle relationship issues in such situations, this may be impossible despite vigorous attempts by the therapist to engage the partner.

In many men there is a resistance to psychological explanations and interventions, which are perceived as 'not taking the problem seriously' (in spite of the time and effort devoted by therapists). In many such patients, the use of IIVD provides an opportunity to engage the patient in a therapeutic relationship. The skilled therapist can then use this relationship to introduce psychological concepts and interventions, rather than simply reinforcing the patient's medicalization of his problem. This may be limited to a discussion about the ways in which the mind and body interact, or may lead into more extensive couple therapy. It is often useful in such cases to state clearly that the 'physical problem' is unquestionably there, but that it is caused by problems in the 'control system', which is, of course, in the brain and can be influenced by any other processes going on in the brain. Many patients also understand the concept of 'mind over matter'. However, the comment 'it's all in the mind' should be avoided at all costs as it is frequently perceived as dismissive and even derogatory.

Limited IIVD may also be indicated in patients who have undergone sex therapy with little or no benefit. However, their chances of success are probably slim, and they may well have to continue using IIVD on a long term basis or turn to another form of treatment.

The use of IIVD in men with no partner presents particular problems, which are discussed in Chapter 15.

Procedure

Treatment with IIVD should not be commenced until the practitioner is confident that the patient has chosen this treatment in the light of the available choices and the doctor's recommendations. The patient should be aware of the nature and frequency of known side effects (see pp 171–174) and the uncertainty about long term side effects (the treatment has only been in use since 1983).

Some authors have recommended that all patients give written consent to the treatment (e.g. Sidi et al 1988). This practice is considered unnecessary by many clinicians, as long as the above information is given to the patients and this is recorded in the notes.

Choice of drug

Various drug combinations and dosage regimes have been recommended in the literature, including papaverine alone (Brindley 1986) papaverine and phentolamine mixture (Sidi 1988) and prostaglandin E1 (Stackl et al 1988). There is no evidence of any clear superiority of the papaverine and phentolamine mixture over papaverine alone. Prostaglandin E1 may be effective in more patients and has a lower rate of side effects. If the longer term follow-up data on the use of prostaglandins confirm this low level of side effects, greater effectiveness and reduced tolerance effects, its use is likely to replace that of papaverine. Probably the most important single advantage of prostaglandin E1 is the apparently very low rate of priapism. This permits the use of a standard dose and eliminates the need for the dose titration procedure. At present, however, papaverine continues to be widely used as a generally effective, cheap and easily available drug. When papaverine is to be used therapeutically, the minimum effective dose must be titrated to reduce the risk of priapism and possibly also of fibrosis. Although the procedure appears time consuming, it in fact adds little time to the simultaneous process of training the patient to inject himself to a safe level of competence.

Titrating the dose of papaverine

Titration of the minimum effective dose of papaverine for each individual undoubtedly minimizes the risk of priapism and may also reduce the incidence of fibrosis. In a study of the side effects of papaverine and phentolamine administration, Lakin et al (1990) demonstrated that patients who developed plaques or nodules had used a significantly higher mean number of injections and total dosage of either drug. It is not clear whether these factors act independently, but on present information it would seem sensible to keep dosage to a minimum effective level.

Dosage titration may involve up to three test injections in the clinic. This process also allows for adequate training and supervision of the patients' injection technique. I recommend the following procedure.

Equipment required: drug, appropriate volume syringe and 15 mm 27–30 gauge needle (a U100 insulin syringe and needle is ideal for volumes of 1 ml or less). For his own protection, the clinician should wear disposable gloves as blood contact on injection frequently occurs.

1. 1st clinic injection: 20 mg papaverine sulphate. Explain and demonstrate sterile technique to the patient, and demonstrate the procedure involved in drawing up the drug into the syringe and the elimination of air bubbles.

The patient can be injected standing, sitting or lying down. It is advisable to have a couch in the room in case he feels dizzy or faint following an injection. Such a reaction may not be apparent if the patient is supine and I therefore generally ask the patient to stand next to a couch during the injection.

The site of injection is then explained to the patient. He should be aiming for the centre of the cavernous bodies and should avoid the urethra, glans and subcutaneous tissues. To achieve this, the needle is inserted at right angles to the shaft in an area halfway down its lateral aspect. It is important to advise the patient to spend some time in good light carefully choosing the site of injection. Avoiding puncturing veins during the injection greatly reduces the likelihood and severity of bruising and bleeding. Some men who are able to induce partial tumescence by masturbation find this makes the area more visible and accessible.

With 15 mm needles, the needle can be inserted up to the hilt and the patient reassured that he can not push it too far. Rapid insertion of the needle minimizes the discomfort. Only minimal resistance should be encountered to needle insertion.

The drug is then injected and again only minimal resistance to this should be felt. At this point, patients frequently describe an unpleasant burning sensation which disappears after 30 seconds. Severe pain and resistance to drug injection suggest that the needle tip may be in subcutaneous tissues, and it should be resited.

Following withdrawal of the needle from a well sited injection, there should be no evidence of bleeding or bruising. Seeing no mark on the penis usually greatly encourages patients. Inevitably, however carefully one sites the injection, bleeding or haematoma formation will sometimes occur. If this is observed, firm pressure on the injection site in the usual manner will minimize its extent.

Massaging the penis following injection to 'mix' the drug around the cavernosal bodies is sometimes recommended (Brindley 1987). It is not clear whether this makes any difference to the effect of the injection. Following injection the effect is observed at 5, 10 and 15 minutes and the degree of tumescence noted. The key indicator of adequacy of the erection for sexual intercourse is 'bendability'. This is simply assessed in the clinical situation by attempting to bend the shaft of the penis laterally. If this is not easily possible, the erection is adequate for sexual intercourse.

In busy clinics patients are frequently left alone or sent back to the waiting room for 5 to 15 minutes while the response is awaited. Although this practice may be necessary in less than ideal conditions, it is preferable for the doctor to stay with the patient. The time can then be used for discussion and counselling, often to the great benefit of the patient. In some cases this may be the only way of engaging a man in a discussion about the psychological aspects of his sexual relationship (see Ch 10 & 15).

Duration of the effect is obviously also important to assess. An adequate response in the clinic may be further enhanced in the home situation by the addition of sexual stimulation. Patients who are not entirely satisfied, despite a response which the clinician considers adequate, should be asked to try the same dose at home before an increase is considered.

Should the effect after 15 to 20 minutes be inadequate, the patient is asked to return for a further injection at a higher dose.

2. 2nd clinic injection: up to 40 mg papaverine sulphate. When the patient returns, he should be asked about:

1. Any improvement in the pharmacologically induced erection following the last appointment.
2. The total duration of the tumescence.
3. Any side effects.
4. Any improvement in erections at other times.

Assuming that he and his partner are happy to continue, the above information will decide the next step. If a delayed, adequate response was obtained after the patient had left the clinic, 20 mg would be the required dose for this patient. If the erection lasted 2–3 hours or more the dose will need to be reduced. Inadequate tumescence or duration (less than 10–15 minutes) will require an increased dose, usually to 40 mg.

The same procedure as with the first injection is repeated, except that the patient may feel confident enough to attempt autoinjection under the doctor's supervision. The doctor will usually need to talk him through the procedure on this occasion.

If both the response and the patient's technique are considered adequate, a prescription can be given for home injection. However, the patient should be warned not to proceed with this if his erection lasts three hours or more in response to the 40 mg injection of papaverine. He should contact the doctor regarding a dose reduction if this happens. If either the erection or the patient's technique are inadequate, the patient will need to return.

3. Session 3: autoinjection of up to 80 mg papaverine sulphate. Again, the same procedure as in session 2 is repeated, with any dosage adjustments as required. At this stage the patient should be able to carry out the entire procedure without guidance from the physician.

If there is little response to 80 mg, it is unlikely that any further increase in dose will produce an adequate erection. If, however, 80 mg of papaverine sulphate results in a nearly but not quite adequate erection, an increase to 120 mg may enhance the response just enough. Increasing the dose above 120 mg does not lead to any worthwhile added benefit.

Follow-up

Once the dose has been established and the physician is confident that the patient is able to carry out autoinjection at home, many patients can be discharged back to the care of their general practitioner for continued prescription and follow-up. Some authors (e.g. Sidi et al 1988; Zorgniotti & Lefleur 1985) recommend indefinite follow-up in a specialist clinic, so that any side effects can be detected. I question both the theoretical need for this and indeed the practical feasibility of such a policy, given the high demand for the limited amount of specialist time in this area. The side effects which are currently known about are easily detectable, not only by well briefed general practitioners, but indeed by the patient himself. The occurrence of side effects may require specialist advice, but screening for them does not. Possible, unknown, long term side effects may of course arise with this treatment but this situation is no different to that which arises with countless other medical interventions. Knowledge about the treatment and its side effects can be effectively relayed to the general practitioner in a standard discharge letter, explaining the treatment, its effects and side effects.

Patients should always be supplied with a handout explaining the treatment technique and containing a warning about the possibility of priapism and clear instructions for what to do if this occurs. I stress to all patients, both verbally and in writing,

the importance of obtaining help within 12 hours, or before, if the erection becomes painful. Accident and emergency departments are well suited to dealing with such situations (which can obviously occur at any time of the day or night). Not all doctors are aware of the detumescence procedure (Gregoire 1990), and to avoid long delays or inappropriate treatment, the patient should be issued with an instruction sheet for doctors (Appendix 11.1), which he can give to the casualty officer. This should explain the detumescence procedure in detail, as well as giving details of the doctor prescribing treatment so that he can be contacted if necessary.

Contraindications

The only generally agreed contraindication to IIVD usage is sickle disease. This arises from the theoretical risk of priapism and induction of sickle crisis. There are no known interactions with other drugs.

There are, however, a number of relative contraindications which relate to the procedure rather than the drug itself. The clinician prescribing for autoinjection at home has a responsibility to ensure that the patient (or whoever is doing the injecting) understands the procedure involved and is able to follow it. Patients who, despite being trained by clinic staff, cannot reach an adequate level of competence in the procedure should not be prescribed this treatment for autoinjection. Given the relative simplicity of the procedure, this situation is rare. Occasionally, clinicians encounter patients whose overenthusiasm with their new toy leads them to increase the dose or the recommended frequency. Patients should be warned against such a practice, but it is difficult to predict in advance those who will intentionally behave in this way.

Some patients are hampered by physical disability, such as the immobility and deformity of arthritis or the tremor of Parkinson's disease. If the patient's partner is similarly affected or is unwilling to carry out the injections, the treatment may be impossible. Obese patients who cannot see their genitals will also find autoinjection very difficult. This situation provides the clinician with a good opportunity to recommend a reducing diet!

Similarly, blind patients are unable to prepare the syringe and even the partially sighted may have difficulty in avoiding veins during injection, thus experiencing more bleeding and bruising.

Men who have partners but refuse to inform them about the treatment pose a difficult problem. It is almost impossible, and psychologically very undesirable, for men to use IIVD without their partner's knowledge. Although some clinicians are prepared to collude in such a deception, I believe that this practice is not in the patient's best interest. I have encountered several couples who have experienced this situation, some with disastrous effect.

Some men attend alone, claiming that their partner does not wish to attend but agrees to the treatment. Whether clinicians are prepared to trust and treat such men is a matter for their own judgement. I believe that in such situations a flexible approach, guided by the individual circumstances, is the most useful one.

Treating men without seeing their partners involves a number of other difficulties. Occasionally men who respond with good erections to clinic injections complain that the effect is no better than they can get anyway, despite having given a history of inadequate erections and inability to have sexual intercourse. Clearly, in such cases the problem does not lie in the penis but in the intrapersonal or interpersonal factors leading to his dissatisfaction with, or altered perception of his penile function. In some such cases it may be that the drug induced erection is instrumental in uncovering a problem which may not otherwise have become apparent.

Acceptability

A crude impression of acceptability can be gained from some of the published studies, but because samples are often highly selected, or biased in other ways, the results should be interpreted with caution. Sidi et al (1988) studied a sample of 372 men with impotence of mainly organic origin, of whom half dropped out at various stages of treatment. Of those patients using treatment at follow-up 78.2% were generally satisfied. In a study of 78 men with impotence of various causes who were selected as 'appropriate' for injection, Girdley et al (1988) found that 22 of 76 patients followed up considered the treatment unacceptable. The remainder reported varying degrees of satisfaction. Acceptability to partners is also important but has not been studied systematically, although partner refusal is reported in the above two studies.

Side effects

Several unwanted effects of IIVD treatment have been described, some of which are clearly understood, others not. Although descriptions of the nature of unwanted effects are consistent, their reported incidence varies greatly. The rates of haematomas (3–47%) and fibrosis of cavernosal tissue (0–57%) are the most extreme examples (see Table 11.1). This variation is probably mainly accounted for by differences in frequency and duration of use. Thus the reader should be wary of too literal an interpretation of the figures quoted in the following discussion.

1. Systemic side effects

Dizziness, faints, postural hypotension. These effects have been reported by several authors, occurring in approximately 2–3% of samples during long term use (Brindley 1986; Sidi et al 1986). Patients describe rapid onset following injection of feelings of dizziness and light headedness which can lead to brief loss of consciousness, but resolve rapidly on lying down. These may be accompanied by flushing and sweating. This reaction matches well the description of vasovagal attacks or psychogenic reactions to injections, or intrauterine contraceptive device insertions. Given the psychologically sensitive nature of the area being injected, it would be surprising if such psychogenic responses were not observed. An alternative, or additional explanation for the phenomenon has been suggested: that it may be the result of the vasodilator effect of the drugs released rapidly into the general circulation in the presence of venous leakage (Wespes & Shulman 1988). However, injection of 80 mg of papaverine intravenously produced no significant drop in blood pressure or dizziness in one subject (Brindley G S, personal communication). In addition there is little evidence that men with venous leakage are more likely to

Table 11.1   Studies describing side effects of IIVD. (From Gregoire 1992)

Authors	Sample	Treatment	Duration of follow-up	Side effects	Discontinued
Sidi et al 1986	100	Papaverine + phentolamine <37 mg + 1.25 mg	1–8 months	Dizziness: 2/100 Haematoma: 3/100 Burning: 2/100 Priapism (8–12 hrs): 4/100 [1 stopped treatment as a result] 'No major complications on follow-up.'	
Brindley 1986	127	Phenoxybenzamine + papaverine	1–3 years	Pain on injection: 'most patients' Haematoma: 'small minority' Injection into urethra: 1/127 Priapism (>12 hrs): 11/127 Faints: 2/127 Fibrosis: 1/127	
Kiely et al 1987b	67	Papaverine + phentolamine	Not specified	Postural hypotension: 2/67 Priapism (> 4 hrs): 2/67 Fibrosis: 0/67	
Williams et al 1987	125	Autoinjection, papaverine + phentolamine	1–24 months	Priapism (> 4 hrs): 34/3513 injections Infection: 0/125 Fibrosis: 0/125 Pain: 18/125 Bruising: 27/125 Abnormal liver function: 0/128	
Stackl et al 1988	112	Autoinjection, PgE1	8 months (mean 4.5 months)	Priapism: 0/112 Pain on erection: 0/112 Bruising: 11/112 Fibrosis: 0/112	Partners considered the treatment 'unnatural': 2/112
Girdley et al 1988	78	Autoinjection, papaverine + phentolamine	1–27 months (mean 9.8 months)	Induration: 13/78 Reduced quality: 27% Variability of response: 49% Pain on injection: 78% Bruising: 47% Lateral deviation: 18% Priapism (> 12 hrs): 8%	Poor health: 13/78 Partner dissatisfied: 7/78 Fibrosis: 2/78
Sidi et al 1988	372	Autoinjection, drug N/S	11.6 (± 5) months	Not specified (resulted in 15 patients dropping out in total)	At dosage determination: 9.7% At injection training: 8.4% During home injection: 31.4%
Levine et al 1989	111	Papaverine + phentolamine	1, 3, 6, 12 and 24 months	Priapism: 2/329 Increased dose needed: 41% Nodule development: 57% at 12/12 (proportional to total no. of injections) Variability in response: 75%	27% at dosage determination 41% total in 12/12
Watters et al 1988	62	Phenoxybenzamine, papaverine + phentolamine	3–21 months (mean 9 months)	Pain: 11/62 Haematoma: 37/62 Priapism: 7/62 Systemic SEs: 4/62	25/62 discontinued 'Cured': 4 Tolerance: 8 Priapism: 3 Haematomas: 5 Did not like: 5
Ishii et al 1989	135	Prostaglandin E1, 20 mg	None	Pain: 0 Priapism: 0	
Lakin et al 1990	81	Papaverine ± phentolamine	1–20 months	Haematoma: 17(21%) Mild discomfort: 11(14%) Priapism: 0 Fibrotic lesions: 15(19%)	

feel faint or dizzy following intracavernosal injection. On present evidence, it seems reasonable to suggest that the effect occurs as a response to the drug in certain sensitive individuals, and in some cases may simply be a nonspecific effect ('vaso vagal attack') associated with injection into a psychologically sensitive area.

The possibility of severe hypotensive episodes raises the theoretical risk of ischaemic cerebral vascular events. As yet, no such events have been described in the literature in association with the use of IIVD.

Mild, nonspecific changes in liver function tests have long been known as a side effect of papaverine use before the days of IIVD. Such changes have been described (Williams et al 1987) but no cases of severe effects on liver function from the use of papaverine for IIVD have been described.

2. Local side effects

Pain. This is common (Brindley 1986; Girdley et al 1988) and occurs both on needle puncture and on injection of the drug. The pain experienced as the needle is pushed in is usually only slight, often to the patient's surprise as this is frequently what they fear most on starting treatment. Complaints of pain or burning sensation on injection of the drugs are very variable, and rarely so severe that the patient stops using the treatment. This pain lasts under a minute. It has been suggested that it is caused by the high acidity of papaverine solution.

Bruising and bleeding. Haematoma formation produces bruises which can be extensive and unsightly, sometimes causing alarm to patients. They are rarely painful or even sore and gradually disappear over several days. Patients can usually proceed with intercourse without particular discomfort. Bleeding of any significance is a rare event. Both can usually be prevented by carefully siting the injection away from visible veins. This will often lead to there being no trace of the injection once the needle has been withdrawn. Should bleeding and bruising be apparent at this stage, pressure applied to the injection site in the usual manner will minimize its extent.

The important contribution of injection technique in minimizing this unwanted effect is prob-

ably the main cause for the great variability in the reported frequency of haematomas. The occurrence of haematomas or bruising in several studies of long term use varies from 3% to 47% (Sidi et al 1986; Girdley et al 1988). Patients rarely stop using the treatment because of this side effect, but they may seek reassurance that it is not causing any permanent damage.

Infection. Although infection was considered as a possible risk of intracavernosal injection at an early stage (Brindley 1983), particularly with home use and in diabetes, the subsequent literature indicates that this, at worst, is an extremely rare occurrence. Careful use of sterile techniques by both doctor and patient will continue to eliminate this risk.

Fibrosis, plaque or nodule formation. The development of lumpiness in the tissues of the corpora cavernosa is a well described complication of IIVD. Initially, this was thought to be an uncommon complication, but there is now evidence, at least with papaverine, that with long term use the risk is substantial.

Levine et al (1989) studied prospectively a group of 111 men embarking on intracavernosal autoinjections of papaverine and phentolamine. Amongst those who continued to use the treatment at follow-up, an almost linear increase in the occurrence of nodules over time was noted. By 12 months, 57% of patients had developed fibrosis. In none of these patient were the nodules felt to be severe enough to end treatment. Only 3 men reported erection distortion. Men who developed nodules, when compared to those who did not, showed significantly higher mean number of injections, significantly higher dosages of papaverine and phentolamine and had been using injections more frequently. Lakin et al (1990) have described very similar results. It is not possible from either of these studies to conclude which, if any, of the factors identified is primary. A number of hypotheses remain as to the cause of nodule formation:

1. Tissue reaction to the chemical injected: the low pH of papaverine, which is thought to account for the burning sensation on injection, has been blamed. The nociception may be associated with tissue damage leading to fibrosis.

2. Fibrosis resulting from scar tissue produced by the trauma of repeated needle puncture.
3. Thrombosis in cavernosal tissues.

Experimental work in monkeys has demonstrated that fibrosis occurs at the site of injection, and smooth muscle hypertrophy is found throughout the corpora on repeated papaverine injection (Abozeid et al 1987).

IIVD using prostaglandin E1 appears to result in lower rates of nodule formation, suggesting that nodules are more likely to be the result of a drug effect than repeated trauma of needle puncture (Stackl et al 1988; Schramek et al 1990).

Delayed ejaculation. It is not uncommon for patients using IIVD to describe delayed ejaculation and in some cases to complain of inability to achieve ejaculation. This phenomenon has also been reported with the use of vacuum devices (Riley 1990; see Ch. 12). Two processes are likely to be involved:

1. Premature ejaculation commonly accompanies erectile dysfunction (Bancroft 1989). Anxiety induced premature ejaculation will show an improvement when the anxiety which surrounds erectile failure is diminished by effective treatment. A significant therapeutic effect on premature ejaculation in the man with psychogenic erectile dysfunction occurs with the use of limited IIVD (Gregoire 1991a). Indeed this therapeutic effect is better maintained at follow-up than that on erectile function.
2. IIVD treatment (and the use of vacuum devices) permits the patient to achieve erections in the absence of physical stimulation and sexual arousal. In men who have been sexually inactive for some time (as indeed many patients have), the habit and pleasures of engaging in foreplay may have been forgotten. In such situations it is not surprising that attempted intercourse without prior physical and psychological stimulation can lead to very delayed or absent ejaculation. Patients should be warned at the outset that these treatments only provide erections; achieving the arousal needed for sexual satisfaction is still up to the patient and his partner.

Priapism. Priapism can be defined as prolonged erection in the absence of continued sexual stimulation. There is little agreement about the exact meaning of 'prolonged' in this context or the amount of time which should be allowed before a detumescence procedure is carried out.

Two types of priapism are defined according to haemodynamic conditions in the corpora: stasis priapism and high flow priapism. Necrosis of cavernosal tissue in cases where stasis priapism has persisted for over 24 hours has been demonstrated (Spycher & Hauri 1986). In contrast, high flow priapism may last for days without any discernible tissue effects. Although the functional significance of such histological changes is not entirely clear, a significant risk of impotence undoubtedly accompanies such tissue damage. The necrosis seen in stasis priapism is a result of tissue hypoxia and is associated with pain. High flow priapism is generally painless (Spycher & Hauri 1986). It is at present not clear whether iatrogenic priapism following IIVD is predominantly of the high flow or stasis type, although blood gas studies suggest hypoxemia after 4 hours (Virag 1985). Cases of deterioration in erectile function have been reported following iatrogenic priapism lasting more than 12 hours (Girdley et al 1988; Virag 1985). However, many patients describe no such deterioration — in one case I have seen, this applied even after 36 hours. Recommendations regarding the maximum time which should be allowed to elapse before detumescence is carried out vary from 4 to 12 hours. Given the evidence cited above, allowing durations of greater than 12 hours would seem unwise and patients should always be advised to seek detumescence immediately should the prolonged erection become painful.

Treatment of iatrogenic priapism. This can be undertaken by the clinic prescribing the IIVD treatment but patients should always be told to seek rapid treatment at a suitable centre local to wherever they may be at the time. Because some accident and emergency departments are still unaware of the appropriate treatment for this condition, patients should be given an instruction sheet for doctors which they can take with them (see Appendix 11.1).

The first step involves aspiration of blood from the corpora to relieve intracavernous pressure.

Table 11.2 Drugs used in the treatment of iatrogenic priapism.

Drug	Recommended dose	Reference
Phenylephrine	10 mg	Sidi et al 1986
Metaraminol	1–2 mg	Brindley 1984
Adrenaline	15 µg	Sidi et al 1986
Dopamine	not specified	Lue & Tanagho 1987

This will also relieve pain and may be sufficient in itself to achieve adequate detumescence. A 23 gauge butterfly needle is inserted into the corpus cavernosum and blood removed until flaccidity is achieved. The removal of 60 ml of blood can be alarming to the patient who should be reassured. If this is not successful in producing detumescence, a vasoconstrictor agent can be administered through the same needle. Drugs which have been used for this purpose are listed in Table 11.2. As these drugs may have hypertensive effects when released into the general circulation, they should be administered gradually with simultaneous monitoring of blood pressure.

Should the procedure be unsuccessful, it can be repeated after one hour. Persistent priapism after this will require a shunting procedure.

Outcome

Studies of outcome with IIVD treatment are based on follow-ups of clinic populations and are usually retrospective. All use different, sometimes undefined measures of outcome in uncontrolled series of patients. Few provide sufficient information about the aetiologies and none clearly defines inclusion criteria. Furthermore, most studies fail to specify the severity of the dysfunction at baseline. Possibly most importantly, the period of follow-up in most of these studies is inadequate. Thus firm conclusions about the effectiveness, acceptability and benefits of IIVD are difficult to make. Nevertheless an examination of the best of the available data (Table 11.3) yields some useful generalizations.

1. Effectiveness of IIVD in inducing erection

Between 75% and 89% of patients respond to IIVD at some dose with an adequate erection (Sidi 1988; Brindley 1986). Clearly, these results

depend on the type of cases being treated in the clinics concerned. The type of drug used and the maximum dosage tried would also affect the results.

2. Reliability of response

It is becoming increasingly apparent that a proportion of patients using IIVD experience an unreliable and unpredictable erectile response. In some patients this becomes so problematic that they can no longer continue with treatment. This may be because of the frustration of repeated failure to respond or due to episodes of priapism or both. Presumably, such individuals, for reasons currently unknown, have a very small therapeutic window, above which priapism occurs and below which the response is inadequate. Alternatively, another powerful and variable factor may be influencing the response. Known factors which may alter the response to intercavernosal injections from one occasion to another include severe anxiety and smoking. In a few cases, an apparent unreliability in response is in fact caused by the patient's ability to inject the correct dose in the correct place each time. Thus a clinic assessment of the patient's injection and preparation technique should be carried out. Unreliability of response appears to be restricted to IIVD using papaverine and has not yet been described in patients using prostaglandin E1.

Similarly, decreased effectiveness of papaverine over time has also been described. It is not clear whether this is due to tolerance developing or gradual deterioration in the underlying pathology. The latter explanation is suggested by the fact that it is patients with organic pathology rather than psychogenic dysfunction who most commonly experience this effect.

Continued use at follow-up

In the order of 40–50% of patients continue to use injections when followed up for nine months or more (Watters et al 1988; Lakin 1990). The reasons for discontinuing use are only documented in a few studies. They appear to be variable and numerous, but mainly related to side effects rather than a dissatisfaction with effectiveness. In a study

Table 11.3   Outcome studies of treatment with intracavernosal injections of vasoactive drugs. (From Gregoire 1992)

Authors	Sample/aetiology	Treatment	Outcome criteria	Results	Follow-up
Cameron & Woodruff 1985	13 'intractable 3 diabetic	Papaverine + phentolamine	'Excellent results' 'No longer needed injections after course of 6'	11/13 4/13	Not specified
Zorgniotti & Lefleur 1985	62 vascular	Papaverine + phentolamine	Coitus at home (within 2 hrs of clinic injection) Coitus using injections: >12 months <12 months	59/62 5/18 13/18	1 year
Sidi et al 1986	100 organic	Papaverine + phentolamine	Responded to injection Chose autoinjections Refused autoinjections	83/100 66/83 17/83	1–8 months
Brindley 1986	127 mixed aetiology	Phenoxybenzamine, papaverine	Stiff enough for coitus Chose autoinjection Stopped autoinjection Stopped autoinjection because of improvement Decreased effectiveness	113/127 73/113 19/73 3/19 (all 'incomplete' impotence) 4/113	1–3 years
Kiely et al 1987b	29 psychogenic 38 organic	Papaverine + phentolamine in clinic	*Psychogenic:* Returned for follow-up Return of erectile function *Organic:* Returned for follow-up Return of erectile function for: 1 month 1 week	24/29 19/24 35/38 4/35 14/35	Not specified
Williams et al 1987	23 psychogenic 102 organic	Autoinjection, papaverine + phentolamine	Returned potency Stopped use Lost partner	11/125 20/125 5/125	1–24 months
Girdley et al 1988	78 mixed specified Selected for 'appropriateness for autoinjection'	Autoinjection, papaverine + phentolamine	Postal questionnaire	Very satisfied: 9/76 Satisfied: 20/76 Acceptable: 15/76 Not acceptable: 22/76	1–27 months
Sidi et al 1988	170 organic	Autoinjection, drug not specified	*Overall:* Satisfied Neutral Dissatisfied *Penile rigidity:* Satisfied Neutral Dissatisfied *Duration:* Satisfied Neutral Dissatisfied	78.2% 13.0% 8.8% 75.3% 16.3% 8.4% 80.0% 12.0% 8.0%	11.6 ± 6.5 months
Watters et al 1988	62 organic 32 psychogenic 30 mixed	Phenoxybenzamine/ papaverine + phentolamine	Continued treatment: 'Cured' 'Nearly cured'	42.0% 4/62} all 4/62} psychogenic	3–21 months
Ishii et al 1989	135 Psychogenic & organic	Prostaglandin E1 20 mg	Erection: Complete Incomplete Tumescence None	83 (62%) 33 (24%) 12 (9%) 7 (5%)	None
Lakin et al 1990	100 Self-selected Mixed Mainly organic	Papaverine ± phentolamine	Continued use Discontinued use: Reason unknown Inadequate erection Improved	50/100 50/100 21/50 13/50 3/50	0–20 months

of 62 men by Watters et al (1988), 25 out of 62 discontinued treatment at a mean follow-up of nine months. In 4 cases this was because they considered themselves 'cured'. Tolerance accounted for 8 drop outs, priapism for 3, haematomas 5, and 5 patients discontinued because they simply did not like the treatment. In the study by Girdley et al (1988), follow-up of between 1 and 27 months revealed that 22 out of 78 patients had discontinued treatment, 13 because of poor health, 7 because the partner was dissatisfied and 2 because of fibrosis.

Acceptability and satisfaction with the treatment

Overall satisfaction rates with IIVD vary from 58 to 78% (Girdley et al 1988; Sidi et al 1988). Satisfaction or acceptability are generally measured in simple ways using 3 or 4 point scales and can do no more than give an overall impression that the treatment seems reasonably acceptable to the majority of patients, although a substantial minority are not satisfied with the treatment. It should be remembered that these satisfaction rates are assessed in the context of there being little else on offer for many of these patients.

Sexual functioning and satisfaction

Virtually no attempt has been made to assess in any reliable way the effects on the man's general sexual functioning and satisfaction or indeed his partner's. Assessment of these features of outcome demands the use of standardized instruments, such as those discussed in Chapter 7. As improvement in sexual satisfaction for a couple is the ultimate goal of any treatment for sexual dysfunction, research examining this central aspect of outcome is now overdue.

TOPICAL DRUGS

Since intracavernosal injections of vasodilators have obvious drawbacks, more 'user friendly' methods of administration have been investigated. That topical application to the penis led to erections adequate for sexual intercourse was first noted by Talley & Crawley (1985) in a patient using transdermal nitrate patches for angina. The patient had tried applying the patches to the penile shaft and found a beneficial effect on erections. Unfortunately, his wife developed a severe headache following intercourse due to the transvaginal absorption of the drug. As a result of this side effect, the authors state that they 'personally doubt that further research in this area will be done'.

Undaunted by this statement, Morales et al (1988) conducted a double-blind placebo-controlled cross-over study of nitroglycerine paste administered to the penis in 30 subjects with erectile failure. The severities and aetiologies of their problems are not described. They measured erectile response to erotic videos using a polygraph starting 10 minutes after application of the paste. In 75% of subjects the quality of erection was at least 50% better with active compared to placebo paste. The level of statistical significance of these findings is not reported. The study did not go on to examine the effects of nitroglycerine paste used with either masturbation or sexual activity with a partner. However, the authors state that further work is planned.

Using ultrasound measurements of penile arterial diameter, Heaton et al (1990) demonstrated dilation in impotent men in response to topical glyceryltrinitrate administration.

I have seen one patient who gets a satisfactory response from spraying the penis with sublingual glyceryl trinitrate spray.

These limited results suggest that topical vasodilators may have a role to play in treating some men with impotence. The problem of transvaginal absorption by the partner could possibly be overcome by the man wearing a condom. This might, of course, have a detrimental effect on erections, as it does in many men, which might eliminate the beneficial effect of the nitrates. Formal testing of this possibility is required. Further investigation of the topical route for the administration of vasodilators is clearly warranted, as it provides a simple and more acceptable alternative to the injected route.

ORAL DRUGS

Three groups of oral drugs have been identified as potentially valuable in the treatment of impotence: alpha$_2$-adrenoceptor antagonists, opiate antagonists and the dopamine agonist, bromocriptine. None of these is yet in common clinical use for the treatment of impotence. The correction of endocrine abnormalities is considered on p. 180.

Alpha$_2$-adrenoceptor antagonists

This group of drugs, which includes idazoxan and yohimbine, appears to have significant facilitatory effects on human penile sensation and on the erectile response to physical stimulation when tested on men with normal erectile function (Murphy & Brindley, personal communication). The action of these drugs on sexual function appears to be mediated largely by their central alpha$_2$-adrenoceptor blocking effects (see Ch. 5). No clinical studies of idazoxan treatment have yet been reported, but several publications have examined the therapeutic effects of yohimbine, mainly using subjective measures in clinical trials. One study has measured erectile response in normal men objectively using plethysmography to monitor penile circumference with or without visual erotic stimulation (Danjou et al 1988). In this double-blind, placebo-controlled experiment, yohimbine did not significantly alter the responses.

Several randomized, double-blind, placebo-controlled trials of yohimbine in impotent men have been reported. Reid et al (1987) claimed significant improvement in erections with yohimbine in 48 subjects with psychogenic impotence. They used a fixed dose of 18 mg and continued treatment for 10 weeks. A response latency of 2–3 weeks was noted in this study. This is difficult to explain as it is not compatible with the known effects of yohimbine, nor was the frequency of administration such as to allow drug accumulation. Although the overall response rate to yohimbine was 46% (compared to 15% placebo), the restoration of erections adequate for penetration only occurred in 25% (5% in placebo group). Somewhat confusingly, results from the same study have been published elsewhere without reference to this paper (Morales et al 1988). Results for an unspecified number of men with organic impotence given the same treatment are also described. In these subjects no significant improvement with yohimbine compared to placebo occurred.

Using a similar design, Susset et al (1989) studied the response to yohimbine in 82 men with impotence of various aetiologies. Instead of using a fixed dose, they titrated the dose according to response (in both active and placebo groups) up to a maximum dose of 43.2 mg daily over a one month period. 65% of subjects reported no improvement on active treatment; 21% noted some response and 14% reported restoration of full and sustained erections. Only 3 subjects reported a response to placebo. The proportion that this represents is unclear because the study used a partial cross-over design and the number of subjects receiving placebo was not stated.

The authors carried out a useful comparison of responders versus non-responders with respect to a number of baseline variables. Factors significantly improving outcome included: self-reported duration of dysfunction of less than 2 years, normal penile-brachial index and high-normal testosterone levels.

The double-blind multicentre trial conducted by Riley et al (1989) obtained data on 61 men with impotence of various aetiologies randomized to yohimbine or placebo. The daily dose used (16.2 mg) was slightly less than that given by Reid et al (18 mg). By 8 weeks, a significant increase in the number of men experiencing adequate stimulated erections was noted in the active treatment group compared to those taking placebo. Furthermore, on crossing over from placebo to yohimbine the number of subjects experiencing adequate stimulated erections increased significantly compared to the group changing from yohimbine to placebo. The proportion of men experiencing this improvement was in the order of 30–40%. No change was found in sexual interest or non-stimulated erections. The latter observation is important and confirms the physiological data presented by Danjou et al (1988) described above.

In another double-blind cross-over study of yohimbine vs. placebo in 40 patients, 11 of 33 patients (33%) who completed the study reported improvement of erectile function on yohimbine alone; 5 of 33 (15%) responded while taking both yohimbine and placebo and 5 of 33 (15%) responded to placebo alone. 12 of 33 (36%) reported no response to either. Of 215 impotent patients subsequently treated with yohimbine, 38% reported some subjective improvement, but only 5% were 'satisfied' with treatment (Sonda et al 1990).

Follow-up data are not available from any of these studies. Despite the statistical significance of the results, the proportion of men showing a significant improvement is not substantial. Thus, the results obtained to date do not give rise to much optimism about the therapeutic impact of this treatment. However, more work on dosage and regimes is warranted as the effects on receptors appear to alter with increasing dosages (see Ch. 5).

Few side effects have so far been reported. Minor increases in blood pressure occur in a few patients. Probably the most common side effect is anxiety, although agitation and even manic symptoms have been described with the use of yohimbine (Charney et al 1982, 1983; Price et al 1984). Dizziness, headaches, nausea and even vomiting have also been reported (Susset et al 1989). These disappear when the drug is discontinued.

Opiate antagonists

The fact that opiate agonists depress sexual function in both sexes (Mintz et al 1974) has stimulated much research into the role of opiates in the control of mammalian sexual behaviour. Opiate antagonists have been found to block the opiate induced decreases in male rat sexual activity (Gessa et al 1979). Furthermore, administration of both naloxone and naltrexone appears to increase sexual activity in normal male rats who have not been exposed to opiates (Myers & Baum 1979) (for a more detailed discussion, see Ch. 5).

Similar effects have been found in man. Goldstein & Hansteen (1977) found that i.v. naloxone had no effect on arousal in a normal subject. Intravenous naloxone, compared in a double-blind fashion to placebo had no significant effect on erection in normal men (Murphy et al 1990). However, the longer acting and more potent opiate antagonist, naltrexone, has been reported to produce spontaneous penile erections in normal men (Mendelson et al 1979) and produced a full return of erectile function in 6 impotent men (Goldstein 1986). Fabbri et al (1989) carried out a placebo controlled trial of naltrexone (50 mg/day) in 30 men with psychogenic impotence. Over the two week treatment period, there was a significant improvement in spontaneous erections, morning erections and frequency of full intercourse in 11 of the 15 treated patients, whereas the placebo group showed no significant change. These results suggest that there may be a tonic overactivity of central opiate pathways in some men with impotence (Fabbri et al 1989).

At 2 month post-treatment follow-up, 5 of the 15 index group showed a return to normal erectile function, but the other 10 had returned to their pre-treatment state. It is unlikely that the sustained improvement seen in these 5 subjects was due to a pharmacological effect. The proportion (30%) of subjects showing such improvement is similar to that seen in studies of other physical treatments (Gregoire 1989).

No significant side effects were reported in this relatively small study, although naltrexone is known to produce abdominal discomfort, vomiting and muscle pain in withdrawn opiate addicts (Martindale 1989). However, it is difficult to generalize side effects in this group to men with no history of opiate abuse. The effect of combining naloxone with yohimbine has been investigated in normal men (Charney & Heninger 1986). Although naloxone alone had only minimal effects on erection in 6 volunteers and yohimbine alone none at all, the combination produced a full erection lasting at least 60 minutes in all 6. Unfortunately, the combination also produced significant anxiety symptoms, casting serious doubt over the clinical usefulness of the regime as administered.

Dopamine agonists

Apomorphine, a dopamine receptor agonist, has been shown to increase penile erection in both rats and humans. (Benassi-Benelli et al 1979; Schlatter & Lal 1972; Lal et al 1984). This finding has important implications for research into dopaminergic systems, as penile erection is a relatively easily measured effect, particularly in rats. Insights into the differentiation of subtypes of dopamine receptors (Costentin et al 1983) and dopamine-opiate receptor interactions (Berendsen & Gower 1986) have been gained by exploiting this effect. The therapeutic potential of apomorphine in erectile impotence is limited by its relatively short duration of action and unpleasant side effects, including nausea, drowsiness, flushing and dizziness. Furthermore, its effects appear to be inconsistent: on repeated testing in the same subjects it produces good erections on some occasions but not on others (Murphy M, personal communication).

In a study of 9 healthy men with normal erectile function, tested with various doses of apomorphine, 7 experienced penile erections (Lal et al 1987). Only 1 out of 9 experienced erection in response to placebo. Yawning, drowsiness and nausea were common.

In a further study, this time of 28 impotent subjects, Lal et al (1989) provide clear evidence that a subgroup of men with impotence experience erection in response to apomorphine. The effect was not blocked in two patients who were on lithium treatment. As lithium inhibits dopamine-induced cyclic AMP accumulation, this finding suggests that the erectile response is mediated by D_2 receptors which are not linked to adenylate cyclase (Kebabian & Calne 1979).

In a second phase of this study, 9 subjects who responded to apomorphine were treated with bromocriptine, a longer acting dopamine agonist with mainly D_2 agonist effects. 6 of the 9 subjects reported improvement in potency. This encouraging result differed from previous studies of the effects of bromocriptine in impotence (Ambrosi et al 1977; Legros et al 1980). Hitherto, only subjects with hyperprolactinaemia had been found to respond to treatment (Thorner et al 1974).

The favourable response rate in the study reported by Lal et al (1989) is likely to be a consequence of the selection of subjects who responded to apomorphine. In addition, the authors suggest that the doses of bromocriptine used in previous studies may have been too high. Higher doses of apomorphine and bromocriptine have been shown to be less effective in inducing erection than lower doses (Holmgren et al 1985, Costentin et al 1983). Furthermore, 4 men with Parkinson's disease in whom impotence was induced by increasing doses of bromocriptine were described by Cleeves & Findley (1987). The likely explanation for this effect is that both apomorphine and bromocriptine have effects on different DA receptors at different concentrations (Kebabian & Calne 1979). The stimulant effect on D_2 receptors

which occurs only at lower doses can therefore be postulated as mediating the positive effect on erections (for a more detailed discussion, see Ch. 5).

Thus it appears that response to apomorphine might be useful in predicting beneficial response to bromocriptine treatment in a subgroup of impotent men. If this approach is to be used clinically patients must obviously be warned of the substantial risk of nausea and vomiting for up to 30 minutes after such a test injection is given.

ENDOCRINE TREATMENT

Endocrine treatments differ from those described above in that their aim is to correct an abnormality which may be the cause of the erectile dysfunction; they are not simply a method of inducing erections.

Hypogonadism

Although there is a popular notion amongst many patients and some clinicians that testosterone can be used as a treatment for erectile problems, irrespective of documented hypogonadism, evidence from trials indicates this is not the case (Benkert et al 1979; O'Carrol & Bancroft 1984). Although erectile dysfunction does not appear to respond to testosterone treatment, there is some evidence that loss of sexual interest does.

The evidence for an improvement in erections in men with documented hypogonadism is more conclusive. Again it is clear that sexual interest improves within two weeks of androgen replacement and that this effect can be reversed by subsequent androgen withdrawal (Davidson et al 1979). Furthermore, this effect has been shown to be dose related (O'Carrol et al 1985). Erectile response measured by nocturnal penile tumescence has been shown to respond to androgen replacement (Kwan et al 1983; O'Carrol et al 1985). However, when erections in response to internal and external erotic stimuli have been considered, the results have been inconsistent. Although Bancroft & Wu (1983) noted effects on erections occurring in response to erotic fantasy, Kwan et al 1983 were unable to demonstrate any such effects.

Despite the current scanty evidence for the effectiveness of androgen replacement for erectile failure specifically, it is an appropriate treatment for men with hypogonadism, particularly if this is accompanied by diminished sexual interest. Before commencing androgen replacement, prostatic carcinoma should always be excluded as this malignancy is androgen dependent. Benign prostatic enlargement may also be increased, leading to obstructive symptoms which may require cessation of therapy. Testosterone can be given in a number of forms, which can broadly be divided into longer acting injectable preparations and sublingual or oral preparations. Transdermal patches may become available in the future. In general, depot injectable preparations containing esterified testosterone derivatives are preferable for replacement therapy. Shorter acting forms, such as testosterone propionate, require injection two to three times a week and may be appropriate when initiating therapy in elderly patients with some prostatic enlargement, as withdrawal can be achieved quickly if obstructive symptoms occur. For maintenance therapy, longer acting preparations, such as testosterone enanthate or preparatory mixtures of testosterone esters, can be administered every three to six weeks. Oral preparations such as mesterolone are generally more acceptable to patients but are absorbed erratically.

In addition to the contraindication of prostatic carcinoma, prescribers should be cautious if there is any history or evidence of hepatic impairment, as hepatic toxicity has been described with some preparations, although esterified derivatives and mesterolone appear to be less hepatotoxic (Wilson & Griffin 1982). Sodium and fluid retention may cause problems when treating patients with heart failure. It is worth warning patients that they may experience a decrease in testicular size which is caused by the depression of gonadotrophin release.

Hyperprolactinaemia

In a large proportion of patients with hyperprolactinaemia the deficiency is the result of the side effects of drugs such as phenothiazines or methyldopa. In such cases, the first line pharmacological intervention is obviously to reduce or change the medication wherever possible. The other main cause of hyperprolactinaemia is the benign prolactin secreting pituitary adenoma. Unless such adenomas are large, treatment with bromocriptine is preferred to surgery and is usually effective.

Cunningham et al (1982) have demonstrated impaired nocturnal penile tumescence in hyperprolactinaemic men. This improves with bromocriptine treatment (Marrama et al 1984) and there is also evidence that stimulated erectile function may improve (Thorner et al 1974).

SUMMARY

The development of effective pharmacological means of inducing erections has revolutionized the treatment of erectile dysfunction, but has in no way produced a panacea.

The most widely used of these developments is the intracavernosal injection of vasoactive drugs. The effectiveness of this method of inducing erections is unquestionable but its acceptability and side effects with long term use make development of more 'user friendly' treatments desirable. At present three main groups of oral treatments have been studied: alpha$_2$-adrenoceptor antagonists, such as yohimbine; opiate antagonists, such as naltrexone; and the dopamine antagonist, bromocriptine. More positive data on the effects of these preparations are required before their more widespread use can be recommended. Current evidence on the use of topical vasodilators suggests that these may be an adequate treatment option in a subgroup of men with erectile problems.

The use of endocrine treatments is only appropriate in cases of documented hormonal abnormality.

APPENDIX 11.1

Treatment of iatrogenic priapism – Guidance notes for doctors:
- The following technique is usually successful in producing detumescence.
- If unsuccessful the procedure can be repeated after one hour.
- Normal aseptic technique should be employed.
- You will need:

– 1 ml (10 mg) ampoule of phenylephrine (an alpha-adrenergic agent).
– 1 ml syringe, filled with 0.5 ml (5 mg) of phenylephrine. (Metaraminol 2 mg may also be used if phenylephrine is not available).
– 60 ml syringe
– 21–23 gauge butterfly needle.
1. Insert butterfly needle into either corpus cavernosum as shown (using usual aseptic technique and avoiding superficial veins).

2. Withdraw 40–60 ml of blood using syringe (this will usually relieve any pain).
3. Inject 1 mg phenylephrine, monitor blood pressure. If no hypertension inject further 4 mg (ie: total 5 mg).
4. Massage the penis gently (often painful).
5. Observe patient for at least one hour after (P + BP).
6. Discharge if all well.
7. Advise no further intracavernosal injections until patient has consulted this clinic.

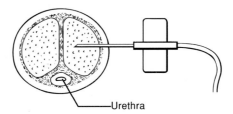
—Urethra

REFERENCES

Abozeid M, Juenemann K P, Luo J A, Lue T F, Yen T S B, Tanagho E A, 1987 Chronic papaverine treatment: the effect of repeated injections on the simian erectile response and penile tissue. Journal of Urology 138: 1263

Ambrosi B, Bara R, Travaglini P, Weber G, Beck Peccoz P, Rondena M, Elli R, Faglia G 1977 Study of the effects of bromocriptine on sexual impotence. Clinical Endocrinology 7: 417–421

Bancroft J 1989 Human sexuality and its problems, 2nd edn. Churchill Livingstone, Edinburgh

Bancroft J, Wu F C W 1983 Changes in erectile responsiveness during androgen therapy. Archives of Sexual Behaviour 12: 59–66

Benassi-Benelli A, Ferrari F, Pellegrini-Quarantotti B 1979 Penile erection induced by apomorphine and N-n-propyl-noraporphine in rats. Archives of International Pharmacodynamic Therapy 242: 241–247

Benkert O, Witt W, Adam W, Leitz A 1979 Effects of testosterone undecanoate on sexual potency and the hypothalamic-pituitary-gonadal axis of impotent males. Archives of Sexual Behaviour 8: 471–480

Berendsen H H G, Gower A J, 1986 Opiate-androgen interactions in drug-induced yawning and penile erections in the rat. Neuroendocrinology 42: 185–190

Brindley G S 1983 Cavernosal alpha-blockade: a new technique for investigating and treating erectile impotence. British Journal of Psychiatry 143: 332–337

Brindley G S 1984 New treatment for priapism. Lancet ii: 220–221

Brindley G S 1986 Maintenance treatment of erectile impotence by cavernosal unstriated muscle relaxant injection. British Journal of Psychiatry 149: 210–215

Brindley G S 1987 Treatment of erectile impotence by intracavernosal injection. Recent Advances in Urology/Andrology 263–267

Cameron L, Woodruff P 1985 Cavernosal alpha blockade: a treatment for erectile impotence. British Journal of Psychiatry 147: 107

Charney D S, Heninger G 1986 Alpha$_2$-adrenergic and opiate receptor blockade. Archives of General Psychiatry 43: 1037–1041

Charney D S, Heninger G R, Redmond D E Jr 1983 Yohimbine induced anxiety and increased noradrenergic function in humans: effects of diazepam and clonidine. Life Sciences 33: 19–29

Charney D S, Heninger G R, Sternberg D E 1982 Assessment of alpha2-adrenergic autoregulator function in humans: effects of oral yohimbine. Life Sciences 30: 2033–2041

Cleeves L, Findley L J 1987 Bromocriptine induced impotence in Parkinson's disease. British Medical Journal 295: 367–368

Costentin J, Dubuc I, Protais P 1983 Behavioural data suggesting the plurality of central dopamine receptors. In: Mangel P, Defeudis F V (eds) CNS receptors — from molecular pharmacology to behaviour. Raven Press, New York

Cunningham G R, Karacan I, Ware J C, Lantz C D, Thornby J I 1982 The relationship between serum testosterone and prolactin levels and nocturnal penile tumescence (NPT) in impotent men. Journal of Andrology 3: 241–247

Danjou P, Alexandre L, Warot D, Lacomblez L, Puech A J 1988 Assessment of erectogenic properties of apomorphine and yohimbine in man. British Journal of Clinical Pharmacology 26(6): 733–739

Davidson J M, Camargo C A, Smith E R 1979 Effects of androgens on sexual behaviour of hypogonadal men. Journal of Clinical Endocrinology and Metabolism 48: 955–958

Fabbri A, Jannini E A, Gnessi L, Moretti C, Ulisse S, Franzese A et al 1989 Endorphins in male impotence: evidence for naltrexone stimulation of erectile activity in patient therapy. Psychoneuroendocrinology 141(1, 2): 103–111

Gessa G L, Paglietti E, Pellegrini-Quarantotti B 1979 Induction of copulatory behaviour in sexually inactive rats by naloxone. Science 204: 203–205

Girdley F M, Bruskewitz R C, Feyzi J, Graversen P H, Gasser T C 1988 Intracavernous self-injection for impotence; a long-term therapeutic option? Experience in 78 patients. Journal of Urology 140: 972–974

Goldstein A, Hansteen R W 1977 Evidence against involvement of endorphin in sexual arousal and orgasm in man. Archives General Psychiatry 34: 1179–1180

Goldstein J A 1986 Erectile function and naltrexone. Annals of Internal Medicine 105(5): 799

Gregoire A 1989 Psychological implications of physical treatments for impotence. Paper presented at annual conference for Society of Psychosomatic Research: 'Mind/ Body in Sexuality and Reproduction'. London, December 1989

Gregoire A 1990 Self-injection treatment for impotence. British Medical Journal 300: 357

Gregoire A 1991a A randomised controlled trial of limited use of intra-cavernosal injections versus sex therapy in the treatment of psychogenic impotence. Psychiatric Bulletin 15: Suppl. 4: 93

Gregoire A 1992 New treatments for erectile impotence. British Journal of Psychiatry 160: 315–326

Hawton K, Catalan J 1986 Prognostic factors in sex therapy. Behaviour Research and Therapy 24: 377–385

Heaton J P W, Morales A, Owen J, Saunders F W, Fenemore J 1990 Topical glyceryltrinitrate causes measurable penile arterial dilation in impotent men. Journal of Urology 143: 729–731

Holmgren B, Urba-Holmgren R, Trucios N, Zermeno M, Eguibar J R 1985 Association of spontaneous and dopaminergic-induced yawning and penile erections in rat. Pharmacological and Biochemical Behaviour 22: 31–35

Ishii N, Watanabe H, Irisawa C, Kikuchhi Y, Kubota Y, Kawamura S, Suzuki K, Chiba R, Tokiwa M, Shirai M 1989 Intracavernous injection of prostaglandin E1 for the treatment of erectile impotence. Journal of Urology 141: 323–325

Kebabian J W, Calne D B 1979 Multiple receptors for dopamine. Nature 277: 93–96

Kiely E A, Bloom S R, Williams G 1989 Penile response to intracavernosal vasoactive intestinal polypeptide alone and in combination with other vasoactive agents. British Journal of Urology 64: 191–194

Kiely E A, Ignotus P, Williams G 1987a Penile function following intravavernosal injection of vasoactive agents or saline. British Journal of Urology 59: 473–476

Kiely E A, Williams G, Goldie L 1987b Assessment of the immediate and long-term effects of pharmacologically induced penile erections in the treatment of psychogenic and organic impotence. British Journal of Urology 59: 164–169

Kwan M, Greenleaf W J, Mann J, Crapo L, Davidson J M 1983 The nature of androgen action on male sexuality: a combined laboratory and self report study in hypogonadal men. Journal of Clinical Endocrinology and Metabolism 57: 557–562

Lakin M M, Montague D K, Vanderbrug Medendorp S, Tesar L, Schover L R 1990 Intracavernous injection therapy: analysis of results and complications. Journal of Urology 143: 1138–1141

Lal S, Ackman D, Thavundyil J N, Kiely M E, Etienne P 1984 Effect of apomorphine, a dopamine receptor agonist, on penile tumescence in normal subjects. Neuro-Psychopharmacological and Biological Psychiatry 8: 695–699

Lal S, Labyea E, Thavundayil J K, Vasavan Nair N P, Negrete J, Ackman D, Blundell P, Gardiner R J 1987 Apormorphine induced penile tumescence in impotent patients — preliminary findings. Neuro-Psychopharmacological and Biological Psychiatry 11: 235–242

Lal S, Tesfaye Y, Thavundayil J K, Thompson T R, Kiely M E, Nair N P, Grassino A, Dubrovsky B 1989 Apomorphine: clinical studies on erectile impotence and yawning. Neuro-Psychopharmacological and Biological Psychiatry 13: 329–339.

Legros J J, Chiodera P, Mormont C, Servais J 1980 A psycho-neuroendocrinological study of sexual impotence in patients with abnormal reaction to a glucose tolerance test. Advances in Biological Psychiatry 5: 117–124

Levine S B, Althof S E, Turner L A, Risen C B, Bodner D R, Kursh E D, Resnick M I 1989 Side effects of self-administration of intracavernous papaverine and phentolamine for the treatment of impotence. Journal of Urology 141: 54–57

Lue T F 1988 Office treatment — papaverine injections for impotence. In: Tanagho E A, Lue T F, McClure R D (eds) Contemporary management of impotence and infertility. Williams and Wilkins, Baltimore

Lue T F, Hellstrom W J G, McAninch J W, Tanagho E A 1986 Priapism: a refined approach to diagnosis and treatment. Journal of Urology 136: 104–108

Lue T F, Tanagho E A 1987 Physiology of erection and pharmacological management of impotence. Journal of Urology 137: 829–836

Marrama P, Carani C, Montamini V 1984 Gonadal function: sexual behaviour in bromocriptine treated men with prolactinoma. In: Segraves T, Haeberle E (eds) Emerging dimensions of sexology. Praeger, New York

Martindale 1989 Naltrexone hydrochloride. In: The extra pharmacopea, 29th edn. Pharmaceutical Press, London, p 486–7

Masters W, Johnson V 1970 Human sexual inadequacy. Little, Brown, Philadelphia

Mendelson J, Ellingboe J, Keuhnle J, Mello N 1979 Effects of naltrexone on mood and neuroendocrine function in normal adult males. Psychoneuroendocrinology 3: 231–236

Mintz J, O'Hare K, O'Brien C P, Goldschmidt J 1974 Sexual problems of heroin addicts. Archives of General Psychiatry 31: 700–703

Morales A, Condra M, Owen J A, Fenemore J, Surridge D H 1988 Oral and transcutaneous pharmacological agents for the treatment of impotence. In: Tanagho E A, Lue T F, McClure K D (eds) Contemporary management of impotence and infertility. Williams and Wilkins, Baltimore

Murphy M R, Checkley S A, Seckl J R, Lightman S L 1990 Naloxone inhibits oxytocin release at orgasm in man. Journal of Clinical Endocrinology and Metabolism 71(4): 1056–1058

Myers B M, Baum M J 1979 Facilitation by opiate antagonists of sexual performance in the male rat. Biochemical Behaviour 10: 615–618

O'Carroll R, Bancroft J 1984 Testosterone therapy for low sexual interest and erectile dysfunction in men: a controlled study. British Journal of Psychiatry 145: 146–151

O'Carroll R, Shapiro C, Bancroft J 1985 Androgens, behaviour and noctural erections in hypogonadal men: the effect of varying the replacement dose. Clinical Endocrinology 23: 527–538

Price L H, Charney D S, Heninger G R 1984 Three cases of manic symptoms following yohimbine administration. American Journal of Psychiatry 141: 1267–1268

Reid K, Morales A, Harris C, Surridge D H C, Condra M, Owen J, Fenemore J 1987 Double-blind trial of yohimbine in treatment of psychogenic impotence. Lancet i: 421–423

Riley A J, Goodman R E, Kellett J M, Orr R 1989 Double-blind trial of yohimbine hydrochloride in the treatment of erection inadequacy. Sexual and Marital Therapy 4(1): 17–26

Riley A J 1990 Erection assisting devices. British Journal of Sexual Medicine 17(6): 175–177

Schlatter E K E, Lal S 1972 Treatment of alcoholism using Dent's oral apomorphine method. Quarterly Journal for the Study of Alcoholism 33: 430–436

Schramek P, Dorninger R, Waldhauser M, Konecny P, Porpaczy P 1990 Prostaglandin E1 in erectile dysfunction. British Journal of Urology 65(i): 68–71

Sidi A A, Cameron J S, Duffy L M, Lange P H 1986 Intracavernous drug-induced erections in the management of male erectile dysfunction: experience with 100 patients. Journal of Urology 135: 704–706

Sidi A A, Reddy P A, Chen K K 1988 Patient acceptance of and satisfaction with vasoactive intracavernous pharmacotherapy for impotence. Journal of Urology 140: 293–294

Sonda L P, Mazo R, Chancellor M B 1990 The role of yohimbine for the treatment of erectile impotence. Journal of Sexual Marital Therapy 16(1): 15–21

Spycher M A, Hauri D 1986 The ultrastructure of erectile tissue in priapism. Journal of Urology 135: 142–147

Stackl W, Hasun R, Marberger M 1988 Intravacernous injection of prostaglandin E1 in impotent men. Journal of Urology 140: 66–68

Susset J G, Tessier C D, Wincze J, Bansal S, Malhotra C, Schwacha M G 1989 Effect of yohimbine hydrochloride on erectile impotence: a double-blind study. Journal of Urology 141: 1360–1363

Talley J D, Crawley I S 1985 Transdermal nitrate, penile erection and spousal headache. Annals of Internal Medicine 103(5): 804

Thorner M O, McNeilly A S, Hagan C, Besser G M 1974 Long-term treatment of galactorrhoea and hypogonadism with bromocriptine. British Medical Journal 2: 419–422

Virag R 1982 Intracavernous injection of papaverine for erectile failure. Lancet ii: 938

Virag R 1985 About pharmacologically induced prolonged erection. Lancet 1: 519

Virag R, Frydman D, Legman M, Virag H 1984 Intracavernous injection of papaverine as a diagnostic and therapeutic method in erectile failure. Angiology 35: 79–87

Watters G R, Keogh E J, Earle C M, Carati C J, Wisniewski Z S, Tulloch A G S, Lord D J 1988 Experience in the management of erectile dysfunction using the intracavernosal self-injection of vasoactive drugs. Journal of Urology 140: 1417–1419

Wespes E, Shulman C C 1988 Systemic complication of intracavernous papaverine injection in patients with venous leakage. Urology 31(2): 114–115

Williams G, Mulcahy M J, Kiely E A 1987 Impotence: treatment by autoinjection of vasoactive drugs. British Medical Journal 295: 595–596

Wilson J D, Griffin J E 1982 The use and misuse of androgens. Metabolism 29: 1278

Zorgniotti A W, Lefleur R S 1985 Autoinjection of the corpus cavernosum with a vasoactive drug combination for vasculogenic impotence. Journal of Urology 133: 39–41

12. External vacuum devices for the treatment of impotence

Alain Gregoire

There are many patients with erectile dysfunction who require a physical treatment but who are not suitable for, or do not want, IIVD or implants. Thus there will always be a role for non-invasive, non-pharmacological physical solutions to erectile failure. Effective devices which fit this description were first patented in the USA over 70 years ago (Nadig et al 1986) but have received little attention until recently. A variety of devices are now commercially available (see Appendix 12.1).

RANGE OF DEVICES

All the external vacuum devices currently avail-

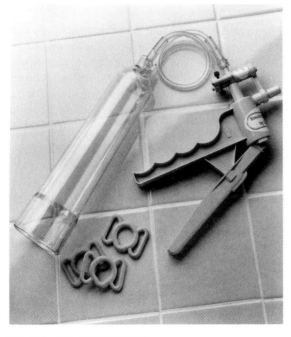

Fig. 12.1 The ErecAid device.

able work on the same basic principle: a vacuum created around the penis draws blood into the corpora, producing tumescence and some rigidity. Three of the devices, the ErecAid (Fig. 12.1) the Pos-T-Vac (Fig. 12.2) and the Active (Fig. 12.3) are very similar, differing only in details of design and appearance. They consist of a rigid plastic tube connected to a handpump at one end, and with an opening at the other end into which the flaccid penis is inserted. Before this is done, the penis and tube need to be well lubricated, and a rubber constriction band is placed around the open end of the tube.

With the penis in the tube, air is pumped out, and the resulting negative pressure draws blood into the corpora, producing an erection. Once this has been achieved, the constriction band can be slipped off the plastic tube so that it surrounds the base of the penis, limiting venous outflow. This maintains the erection and allows the release of the negative pressure and removal of the plastic tube. The constriction band can be left on for up to 30 minutes to permit intercourse, but must then be removed to restore adequate circulation of blood to the tissues.

The Correctaid system (Fig. 12.4), although working on the same principle, differs in that the device, which consists of a sheath made of transparent silicon rubber, remains on the penis during intercourse. Suction is applied by mouth to a fine tube which enters the rubber sheath at its base and passes through it to open on the inside of the tip of the sheath. The sheath is designed to fit around the erect penis and is therefore supplied in various sizes. Patients ordering the device supply the manufacturer with the length and circumference of the stretched penis.

185

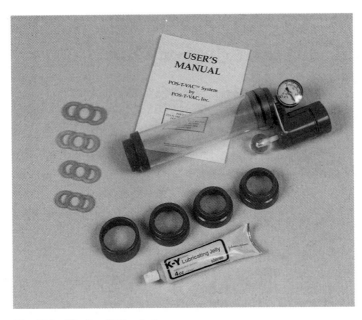

Fig. 12.2 The Pos-T-Vac device.

Several suppliers of 'marital aids' and sex shops also stock similar appliances, sometimes called 'penis developers', usually at a much lower price than the above devices. However, the effectiveness of these devices has not been formally studied. One patient attending the author's sexual problems clinic has described the successful use of the suction pipe on his vacuum cleaner. Given the varied size of such equipment and the considerable power of some vacuum cleaners, this method of achieving erections is not to be recommended.

The involvement of the clinician in the choice of device should be limited to impartial descriptions of the products, their pros and cons and, if possible, allowing the patient to see demonstration models. It is useful to provide interested patients with the information sheets available from the suppliers.

Indications

The manufacturers state that the devices are suitable for men with impotence of almost any cause, although a medical prescription or recommendation is required by some of the manufacturers. In theory, this is a responsible attitude, although there are, in fact, no useful data to guide clinicians

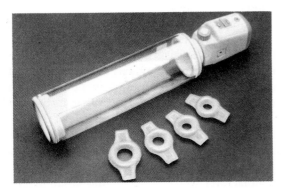

Fig. 12.3 The Active device.

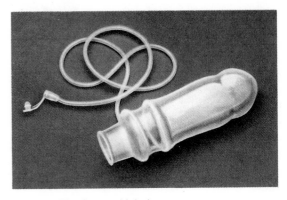

Fig. 12.4 The Correctaid device.

on appropriate indications or contraindications. Although some patients may find it difficult, or indeed impossible, to use the devices, there are no specific medical reasons why any man with impotence who would like to try such a device should not do so. Thus a major factor in selecting this form of treatment is the patient's choice in preference to the other treatments presented by the clinician.

Two specific situations in which vacuum devices may be particularly useful have been described: combination use with intracavernosal injections and the explanted penile prosthesis patient.

In a study of 22 patients who obtained only partial responses to intracavernosal injections of vasoactive drugs, Marmar et al (1988) investigated the effects of combining IIVD with the use of a vacuum constrictor device. Their findings suggest that a combination of these two treatment methods is more effective than either of the treatments alone.

Complication rates requiring explantation of penile prostheses occur at a relatively consistent rate of approximately 5% (See Ch. 14). This population presents particular problems, as they are rarely suitable for reimplantation of new prostheses and the severity of the original problem added to the tissue destruction makes it unlikely that pharmacological treatments will succeed. 14 patients who had had their penile prosthesis removed because of physical complications were offered the use of a negative pressure device in an attempt to restore erections (Moul & McLeod 1989). 11 patients agreed to try using the device at home and 10 of these reported at least satisfactory erections leading to intercourse.

The authors point out that the quality of erection and satisfaction improve with time, which they attribute to a resolution of corporeal scarring and the well documented learning curve which occurs with the use of these devices. All patients in this study commented that they would like to have been offered the vacuum devices prior to receiving their prosthesis. Although in a sense this is not surprising as their prosthesis failed, the important lesson is that all available treatments should be presented to the patients in an impartial way to allow them to make an informed choice before proceeding with any one treatment.

Usage

Although simple in principle, success with these devices does depend on a level of skill which requires instruction and practice. The manufacturers provide written instructions with each device supplied. These are generally easy to understand, clearly illustrated step-by-step guides to the safe and effective use of the devices. Back-up advice over the telephone is also available from the manufacturers. Videos which can be shown to patients are also available to professionals from the manufacturers. Alongside these forms of instruction it is essential that the clinician use a demonstration model and give a verbal account to the patient on the use and misuse of the devices. In some cases, supervision in the clinic may also be needed.

In surveys of users, the time required to master the use of these devices ranged from 1 day to 6 weeks, and from 1 to 12 practice sessions (Witherington 1989; Sidi et al 1990). It is, therefore, important to warn patients that it may take some time before good results are obtained and they should not be discouraged after the first or second unsuccessful attempt. Once the patient has become accustomed to using the device, it takes from 30 seconds to 7 minutes to achieve an adequate erection.

Outcome and patient satisfaction

The three devices described above produce erections which are generally adequate for penetration in up to 90% of men with erectile dysfunction, although this is often not a full rigid erection. Furthermore, cavernosal tissue proximal to the constriction band is not engorged by the devices and the erection obtained is frequently 'hanging' rather than 'standing up' — sometimes to the dismay of the patient.

Reports from a number of series of mainly elderly patients treated with these devices are quoted by the manufacturers, though only a proportion of these are published in medical journals (Table 12.1).

Nadig et al (1986) reported their observations of 35 men with organic impotence using a rigid cylinder/constriction band type device. Only 4 of these failed to obtain erections adequate for

Table 12.1 Outcome studies of the use of external vacuum devices.

Author	Device	Sample	Outcome	Unwanted effects
Glugla & Draznin 1988	Correctaid	15 diabetic 12 non-diabetic	100% adequate erections 82% satisfied at 3 months	Delayed ejaculation Diminished sensation
Asopa & Williams 1989	Correctaid	20 mixed aetiology, unselected	40% using at 14 months 14 months follow-up	Too complicated Diminished sensation
Nadig et al 1986	ErecAid	35 mixed organic	91% adequate erections 80% using at 10 months follow-up	Discomfort when applying vacuum Painless bruising
Wiles 1988	ErecAid	10 diabetic	100% adequate erections 6/10 regular use + improved sexual and general relationships	
Lloyd et al 1989	ErecAid	17 spinal cord injury	12/17 adequate erections 11/17 intercourse once a week or more	Bruising, discomfort
Witherington 1989	ErecAid	Postal survey of 1700 users (from a total of 15 000)	12% no response 92% adequate erections 77% intercourse > 2 weekly 58% improved self-image	37% bruising with initial use 9% pain on orgasm Pleasant orgasm in only 57%
Turner et al 1990	ErecAid	36 mixed 29 completed 6 months follow-up	89% adequate erections Improved sexual satisfaction in men & women; $p < 0.01$	Blocked ejaculation Bruising Pivoting of erections Discomfort
Korenman et al 1990	ErecAid	20 organic	19/20 adequate erections Coital frequency went from 0 to mean of between 3 & 5 per month over 6 months	No repeated problems
Sidi et al 1990	ErecAid	127 mixed	Satisfaction rate overall 68% Penile rigidity 78% Penile tumescence 83%	22% slight pain 11% moderate pain 2% severe pain & stopped 21% stopped use

intercourse. 24 (80%) of the subjects were satisfied and used the device regularly.

Wiles (1988) described results obtained by 10 diabetic men using the ErecAid device over a 3 month period. All patients achieved adequate erections. One couple were not using the device because of marital disharmony, and 3 others were dissatisfied with the device. The remaining 6 patients and their partners described improvements in both their sexual and marital relationships, as well as self-esteem, on visual analogue scales.

In the only study to allocate unselected subjects to the use of the Correctaid, Asopa & Williams (1989) describe the 'dissatisfaction' rates of over 50%. This rate appears to be higher than with the ErecAid device. Reasons for dissatisfaction resulted mainly from the need for precoital application of the device, which was seen as unnatural and time consuming. Users of the Correctaid device also complain of decreased sensation. The authors conclude that careful selection and coun-

selling of patients is essential to success with these devices.

In a prospective study, 29 of an initial 36 men completed a 6 month follow-up evaluation into the use of the ErecAid device (Turner et al 1990). Adequate erections were produced in 89% of the men and over 6 months 19% of participants dropped out. Statistically significant improvements occurred in erection quality, frequency of intercourse and patient and partner sexual satisfaction.

Unwanted effects

Adverse effects in this study included blocked ejaculation (due to compression of the urethra by the constriction ring). 10 more reported physical discomfort, and 3 men complained of occasional bruising.

The most common complaints made by patients include the devices being unnatural, difficult to use, messy and, in the case of the Correctaid, resulting in decreased sensation. Another effect often described by patients is delayed or absent ejaculation (Riley 1990). There is little mention of this phenomenon in the literature, although in the author's experience it also occurs quite commonly in patients using intracavernosal injections of vasoactive drugs and implants. It is likely that in many men this effect is due to a neglect of foreplay by patients who no longer need to be aroused to achieve erection and penetration. In some men with organic dysfunction it may also be another symptom of the underlying disorder. A problem for many patients not mentioned in these papers is the cost, which is currently high, but may drop as a result of the increase in competing products.

The use of constriction rings alone

The use of constriction rings at the base of the penis in an attempt to prevent venous outflow is probably one of the oldest ways of trying to boost erectile function. A wide variety of such devices have been used, ranging from the simple rubber band to the elaborately carved Chinese ivory rings described by Alex Comfort (1977). Currently available devices are usually made of flexible rubber, although some are made of rigid materials incorporating a hinge device. Some devices have been given an air of increased sophistication by the addition of features which are based on dubious physiological concepts, for example the Blakoe 'energizer', which has metal plates embedded in it. These are said to produce a small electrical current when in contact with the skin. Empirical evidence for the effectiveness of any of these devices is difficult to find. Cooper (1974) compared the Blakoe energizing device with a simple ring of similar appearance and found no difference between the two types of rings, although both appeared to have some beneficial effects.

SUMMARY

External vacuum devices provide a safe and generally effective method of inducing erections in men who wish to avoid the invasiveness of pharmacological or surgical treatments, and who are not suitable for, or do not wish to undertake, a course of sex therapy. A number of devices are available commercially, but with little to choose between them in terms of effectiveness. Their use has also been described in men with explanted failed penile prostheses, and in conjunction with intracavernosal injections when these alone have not given adequate results.

It is important that patients be carefully instructed in the use of these devices and warned that it often takes practice to obtain adequate results.

REFERENCES

Asopa R, Williams G 1989 Use of the 'Correctaid' device in the management of impotence. British Journal of Urology 63: 546–547

Comfort A 1978 The joy of sex. Quartet, London

Cooper A J 1974 A blind evaluation of a penile ring — a sex aid for impotent males. British Journal of Psychiatry 124: 402–406

Glugla M, Draznin B 1988 Treatment of impotence with vacuum-operated erection assistance device. Diabetes Care II: 445–446

Katz P G, Haden H T, Mulligan T, Zasler N 1990 The effect of vacuum devices on penile hemodynamics. Journal of Urology 143: 55–56

Korenman S G, Viosca S P, Kaiser E, Mooradian A D, Morley J E 1990 Use of a vacuum tumescence device in the management of impotence. Journal of the American Geriatrics Society 38: 217–220

Lloyd E E, Toth L L, Perkash I 1989 Vacuum tumescence: an option for spinal cord injured males with erectile dysfunction. Spinal Cord Injury Nursing 6(2): 25–28

Marmar J L, DeBenedictis T J, Praiss D E 1988 The use of a vacuum constrictor device to augment a partial erection following an intracavernous injection. Journal of Urology 140: 975–979

Moul J W, McLeod D G 1989 Negative pressure devices in the explanted penile prosthesis population. Journal of Urology 142: 729–731

Nadig P W, Catesby-Ware J, Blumoff R 1986 Noninvasive device to produce and maintain an erection–like state. Urology 27(2): 126–131

Riley A J 1990 Erection assisting devices. British Journal of Sexual Medicine 17(6): 175–177

Sidi A, Becher E F, Zhang G, Lewis J H 1990 Patient acceptance of and satisfaction with an external negative pressure device for impotence. Journal of Urology 144: 1154–1156

Turner L A, Althof S E, Levine S B, Tobias T R, Kursh E D, Bodner D, Resnick M I 1990 Treating erectile dysfunction with external vacuum devices: impact upon sexual, psychological and marital functioning. Journal of Urology 144: 79–82

Wiles P G 1988 Successful non-invasive management of erectile impotence in diabetic men. British Medical Journal 296: 161–162

Witherington R 1989 Vacuum constriction device for management of erectile impotence. Journal of Urology 141: 320–322

APPENDIX 12.1

Distributors of external vacuum devices.

ErecAid

UK: Cory Bros Co. Ltd
      4 Dollis Park
      London N3 1HG
      UK

USA: Osbon Medical Systems Ltd
      1253 Broad Street
      Augusta, Georgia 30901
      USA

Australia & New Zealand:
      Impotec
      Unit 19, Second Floor
      6 Campbell Street
      Artarmon, Sydney, NSW 2064
      Australia

Pos -T-Vac

UK: EuroSurgical Ltd
      The Common
      Cranleigh, GU6 8LU
      UK

Correctaid

USA: Synergist Institute Inc.
      1610 Fannin, Suite 100
      Houston,
      Texas 77030
      USA

UK & elsewhere:
      Genesis Medical Ltd
      Freepost WD 1242
      London NW3 4YR
      UK

Active

USA (known as 'Plus'):
      Osbon Medical Systems
      1246 Jones St.
      Augusta, Georgia 30901
      USA

UK & elsewhere:
      Genesis Medical Ltd
      Freepost WD 1242
      London NW3 4YR
      UK

13. Surgical procedures to correct erectile dysfunction

John P. Pryor

This chapter deals with surgical procedures to overcome erectile dysfunction. These are mainly concerned with techniques to improve the quality of erection, but first it is useful to cover those techniques which alleviate the conditions listed in Table 8.1 (p. 107).

Phimosis and tight frenulum

A tight frenulum is the cause of pain on erection and may even tear, sometimes with a worrying amount of bleeding. It is sufficient to divide the band transversely under local anaesthesia and sew the wound up longitudinally. Phimosis, and following a paraphimosis, is treated by circumcision.

Table 13.1 Outcome of Nesbit procedure to correct an erectile deformity of congenital origin in 63 men.

		Preoperative	Postoperative
Quality of erection:	normal	59	60
	impaired	4	3
Degree of curvature:	<15°	1	56
	16–30°	15	5
	>15°	47	2
Sexual intercourse:	normal	0	44
	impaired	20	8
	impossible	18	0
	untried	25	11
Mental state:	suicidal	3	1
	depressed	18	3
	severely embarrassed	17	11
	anxious about future sexual performance	21	4
	normal	19	48

Penile curvature

Penile curvature that is associated with hypospadias is best treated by excision of the chordee and reconstruction of the urethra. All other forms of erectile curvature are best treated by the Nesbit technique (Nesbit 1965; Bailey et al 1985; Bailey & Pryor 1987), in which an ellipse of tunica albuginea is excised from the convex side of the curvature of the penis. Excision of small plaques of Peyronie's disease was recommended by Devine & Horton (1974) but often gives disappointing results (Melman & Holland 1978).

The results obtained with the Nesbit technique in congenital deformities and Peyronie's disease are shown in Tables 13.1 and 13.2. It should be noted that some men with only a slight congenital deformity will require surgical correction as they are afraid that they will be ridiculed by a partner. Medical help had been sought by 21 of the 63 men with congenital erectile deformities and 3 of the men had been 'suicidal'. It is rare for a married man with the acquired erectile deformity

Table 13.2 Results of Nesbit procedure in 174 men with Peyronie's disease.

Outcome	Number	
Excellent: normal sexual function, residual deformity <15°	93	(53%)
Moderate: some impairment of erection or deformity 15°–30°; coitus possible	32	(19%)
Poor: absent erection or deformity >30° coitus impossible	49	(28%)

The poor results increased from 12% at 3 months to 28% at 4 years.

of Peyronie's disease to undergo surgery for a bend of less than 45°. In general, the poor results stem from those men with a poor quality of erection and such patients should be offered the implantation of a penile prosthesis if the problem is vasculogenic in origin — as it often is. The selection of patients for the Nesbit procedure has been facilitated by the use of diagnostic intracorporeal papaverine and colour Doppler ultrasonography.

Satisfactory results were reported in 95% of 186 patients with Peyronie's disease who had undergone prosthetic implants in 12 reported series (Bailey & Pryor 1987).

It is worth mentioning one other congenital erectile deformity. There is a group of men who obtain a stiff erection but the penis does not lie in the normal position due to the lack of the suspensory ligament. Coitus is difficult and the penis has to be placed into the vagina and tends to slip out. Such patients find it difficult to describe the abnormality and it is necessary for the clinician to have a high index of suspicion. The problem may be corrected by placing nonabsorbable sutures between the tunica albuginea of the penis and the symphysis pubis (Pryor & Hill 1979).

ABNORMALITIES OF PENILE SIZE

Some men are born without a penis and the tendency is for them to be reared as girls. There are other men who lose their penis through accidents, or self-mutilation, infection or tumour. Surgical techniques to construct a phallus are difficult. The standard procedure was that of Gillies & Harrison (Gillies & Harrison 1963) which required five procedures. Complications were common and the results often unsatisfactory. I currently use a one stage pubic phalloplasty using the suprapubic skin. Complications still occur but the patients require shorter hospitalization. Coitus is possible and a penile prosthesis may be inserted if necessary (Fig. 13.1).

Some men have a small penis and the glans may be less than 1 cm in diameter; this is often associated with a hypospadias (Fig. 8.1). Mobilization of the crura from the symphysis pubis (Johnson 1974) may give an extra 1–2 cm in length, which is of significance when the penis has a stretched length of 5 cm. In addition, the use of skin flaps

for the urethral reconstruction and the altered position of the penis to the anterior abdominal wall all contribute to a larger appearance (Fig. 8.2). Most men complaining of a small penis would be able to have intercourse normally were it not for their dissatisfaction. Such men are difficult to treat and often fail to respond to psychological help.

In marked contrast, some men present with a penis that is too large. This is usually the result of lymphoedema and penetration is difficult. It is possible to excise the redundant thickened tissue and remodel the penis to a more normal size and one where vaginal penetration and coitus is possible.

VASCULAR ABNORMALITIES

The role of vascular surgery to overcome impotence is the subject of much debate. Sharlip

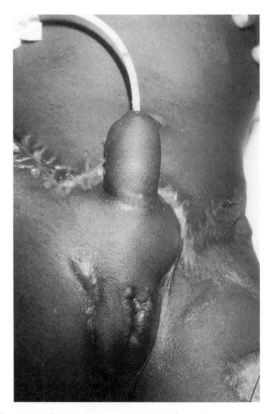

Fig. 13.1 Postoperative photograph of a phalloplasty procedure in a 10-year-old boy who suffered the loss of his penis in a road accident.

(1991) focused on this at the International Society for Impotence Research in his talk entitled 'The incredible results of penile vascular surgery'. Some results are too good to believe and many of the methodological problems stem from the lack of objective assessment of the cause of impotence. The only objective way to exclude a psychogenic cause for the problem is to demonstrate impaired nocturnal penile tumescence, with all the problems of methodology and interpretation which this test entails (Ch. 9). It is not sufficient to diagnose vasculogenic impotence on the basis of the history and impaired response to the intracavernous injection of a vasoactive agent. Nor is the demonstration of a lesion on arteriography sufficient to conclude that it is the cause of the erectile dysfunction. Nevertheless, the enthusiasm for venous leak surgery in the late 1980s was based upon such errors. Penile corrective surgery invariably carries with it a placebo effect which, in the absence of clearly defined aetiologies and control groups, makes the results obtained almost impossible to interpret.

Despite a degree of cynicism it has to be recognized that there is a role for vascular surgery to improve the quality of penile erection. It is the correct selection of patients, together with meticulous surgery and honest assessment of the outcome that is necessary to put the subject into perspective.

ARTERIAL REVASCULARIZATION PROCEDURE

Virag (Virag et al 1985) drew attention to the risk factors for arteriogenic impotence being smoking, diabetes, obesity and hypertension. The risk associated with smoking has also been emphasized by Bornman & du Plessis (1986), Condra et al (1986), Juenemann et al (1987) and Forsberg et al (1989). Such is the importance of the risk factors associated with arterial disease that most surgeons will not perform reconstructive procedures when any of these factors are present or in men more than 40 years old. The effect of such a rigid selection programme is to reduce the number of men eligible for reconstructive surgery, but also it increases the percentage of men who obtain long term benefit from such operations.

Leriche (1923) noted the association between obstruction of the aortic bifurcation and impotence. Most men with aorto-iliac arterial disease present with symptoms of limb ischaemia rather than impotence but nevertheless surgery for major vessel disease may give good results (Virag et al 1981; Michal et al 1979; Dewar et al 1985; de Palma et al 1988). It is necessary to avoid damage to the sympathetic nervous fibres at the time of aorto-iliac surgery in order to prevent postoperative ejaculatory failure (May et al 1969).

More recently, balloon angioplasty has been used successfully for isolated occlusion of internal iliac disease causing impotence (Costandga-Zunica et al 1982; Marsman & Van Unnik 1984).

Suitable candidates for revascularization are those patients who do not have other stigmata of cardiovascular disease (Table 13.3). They will be young, nondiabetic, nonsmokers or prepared to give up smoking, and with a history suggestive of a congenital abnormality or injury. These injuries may be associated with a fractured pelvis or obtained by direct trauma to the perineum, as may occur in basketball (St Louis et al 1983). The response to papaverine will be impaired and duplex colour ultrasonography will confirm the presence of decreased blood flow velocity in the cavernous penile artery. Phalloarteriography (Lurie et al 1988; Rosen et al 1990; Levine et al 1990) will identify the site of arterial obstruction and facilitate the choice of revascularization procedures.

Surgical techniques for microsurgical penile revascularization

The origin of small vessel surgery to restore potency stems from the work of Michal (Michal et al 1973) who performed an end-to-side anastomosis between the inferior epigastric artery and a defect made in the side of the tunica albuginea of the corpus cavernosum (Michal I procedure). Although the initial results with this procedure

Table 13.3 Criteria of suitability for reconstructive surgery

1. Age: less than 40–60 years
2. Absence of diabetes, hypertension or other cardiovascular disease
3. Nonsmokers, or willingness to stop smoking
4. Willingness to undergo reconstructive surgery even though it may fail

were successful (Michal et al 1977; Zorgniotti et al 1980), the technique was subsequently abandoned. It is of interest that many of the patients developed priapism. Attempts to divert blood from the femoral artery to the corpora via a saphenous vein graft also proved to be unsuccessful (Sharlip 1981; Metz & Frimodt-Muller 1983; Hawatmeh et al 1983; Michal et al 1980). Michal turned to direct arterial anastomosis and anastomosed the end of the inferior epigastric artery to the dorsal artery of the penis (Michal II procedure) with good effect (Fig. 13.2).

McDougal & Jeffrey (1983) utilized this technique to such effect that 6 of the 8 patients still benefited from the operation one year later. Crespo et al (1982) operated upon 138 patients with beneficial results in 78% after six months. He also utilized a vein graft between the femoral or external iliac arteries and the dorsal penile or cavernous penile arteries. MacGregor & Konnak (1982) anastomosed the inferior epigastric artery directly to the cavernous artery as did Shaw & Zorgniotti (1984). These procedures have not found widespread acceptance, but there would seem to be a place for anastomosis of the inferior epigastric artery to the proximal end of the dorsal penile artery (Fig. 13.3) where there is an obstruction proximal to the bifurcation of the internal pudendal artery into its cavernous and penile branches (Goldstein 1986; Carmignani et al 1987).

Virag, a vascular surgeon in Paris, performed a series of operations which were designed to revascularize the corpus cavernosum by the retrograde flow of blood through the dorsal vein of the penis (Virag et al 1981). The Virag V procedure (Fig. 13.4) has met with most success and consists of anastomosis of the inferior epigastric artery to the deep dorsal vein of the penis. All the tributaries are ligated and the distal end anastomosed to a window made in the corpus cavernosum. The proximal end of the deep dorsal vein is ligated proximal to the arterio venous anastomosis. This operation is similar to one described by Furlow (Furlow & Fisher 1988) and differs only in that the corpus cavernosum is revascularized through one of the emissary veins. The distal end of the deep dorsal vein is ligated to prevent hyperaemia of the glans.

A similar operation (Fig. 13.5) was devised by Hauri (1986) in which the inferior epigastric artery is anastomosed to the dorsal penile artery

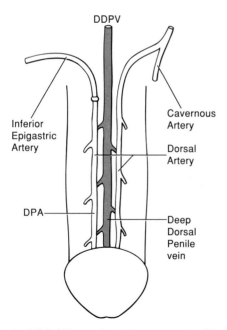

Fig. 13.2   Michal II operation with anastomosis of the inferior epigastric artery to the dorsal penile artery.

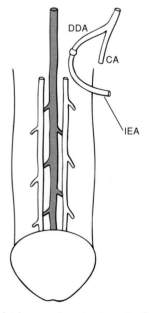

Fig. 13.3   Goldstein operation: anastomosis of the inferior epigastric artery to the proximal end of the dorsal penile artery.

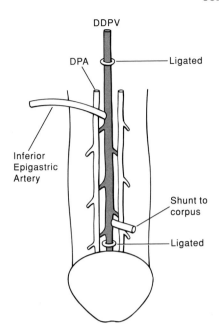

Fig. 13.4 Virag V operation: inferior epigastric artery anastomosed to the deep dorsal penile vein.

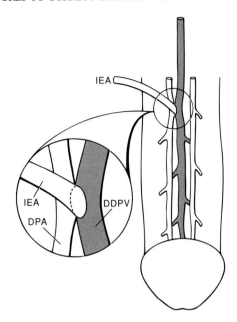

Fig. 13.5 Hauri procedure: inferior epigastric artery anastomosed to the deep dorsal vein and dorsal penile artery.

and deep dorsal veins, which have been joined to create an arteriovenous shunt.

Selection of patients for arterial reconstruction

Many of the issues relating to patient selection have already been discussed. Patients should have been screened from their history and response to intracavernosal drugs. Colour Doppler ultrasonography will identify those with arterial defects and any who are considered suitable for reconstructive surgery will proceed to arteriography. These criteria are shown in Table 13.3. Both de Palma and Borges found only 2% of impotent men suitable for reconstructive surgery (Table 13.4).

Some men will complain of an impaired or suboptimal erection and wish for the restoration of a normal full erection. Where this impairment is due to trauma, then a good result may be expected. In others, where the impairment has been more gradual in onset and is likely to be due to atherosclerosis, then the outcome is less likely to be favourable. Similarly, some surgeons would only consider arterial reconstructive procedures if the quality of erection was such that intercourse was not possible either with or without the

intracavernosal injection of a vasoactive agent. In view of the widespread variation in the selection of patients for operation, it is not surprising that comparison of the outcome will remain difficult.

Choice of revascularization procedures

The aim of reconstructive surgery is to rearterialize the corpus cavernosum. When the obstructive lesion is proximal to the bifurcation of the dorsal penile and cavernous arteries, then a direct anastomosis of the inferior epigastric artery to the proximal end of the dorsal penile artery is indicated. When this is not possible, then it would

Table 13.4 Selection of patients for revascularization and results given by de Palma and Borges at the 7th International Meeting of the Impotence Research Society.

	de Palma		Borges	
Number	770		4702	
Abnormal perfusion	334	(43%)	558	(12%)
Angiography	44	(6%)	169	(4%)
Operation	18	(2%)	105	(2%)
Patent	12	(1.5%)	56	(1.2%)
Follow-up (months)	>12		1–48	
Patency rate		(67%)		(53%)

appear that the Hauri, Virag V and Furlow techniques give similar results. They all rely upon arterialization of the deep dorsal vein.

The operations are usually performed under general anaesthesia and require the use of magnification — preferably an operating microscope — to perform the revascularization procedure. The skin incisions vary. Zorgniotti (1991) prefers a vertical incision from the midline over the symphysis pubis, extending downwards around the base of the penis onto the scrotum, and a separate and higher transverse incision to facilitate access to the inferior epigastric artery. It is also possible to perform the operation through a single oblique incision from the base of the penis, which permits exposure of the deep penile vessels and the inferior epigastric artery. The latter is dissected from its origin at the mid inguinal point from the external iliac artery upwards, along the lateral border of the rectus abdominal muscle to the left of the umbilicus, where it often divides into two major branches. All side branches are ligated. The vascular anastomoses are carried out under magnification using 6–0 to 8–0 nonabsorbable sutures. The techniques of the various operations are illustrated in diagrammatic form.

Complications

General complications as may follow any operation are to be expected, although as the operation is superficial it is rare for them to be serious. Blood loss is rarely of concern and prophylactic antibiotics are always given to prevent infection at the site of the anastomosis. Many surgeons anticoagulate patients for 48 hours and continue with dipyridamole to prevent future graft thrombosis. Short term anticoagulation also reduces the risk of pulmonary embolus. There is often some degree of bruising and if there has been a great deal of oozing then it is sensible to use some form of suction drainage.

The incidence of graft thrombosis varies considerably and was reported to be as low as 8% in 38 patients (Zorgniotti 1991) and as high as 100% by Hawatmeh et al 1983, using saphenous vein grafts from the femoral artery to the cavernosa. Most surgeons prohibit any sexual activity for 4–8 weeks following the operation to prevent

thrombosis but Austoni prefers to give intracorporal injections of vasoactive agents to stimulate blood flow and prevent thrombosis.

Penile shortening may occur when there are adhesions between the corpora and the skin incision. Priapism was a problem in the early operations but this is no longer the case. A similar complication of hyperaemia of the glans, which was painful and caused ulceration and sometimes necrosis, occurred with too great a blood flow going into the glans penis. This may be prevented by ligating the distal end of the dorsal penile artery or vein.

Results

These are difficult to compare as there are many differences, not only in the selection of patients but also in the choice of procedure and the assessment of the results. The 'incredible' nature of the results has already been alluded to (Sharlip 1991). Sohn et al (1990), using a combination of Hauri and Virag techniques in 20 patients, obtained a 95% success rate at 3 months which fell to 83% at 6 months and 80% at 12 months. They defined success as the ability to have 'regular, satisfying sexual intercourse' as the only important subjective parameter. In addition they monitored penile blood flow. In contrast, Zorgniotti (1991) measured success as good when a patient was able to achieve satisfactory erections resulting in intercourse on more than 50% of attempts without employing adjunct intracavernous therapy. In a series of 38 patients the success rate fell from 68% at 3 months to 65% at 6 months, 58% at 12 months and 29% at 2 years. He found similar success rates at one year from both the Virag V and Furlow procedures.

SURGERY FOR VENO-OCCLUSIVE DYSFUNCTION

The net increase in penile blood volume at the time of erection suggests that there might be some alteration to the outflow. That some blood continues to leave the penis during erection is not doubted but debate continues as to the relative importance of active and passive mechanisms of outflow restriction. Regardless of these mechanisms it is logical to suppose that impaired erection might occur as a result of abnormal leakage of blood from the corpora. This may occur as a result of:

1. Failure of the normal drainage mechanisms to close:
   a. neurogenic
   b. musculogenic
   c. valve mechanism
2. Abnormal drainage channels:
   a. congenital
   b. collateral.

Wooten (1902) ligated the deep dorsal vein of the penis in an attempt to improve the quality of the erection but this technique, together with an attempt to improve erections by crural compression (Lowsley & Bray 1935), fell into abeyance. Interest in 'venous leakage' was rekindled by the report of Ebbehoj & Wagner (1979) who described four patients with erectile dysfunction due to a congenital fistula between the corpus cavernosum and corpus spongiosum. Closure of the fistula produced an improvement in the quality of erection. The recent interest in 'venous leakage' stemmed from the application of cavernometry to the diagnosis of the condition (Wespes et al 1984; Virag 1981). This led first to the ligation and stripping of the deep dorsal penile vein and, in an attempt to improve the long term results, the closure of cavernosal and crural veins. The failure of such operations has led to a reappraisal of the mechanisms of venogenic impotence and a change in nomenclature. The condition is now referred to as veno-occlusive dysfunction and with this goes an understanding that the problem may result from the failure of the cavernous smooth muscle to relax fully.

Selection of patients for operation

The men complain of an incomplete erection on all occasions and this may have always been so (primary) or acquired during later life. Veno-occlusive dysfunction is not associated with a failure to maintain an erection either before or after penetration. The response to intracavernous vasoactive agents is incomplete and there should be no arterial deficit — preferably determined by colour Doppler ultrasound scanning. The diagnosis may be confirmed by performing cavernometry after using sufficient papaverine, or equivalent, to produce full relaxation of the cavernous smooth muscle. Cavernosography should be performed at the time of full erection in an attempt to localize the site of the leakage. Candidates for venous surgery should be young and preferably with primary erectile dysfunction of focal leakage from the corpora. Older men, particularly with a history of smoking, diabetes or cardiovascular problems should be excluded as they will probably have an element of arterial and/or cavernous muscle dysfunction. It has been suggested that the cavernous muscle should be biopsied to exclude dysfunction (Wespes 1990; Meuleman et al 1990).

Because of the unpredictable outcome of surgery, patients should choose between venous surgery, with a 30% chance of restoring a normal erection for one year, or a 90–95% chance of being able to have intercourse with a penile prosthesis but without a normal erection.

Operation

It is usual to perform the surgery under general anaesthetic with the patient either supine or with the legs elevated with the hips flexed and abducted, if crural plication is being considered. A transverse (infrapubic) incision at the base of the penis is satisfactory for most procedures and this may be curved downwards around the base of the penis to the root of the scrotum for crural plication. This incision is very similar to the hockey stick incision described by Lue (1989). When the surgery is being confined to the penis, a degloving circumcision may be used.

Diagnosis of the site of leakage is difficult. Cavernosography performed with complete smooth muscle relaxation (be it after intracavernous injection of vasoactive agents or with visible sexual stimuli) is helpful as a focal leak is shown. Infusion of saline, to which methylene blue or contrast medium may be added at operation to facilitate identification, may be beneficial. An attempt may be made to identify the source of the leakage by manual compression of the glans, corpus spongiosum, base of the penis, cavernosal subpubic arch veins and the crura. None of these techniques is entirely reliable.

It is also possible to perform cavernometry at the

commencement of surgery and repeat it throughout the procedure until there is a rapid pressure rise. Intracavernous papaverine is a nuisance as it increases the bleeding and I usually delay giving it until the procedure is completed. A suction drainage tube is often necessary at this stage.

Closure of leakage between the corpus cavernosum and corpus spongiosum. Successful closure of a congenital fistula between the glans and the corpus cavernosum was described by Ebbehoj & Wagner (1979). Such patients are extremely uncommon and it is more usual to find men who have undergone a shunt procedure for priapism. In most of these the corpora are fibrotic and the erection would not improve, but on occasion surgery will be beneficial. At the time of operation care should be taken not to damage the distal penile arteries and cause gangrene of the glans. The dissection should be carried out from the ventrolateral aspect of the penis.

It is possible to dissect the corpus spongiosum from the corpora cavernosa throughout the length of the penile shaft. There are many fine communicating vessels between the two and, rarely, a large communication, or fistula, is the source of leakage.

Dorsal vein ligation/stripping. Wespes & Schulman (1985) and Lewis & Puyau (1986) described techniques for ligating the deep dorsal penile vein near the base of the penis. There were many favourable results quoted but most authors were optimistic and based their results on a short follow-up. Lewis (1988) reviewed the literature and found that only 22% of 549 patients were cured. By this time, it was considered necessary to strip the dorsal vein and to ligate all the tributaries. Puech-Leão (Puech-Leão et al 1987) recommended ligation of the corpus cavernosum proximal to the entry of the cavernosal arteries in an attempt to obstruct the crural veins and Goldstein (1986) and Lue (1989) recommended that the cavernosal as well as the crural veins should be ligated. In order to ligate the cavernosal veins it is necessary to divide, and subsequently resuture, the two elements of the suspensory ligament and dissect under the pubic arch — traction is used to pull the penis downwards and care must be taken not to damage the paired cavernosus nerves and arteries. This is best achieved by taking care not to cause any venous bleeding and, in this respect, it is useful to use vascular clips rather than ties.

Complications

Minor wound complications are common. There is usually some bruising of the invaginated penis and also penile oedema. Haematoma formation is minimized by the use of suction drains.

It is important to close the wound in layers and reconstruct the suspensory ligament to prevent penile instability (lack of the basal part) or penile shortening, due to retraction of the more superficial element that fans out into the subcutaneous tissue.

Results

These are difficult to interpret as selection of patients, choice of operation and assessment of outcome vary. It would seem that approximately 30% of men with inadequate erection due to veno-occlusive dysfunction have a normal erection following operation and are able to have intercourse (Trieber & Gilbert 1989; Wespes 1990; Glina et al 1990). Some men obtain some improvement for a short time (less than a year) or are able to have intercourse with the help of intracavernous injections. The trend towards more extensive operation does not appear to have improved the percentage of cures and attention is now focused on the cavernous muscle.

Other types of venous surgery

In an attempt to improve such matters outlined above some authors have recommended an intrapelvic approach to vein ligation (Wagenknecht 1989) but this type of surgery has not found general acceptance. Finally, surgery to revascularize the corpus cavernosum by arterialization of the dorsal vein of the penis may be considered (Furlow, Virag V or Hauri operations, which are described on p. 194). The rationale for such operations is good but the outcome remains uncertain.

SUMMARY

The success of surgery to correct erectile dysfunction depends upon correct patient selection. This not only depends upon the selection of those men with a penile abnormality that is suitable for correction, but those men who have a realistic expectation for the operation. Deformities of the penis are amenable to correction but strict criteria need to be adopted for those men with arteriogenic or venogenic problems. Young men with congenital or traumatic abnormalities of the

arterial inflow benefit, but the long term results for those men with abnormalities of venous drainage are poor. It is to be hoped that as our understanding of cavernous muscle physiology improves, so may the selection of patients for operation. In those men where reconstructive surgery is unlikely to be of benefit, or when it fails, it is always possible to consider the implantation of a penile prosthesis.

REFERENCES

Bailey M J, Pryor J P 1987 Penile curvature and Peyronie's disease. Problems in Urology 1(2): 259–273
Bailey M J, Yande S, Walmsley B, Pryor J P 1985 Surgery for Peyronie's disease: a review of 200 patients. British Journal of Urology: 746–749
Bornman M S, du Plessis D J 1986 Smoking and vasculogenic impotence, a reason for concern. South African Medical Journal 13: 29–36
Carmignani G, Corbu C, Pirozzi F, de Stefani S, Spano G 1987 Cavernous artery revascularization in vasculogenic impotence: new simplified technique. Urology 30: 23–26
Condra M, Morales A, Owend A, Surridge D H, Fenemore J 1986 Prevalence and significance of tobacco smoking in impotence. Urology 27: 495–498
Costandga-Zunica W R, Smith A, Kaye K 1982 Transluminal angioplasty for treatment of vasculogenic impotence. American Journal of Radiology 139: 371–373
Crespo E, Soltanik E, Bove D, Farrell G 1982 Treatment of vasculogenic sexual impotence by revascularizing cavernous and/or dorsal arteries using microsurgical techniques. Urology 20: 271–275
de Palma R G, Edwards C M, Schwab F J, Steinberg D L 1988 Modern management of impotence associated with aortic surgery. In: Bargan J J, Yao S T (eds) Arterial surgery: new diagnostic and operative techniques. Grune & Stratton, Orlando p 337–348
Devine C J, Horton C E 1974 Surgical treatment of Peyronie's disease with a dermal graft. Journal of Urology 111: 44–49
Dewar M L, Blundell P E, Lidstone D, Herba M J, Chiu R C 1985 Effects of abdominal aneurysmectomy, aortoiliac bypass grafting and angioplasty on male sexual potency, a prospective study. Canadian Journal of Surgery 28: 154–159
Ebbehoj J, Wagner G 1979 Insufficient penile erection due to abnormal drainage of cavernous bodies. Urology 13: 507–510
Forsberg L, Hederstromm E, Olsson A M 1989 Severe arterial insufficiency in impotence confirmed with an improved arteriographic technique: the impact of smoking and some other etiologic factors. European Urology 16: 357–360
Furlow W L, Fisher J 1988 Deep dorsal vein arterialization: clinical experience with a new technique for penile revascularization. Journal of Urology 139: 289A
Gillies H, Harrison R J 1963 Congenital absence of the penis with embryological considerations. British Journal of Plastic Surgery 1: 8–28
Glina S, Puech-Leao P, dos Reis J J M, Reichelt A C, Chao

S 1990 Surgical exclusion of the crural ending of the corpora cavernosa: late results. European Urology 18: 42–44
Goldstein I 1986 Arterial revascularization procedures. Seminars in Urology 4: 252–258
Hauri D 1986, A new operative technique in vasculogenic impotence. World Journal of Urology 4: 237–249
Hawatmeh I S, Houtuin E, Gregory J G, Blair O M, Purcell M H 1983 Diagnosis and surgical management of sexual impotence. Journal of Urology 129: 517–521
Johnson J H 1974 Lengthening of the congenital or acquired short penis. British Journal of Urology 46: 685–687
Juenemann K P, Lue T F, Benowitz N L, Abozeid M, Tanagho E A 1987 The effect of cigarette smoking on penile erection. Journal of Urology 138: 438–441
Leriche R 1923 Des obliterations arterielles hautes causes des insuffisances circulatoires des membres inferieurs. Bulletin et memoires de la societe de chirurgie 49: 1404–1406
Levine F J, Greenfield A J, Goldstein I 1990 Arteriographically determined occlusive disease within the hypogastric-cavernous bed in impotent patients following Journal of Urology blunt perineal and pelvic trauma. 144: 1147–1153
Lewis R W 1988 Venous surgery for importance. Urology Clinics of North America 15: 115–121
Lewis R W, Puyau F A 1986 Procedures for decreasing venous drainage. Seminars in Urology 4: 263–272
Lowsley O S, Bray J C 1935 The surgical relief of impotence: further experiences with a new operative procedure. Journal of the American Medical Association 107: 2029–2035
Lue T F 1989 Penile venous surgery. Urology Clinics of North America 16: 607–611
Lurie Al, Bookstein J J, Kessler W O 1988 Angiography of post traumatic impotence. Cardiovascular and International Radiology 11: 232–236
McDougal W S, Jeffrey R F 1983 Microscopic penile revascularisation. Journal of Urology 129: 517–521
MacGregor R J, Konnak J W 1982 Treatment of vasculogenic erectile dysfunction by direct anastomosis of the infertior epigastric artery to the central artery of corpus cavernosum. Journal of Urology 127: 136–139
Marsman J W P, Van Unnik J G 1984 Impotence due to external ileac steal syndrome treated by percutaneous transluminal angioplasty. Journal of Urology 131: 544–545
May A J, de Weese J A, Rob C G 1969 Changes in sexual function following operation on the abdominal aorta. Surgery 65: 41–47
Melman A, Holland T F 1978 Evaluation of the dermal graft and inlay technique for the surgical treatment of Peyronie's disease. Journal of Urology 120: 421–422
Metz P, Frimodt-Muller C 1983. Epigastrio-cavernous

anastomosis in the treatment of arteriogenic impotence. Scandinarian Journal of Urology and Nephrology 17: 271–275

Meuleman E J H, ten Cate N L, de Wilde P C M Voogs C P, Debruyne F M J 1990 The use of penile biopsies in the detection of end organ disease: a histomorphometric study of the human cavernous body. International journal of Impotence Research 2: 161–166

Michal V, Kramar R, Pospichal J 1973 Direct arterial anastomoses to the cavernous body in the treatment of erectile impotence. Rozhledy V Chirurgii 52: 587–593

Michal V, Kramar R, Pospichal J 1977 Arterial epigastriovenous anastomosis for the treatment of sexual impotence. World Journal of Urology 1: 515–520

Michal V, Kramar R, Hejhal L, Firt P 1979 Aortoiliac occlusive disease. In: Zorgniotti A W, Rossi G (eds) Vasculogenic impotence. Proceedings of the 1st international conference on corpus cavernosum revascularization. Thomas, springfield, Illinois p 203–214

Michal V, Kramar R, Pospichal J 1980 Vascular surgery in the treatment of impotence: its present possibilities and prospects. Czechoslovak Medicine 3: 213–217

Nesbit R M 1965 Congenital curvature of the phallus: report of three cases with description of corrective, operation. Journal of Urology 93: 230–232

Pryor J P, Hill J T 1979 Abnormalities of the suspensory ligament of the penis as a cause for erectile dysfunction. British Journal of Urology 51: 402–403

Puech-Leão P, Reis J M S M, Glina S, Reichelt A C 1987 Leakage through the crural edge of corpus cavernosum. European Journal of Urology 13: 163–165

Rosen M P, Greenfield A J, Walker T G, Grant P, Guben J K, Dubrow J, Bettmann M A, Goldstein I 1990 Arteriogenic impotence: findings in 195 impotent men examined with selective internal pudendal angiography. Radiology 174: 1043–1048

Sharlip I D 1981 Penile revascularisation in the treatment of impotence. Western Journal of Medicine 134: 206–211

Sharlip I D 1991 The incredible results of penile vascular surgery. International Journal of Impotence Research 3: 1–6

Shaw W S, Zorgniotti A W 1984 Surgical techniques in penile revascularisation. Urology 23: 76–78

Sohn M, Sikora R, Bohndorf K, Deutz F-J 1990 Selective microsurgery in arteriogenic erectile failure. World Journal of Urology 5: 104–110

St Louis E L, Jewett M A S, Gray R R, Grossman H 1983 Basketball related injuries. Journal of the American Medical Association 308: 595–596

Trieber U, Gilbert P 1989 Venous surgery in erectile dysfunction: a critical report on 116 patients. Urology 34: 22–27

Virag R 1981 Syndrome d'erection instable par insufficance veineuse — diagnostie et correction chirurgicale a propos de 10 cas. Journal der Maladies Vasculaires, 6: 121–124

Virag R, Zwang G, Dermange H, Legman M 1981 Vasculogenic impotence: a review of 92 cases with 54 surgical operations. Vascular Surgery 15: 9–17

Virag R, Brouilly P, Frydman D 1985 Is impotence an arterial disorder? Lancet 1: 181–184

Wagenknecht L V 1989 Microsurgical arterialization for vascular impotence. European Journal of Urology 16: 262–266

Wespes E 1990 Penile venous surgery for cavernovenous impotence World Journal of Urology 8: 97–100

Wespes E, Schulman C C 1985 Venous leakage: surgical treatment of a curable cause of impotence. Journal of Urology 133: 796–798

Wespes E, Delcour C, Strugven J, Schulman C C 1984 Cavernometry-cavernosography: its role in organic impotence European Journal of Urology 10: 229–232

Wooten J S 1902 Ligation of the dorsal vein of the penis as a cure for atonic impotence. Texas Medical Journal 18: 325–328

Zorgniotti A W 1991 Penile revascularisation. In: Zorgniotti A W, Lizza E F (eds) Diagnosis and management of impotence. B C Decker, Philadelphia p 121–138

Zorgniotti A W, Rossi G, Padula G, Makovsky R D 1980 Diagnosis and therapy of vasculogenic impotence. Journal of Urology 123: 674–677

14. Penile prostheses

John P. Pryor

The implantation of a penile prosthesis is a simple procedure that can restore a man's potency and greatly improve the quality of life for both the patient and his partner. The success of these operations is beyond dispute but depends upon the correct selection of patients who have realistic expectations.

PATIENT SELECTION

Those patients with irreversible organic impotence are the prime candidates for operation, and Table 14.1 summarizes the indications for operation in a collected series of men who have had a prosthesis.

Diabetes is usually the most common aetiological factor. Diabetic men may be impotent for a variety of reasons (see Ch. 8) but in those undergoing operation it is usually due to decreased blood supply. Vasculogenic impotence is diagnosed from the history of impaired erection under all conditions and the failure to respond to a full dose of an intracavernosal vasoactive agent (papaverine, 80 mg or prostaglandin E1, 20 μg). The history should correspond with the outcome of the

Table 14.1 Indications for penile prosthesis in collected series of 3884 men.

Diabetes	25.6%
Vasculogenic causes	19.5%
Peyronie's disease	6.2%
Post priapism	1.0%
Pelvic trauma	7.5%
Pelvic surgery	15.9%
Spinal injury	5.1%
Psychological	7.8%
Other causes	11.8%

injection and if there is any doubt, it is worthwhile monitoring the sleeping erections. Arterial reconstructive surgery or operations for veno-occlusive dysfunction are more appropriate for younger men (see Ch. 13) and some men may prefer a trial with a vacuum device. Penile fibrosis — following papaverine injection or associated with Peyronie's disease — is no contraindication to an implant nor is the extensive penile fibrosis that may occur after a priapism. Men with a neurogenic cause for impotence — paraplegics, multiple sclerosis or following radical pelvic surgery — may wish to avoid another operation and thus prefer a vacuum device or intracorporeal drugs.

Men in whom psychological factors are suspected may benefit from psychological intervention, given by psychosexual counsellors, psychiatrists or psychologists (see Ch. 10). The role of a penile prosthesis in psychogenic impotence remains a matter of debate and surgeons should exercise caution as there is a substantial risk of patient dissatisfaction, in addition to the likelihood of carrying out unnecessary surgery. However, some patients with psychogenic impotence fail to respond adequately to other treatments and these may be considered candidates for the operation. They should not be implanted until they have been thoroughly assessed and treated, preferably by two therapists using different forms of therapy. The decision to implant in such patients is best taken in consultation with the therapist. The operation destroys the normal corpus cavernosum and in younger patients it may be better to implant a single prosthesis in the hope that potency may improve at a later date. Despite these warnings, some patients with psychological impotence can benefit from the procedure.

Thus patients who are judged to have irreversible organic impotence, or who have failed with psychological treatment, are candidates for the implantation of a penile prosthesis. It is rarely necessary to exclude patients on the grounds of fitness to undergo the operation as the procedure may be performed using local or regional anaesthesia. Severe myocardial insufficiency causes the greatest difficulty and yet, even after the risk of further myocardial infarction and death is explained to them, some men prefer to proceed with the operation rather than remain impotent.

Patients should always be informed of alternative methods of management and this includes external aids to assist erection (Ch. 12) and the use of intracavernous drugs where applicable (Ch. 11).

Many patients elect not to proceed with an operation on the grounds that they are too old or unfit, do not wish to have an operation, or that such techniques are unnatural. These factors vary in different societies and are changing constantly as a result of changes in public opinion — usually produced by media attention. There is no purpose in trying to persuade a patient to proceed with an operation. The clinician should restrict himself to providing impartial information and counselling the patient in a non-directive fashion. The patient should usually be seen with his partner before the final decision is made, and it is advisable that there should be an interval between the discussion and the final decision to operate.

In some patients, it is desirable to insert a prosthesis at the time of surgery for malignancy, e.g. radical cystectomy, whilst in others it is useful to insert the reservoir of an inflatable prosthesis whilst closing the abdominal wound.

It is essential for patients to have a realistic expectation of the operation (Berg et al 1984). The penile prosthesis provides sufficient rigidity to permit penetration but it is not possible to guarantee sexual satisfaction (Steege et al 1986). The patient should be informed that the penis remains at its flaccid length and only with an inflatable prosthesis is there any significant increase in girth. Most patients, and their partners, obtain sexual gratification, but there are some who find sexual intercourse with a prosthesis unsatisfying. It is important for the patient to realize that an implant does not restore normality, and this is particularly important in those men with mainly psychogenic impotence or with vasculogenic problems — particularly if coitus is possible but the erection is incomplete or poorly sustained. In a study of 86 consecutive patients seen during a 3 month period at St Peter's Hospital, London, approximately 60% of patients were unable to have intercourse for predominantly psychogenic reasons, although in some of these the quality of erection was less than perfect due to vasculogenic factors. Only 16% of patients elected to proceed with the implantation of a penile prosthesis even though many of the patients were originally referred for consideration of this method of treatment (Cumming & Pryor 1991).

CHOICE OF PROSTHESIS

The first operations to implant a penile prosthesis were carried out on men undergoing reconstructive procedures following traumatic amputation of the penis. Bogarus (1936) and Frumkin (1944) used cartilage to give the phalloplasty rigidity. Autologous tissue was slowly reabsorbed, and in order to overcome this difficulty synthetic materials were implanted into the penis. Goodwin & Scott (1952) reported the use of acrylic to stiffen the penis in two men who underwent penile reconstruction following amputation of the penis in the treatment of a neoplasm. In 1960, Beheri, working in Cairo, reported the technique of implanting polyethylene implants into each corpus cavernosum and by 1966 he was able to report his results in 700 patients: 95% of these implants were carried out in men with psychogenic impotence and in no other series have penile prostheses been used so readily for this condition. He described the technique of dilating the corpora cavernosa with Hegar's dilators in order to place the prosthesis within the erectile tissue rather than in a subcutaneous or subalbugineal plane. This has now become the standard technique.

Acrylic and polyethylene implants were not ideal substances for implantation into the body, as they were rigid and tended to fracture, and their use was abandoned with the discovery of the silicones (Brown et al 1953). In 1964 Lash et al reported the use of silicone for implantations into the body and showed a photograph of its use as a penile implant. The early results with this single prosthesis proved satisfactory (Lash 1968; Loeffler & Iveson 1976) but the shape of the implant was modified to a Y shape in an attempt to stabilize the penis.

The disadvantage of all these prostheses was that the penis remained stiff all the time and it was not until the flexible Small–Carrion prosthesis (Small & Carrion 1975) and the inflatable prosthesis of Scott (Scott et al 1973) were introduced that penile prosthetic surgery became an acceptable form of treatment. There is now a wide choice of prostheses and the selection depends upon financial considerations as well as the preferences of the patient and surgeon, the availability of each and the backup from the distributors. During the period 1975–1990 I have used 370 prostheses, as shown in Table 14.2.

All prostheses that are implanted at the present time are paired and are made, with the exception of the Mentor inflatable ones, of a silicone polymer. This is inert and is well tolerated by the body. The prostheses currently available fall into three main categories: malleable, mechanical and inflatable. The Small–Carrion prosthesis was for many years a popular choice and good results were obtained with its use (Chaikin et al 1981; Small 1987). Its use has now been largely abandoned in favour of the malleable prostheses, which offer similar functional results but with lower capital costs to obtain a complete inventory of sizes, and also permitting better concealment.

Table 14.2 Types of penile prosthesis implanted by the author (1975–1990).

Small–Carrion	162
Finney Flexirod	7
Subrini	5
Jonas	8
AMS 600	59
Mentor malleable	79
Flexiflate	2
Hydroflex	21
Dynaflex	6
GFS Resipump	2
AMS 700	18
Mentor inflatable	1
TOTAL	370

The hinged prostheses of Subrini (1974) and Finney (1977) consist of a firm penile and a softer crural element. This hinge mechanism permits the penis to be folded down to facilitate unobtrusive dressing. The length of the prosthesis is adjusted at the time of surgery by trimming the crural end with a scalpel. These prostheses are still used by some surgeons. The Finney prosthesis is produced by Surgitek and marketed as the Flexirod. It is important to determine the correct length of the more rigid penile part prior to implantation in order that the hinged area is correctly sited. The prosthesis is available in a range of diameters and lengths and the conical tip of the distal end was designed to fit snugly into the distal part of the corpus cavernosum. The prosthesis gives good concealment, is extremely durable and gave good results in the first 763 patients (Finney 1984). The manufacturers state that over a ten year period 20 000 pairs were sold and only 4 were returned for mechanical failure.

Malleable prostheses

These prostheses have an inner metal core that allows the penis to be bent into different positions. This allows the penis to be folded downwards when not required for coitus, although in reality many men continue to dress with the penis against the abdominal wall.

Jonas prosthesis. This prosthesis (Jonas & Jacobi 1980) was the first of the malleable prostheses and was introduced in 1978. It consists of a pair of silicone prostheses with an inner core of ten silver wires, 0.6 mm in diameter, which are surrounded by a Teflon coat. It is available in three diameters and in varying lengths from 16 to 25 cm. It is also available as a 'trimming tip' version in an attempt to reduce the inventory of sizes. The prosthesis was tested in a laboratory prior to its introduction but after some years, fracture of the silver wire was reported by some patients (Tawil & Gregory 1986). The manufacturers believe that the problem has been overcome by modification of the prosthesis.

Jonas (1983) summarized the experience of 309 physicians implanting 1890 prostheses with an overall success rate of 92%, and other favourable reports are quoted by Krane et al (1981), Benson et al (1983) and Rowe & Royle (1983). It should be noted that cheaper 'lookalike' implants are manufactured in some countries and these are less reliable as the silver coil tends to fragment.

American Medical Systems malleable prosthesis (AMS 600). This prosthesis (Fig. 14.1) was introduced by American Medical Systems in 1983 and a report of its use in 56 patients was published in 1986 (Moul & McLoed 1986). It has a core of steel wires which are surrounded by an outer cloth sheath in order to minimize the risk of a fractured wire perforating the surrounding silicone. The prosthesis is manufactured in three lengths (12, 16 and 20 cm) and has rear tip extenders (1, 2 and 3 cm long) which are fitted to the prosthesis at the time of surgery in order to obtain the correct length. The prosthesis is 13 mm in diameter but the outer silicone jacket may be removed at operation to reduce the diameter to 11 mm. This is easily accomplished by carefully sliding the tip of a blunt scissors under the rear portion of the jacket and sliding the scissors along the entire length of the rod. Care is taken not to damage the surface of the white silicone. The outer jacket is then peeled away and discarded.

The manufacturers report that of the first 500 prostheses implanted (1983–1986), there was only one revision for mechanical considerations and there were no mechanical failures in the first 12 000 to 15 000 implanted (Nielsen & Bruskewitz 1989). In 1987 a review of the results obtained in 19 patients showed that 7 prostheses had been removed — usually for erosion (Cumming & Pryor 1991). The prosthesis has been modified to become more flexible and in the period 1988–

1989 only two prostheses were removed and that was for infection. Dorflinger & Bruskewitz (1986) also found a high incidence of complications with this prosthesis.

Mentor malleable prosthesis. The Mentor malleable prosthesis consists of a moulded silicone elastomer incorporating a trimmable tail section of softer silicone. The shaft part of the prosthesis contains a silver wire to give additional rigidity and also limit flexibility. The prosthesis is trimmed to the correct length at the time of operation and the rear cap fitted. Minor adjustment of length may be made by further trimming or adding caps which are 0.5 or 1 cm in length. The prosthesis is available in three diameters (9.5, 11 and 13 mm). Results obtained with this prosthesis have been very satisfactory with no mechanical failures. The Mentor malleable has recently been modified to improve its capacity for concealment — the Acuform. Figure 14.2 compares the resting position of the two prostheses when they had been bent to 90°. It should be noted that the Acuform has 70–80% greater column strength than the Mentor malleable prostheses, but whether or not this is an advantage remains to be seen.

Mechanical prostheses

The OmniPhase (Dacomed Corporation) is a paired prosthesis and each element consists of three main components. The proximal and distal tips are made of medical grade silicone, a flexible body that is encased in polytetrafluoroethylene (PTFE) and a sheath of silicone. The body of the prosthesis is composed of a column of plastic segments, held together by a tension cable which passes

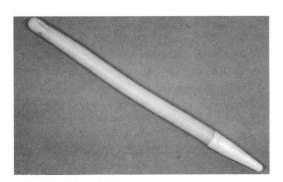

Fig. 14.1   AMS 600 malleable penile prosthesis (courtesy of American Medical Systems).

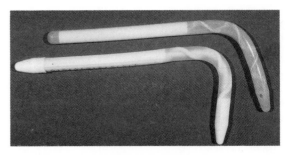

Fig. 14.2   Mentor malleable prosthesis showing that the Acuform (lower) maintains its position better when bent.

through the centre of the column. When the cable is tightened, the prosthesis becomes rigid and on releasing the cable the prosthesis lengthens by 4 mm and the prosthesis may be positioned like a malleable one. A further description of the prosthesis and the results are to be found in the initial report of Krane (1986).

A modification of this prosthesis — the Dura-Phase — does not have an activator mechanism and unlike the OmniPhase, it may be implanted through a penoscrotal incision (Krane 1988). Mulcahy (1989a) described his early experience with the OmniPhase and found that the manufacturers had observed a 7% incidence of mechanical failure in the first 1400 prostheses implanted. Despite this, he concluded that these prostheses have a role because of the ease of the manipulation of the implant by the patient and more recent reports remain optimistic (Mulcahy et al 1990).

Inflatable prostheses

The advantage of these prostheses is that they permit the penis to become flaccid and yet on activation there is sufficient rigidity to permit intercourse. The original prosthesis, designed by Brantley Scott, has undergone many modifications since its introduction but remains the standard against which all others are compared. The past five years have seen the introduction of self-contained and two part (cylinders and combined pump and reservoir) prostheses, and the role of these has yet to be fully evaluated.

The advantage of all the inflatable prostheses has to be offset by the increased risk of a mechanical failure and the increased cost of the prosthesis. It should also be remembered that the prosthesis may give an increasing girth of the penis but, as yet, it does not permit an increase in the length of the penis on inflation, although the recently introduced Ultrex attempts to remedy this problem.

Self-contained inflatable prostheses

In 1985, American Medical Systems introduced the Hydroflex prosthesis (Fishman 1986; Mulcahy 1989b). This prosthesis appeared simple and was often selected by patients when given the choice of

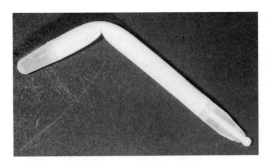

Fig. 14.3 Dynaflex penile prosthesis which becomes mobile when folded over for 10 seconds and rigid when the end is squeezed 6 or 7 times (courtesy of American Medical Systems).

a malleable, self-contained inflatable or a multipart inflatable prosthesis. Squeezing the end of the prosthesis — situated near the glans — produced rigidity, but the deactivation mechanism was more difficult. This led to its replacement by the Dynaflex which is deactivated by being folded over for 10 seconds (Fig. 14.3).

The Flexiflate self-contained inflatable prosthesis was developed by Surgitek in an attempt to provide a simple inflatable prosthesis. The prosthesis is activated by squeezing the distal part and deflation occurs by flexing the prosthesis within the penis. There was a tendency for the initial prosthesis to deflate spontaneously during intercourse (Finney 1986) but this problem has been reduced in the current model from 73% to 58% (Stanisic & Dean 1989). These authors reported a mechanical failure rate of 11.6% due to leakage of fluid.

Two part inflatable prostheses

Uniflate 100. This is the latest prosthesis available from Surgitek and consists of a pair of inflatable penile cylinders which are attached to a combined scrotal pump and reservoir with kink resistant tubing (Fig. 14.4). The prosthesis is prefilled but the final fluid volume may be adjusted at the time of operation. The scrotal reservoir (20 ml) has a small self-sealing port at its base which permits intra- or postoperative adjustment of the fluid volume within the prosthesis. An erection is created by firmly and continuously squeezing the pump/reservoir, located within the scrotum, to transfer fluid to the inner sheath. The

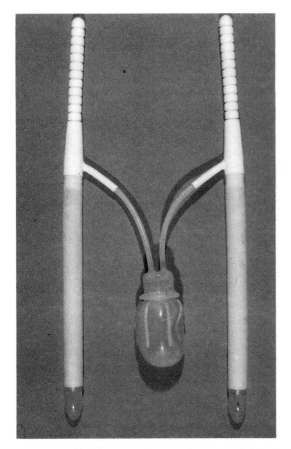

Fig. 14.4 Uniflate prosthesis — manufactured by Surgitek.

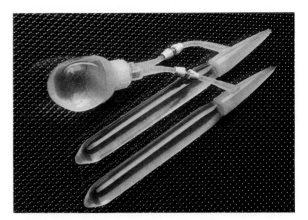

Fig. 14.5 Mentor GFS Mark II inflatable prosthesis.

erection is released by squeezing the release ring at the tip of the pump and this allows fluid to transfer back to the reservoir/pump bulb. As the inner erectile sheath becomes depressurized, the inner sheath softens, allowing the penis to return to a flaccid state.

Mentor Mark II inflatable penile prosthesis with Resipump. The Mentor inflatable penile prostheses differ from all others by being constructed of bioflex polyurethrane elastomer. This is considered to be more durable than silicone polymers, does not have crease fold failures and allows the manufacturers to give a ten year warranty.

The Mark II prosthesis (Fig. 14.5) consists of two inflatable penile cylinders (12 to 22 cm in length at 1 cm intervals) connected to a GFS Resipump of 20 or 25 ml capacity. The system is filled peroperatively and the tubing connected with special snap-lock connectors.

Multipart inflatable prostheses

American Medical Systems AMS 700. This is a development of the original Scott inflatable prosthesis. The original model consisted of two penile cylinders and two pumps and reservoirs, but was soon simplified by the elimination of one pump. The prosthesis has undergone many modifications since its introduction in an attempt to improve its mechanical reliability. The current model is shown in Figure 14.6. Each penile cylinder consists of outer and inner silicone layers with an expandable woven fabric in between which prevents aneurysm formation. Each 700 CX cylinder expands from 12 mm flaccid diameter to 18 mm erect diameter, ensuring that the flaccid penis appears and feels more natural. The small 700 CXM cylinder expands from 9.5 mm flaccid to 14.2 mm when inflated. A recent innovation is the Ultrex cylinder which, on inflation, increases in length as well as girth. The standard cylinders are supplied in four lengths and rear tip extenders are used to obtain the correct length at the time of operation.

It is important that the prosthesis is filled with an isotonic solution, as silicone is semipermeable and fluid is slowly lost from demonstration models. A list of filling solutions is shown in Table 14.3.

The main advantage of this prosthesis is that it gives good flaccidity (Fig. 14.7) and on activation, by squeezing the scrotal pump to transfer fluid from the intra-abdominal reservoir, the penis becomes erect (Fig. 14.8).

Impressive results have been obtained with

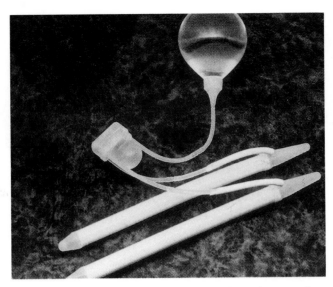

Fig. 14.6 AMS inflatable 700 CX penile prostheses (courtesy of American Medical Systems).

these prostheses (Scott et al 1983; Malloy et al 1987; Furlow & Motley 1988; Scarzella et al 1988) but their long term mechanical reliability is uncertain. Fluid loss can occur from any part of the multiple component inflatable prostheses, necessitating reoperation. The improvements that have been introduced are designed to overcome leaks which were usually from the penile cylinders. CX cylinders have not only reduced the rate of leakage but largely prevented aneurysm formation. The latter may occur due to inherent weakness of the tunica albuginea or as a consequence of weakness where the corporotomy was closed (Diokno 1983).

Table 14.3 Filling solutions for inflatable prostheses.

	Contrast medium (ml)	Sterile water (ml)	Total volume (ml)
Hypaque 25%	50	60	110
Conray 280	20	60	80
Cysto-Conray II	60	15	75
Isopaque-Cysto	60	27	87
Iopamiro 300	47	53	100
Hexabrix	53	47	100
Urografin 30%	49	51	100
Solutrast 300	53	47	100
Conray FL	58	42	100
Telebrix 12	53	47	100

If the patient is sensitive to contrast media then isotonic saline solution should be used.

The site of a leak may be detected by a simple radiograph or, at operation, by testing each component in turn. Silicone is non-conductive and there should be no loss of current from the system when fluid is injected and an ohmmeter is attached to the tubing.

Self-inflation may occur due to raised intra-abdominal pressure or when the space for the reservoir is too small to prevent its expansion. This is avoided at operation by filling it and checking that there is no tendency of the reservoir to empty. It is for this reason that the reservoir is kept filled during the early postoperative period. The penile cylinders may expand by having the fluid forced into them by the pump mechanism but the filling of the reservoir is on a more passive basis.

Mentor Multipart inflatable prosthesis. This is similar in appearance to the AMS 700 prosthesis but is manufactured from bioflex for added durability. The manufacturers are sufficiently confident of its reliability that they offer a ten year replacement policy. The rounded pump has a collar which allows easy release without the need to orientate the scrotal pump. The kink free tubing is readily joined by the use of snap-lock connectors.

The overall satisfactory results with this prosthesis have been summarized by Merrill (1989)

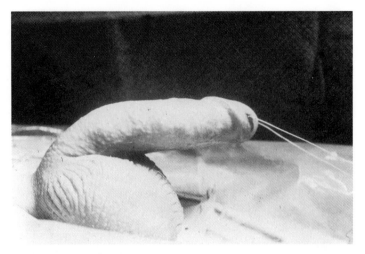

Fig. 14.7   Penis in the flaccid state after insertion of AMS 700 prosthesis (courtesy of American Medical Systems).

but, whereas he had a reoperative rate of 2%, some authors had a reoperative rate as high as 39%.

Which prosthesis?

The ideal prosthesis does not exist. It should be inert when implanted and free from mechanical failures. It should allow the penis to be dependent in the flaccid state and yet be sufficienty rigid to permit intercourse. Inflation of the prosthesis should make the penis expand in both length and girth. The implantation procedure should be simple and the prosthesis cheap.

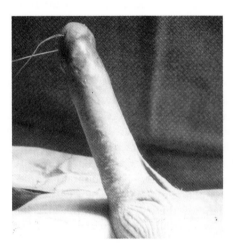

Fig. 14.8   Penis erect following transfer of fluid from the reservoir to the penile cylinders by manipulating the scrotal pump (courtesy of American Medical Systems).

The final choice of prosthesis is far from easy and depends upon reliability, cost, personal preference of both surgeon and patient and also upon availability. In general terms, it is likely that a malleable prosthesis will be cheaper and more reliable, especially as inflatable prostheses are likely to require reoperation in 5–10 years on account of wear. The benefits of the inflatable prosthesis are the flaccidity for those groups who require it and that the tumescence is associated with an increased girth of the penis. Beutler et al (1986) found that patients' and their partners' satisfaction was greater with the inflatable prosthesis, but this issue is far from resolved.

The manufacturers have invested much time and money in an attempt to improve the prostheses. They try to provide an excellent service but the limited number of suppliers makes it difficult to provide this on a worldwide basis. The choice is varied and there is no single 'best buy'.

PREOPERATIVE CONSIDERATIONS

Proper informed consent is essential and, although the meaning of this may vary in different countries, the basic requirements are common to all. The need for operation should have been assessed and the patient advised as to the alternative methods of treatment, his expectation and the risk of complications. It is the latter that most frequently give rise to litigation, and unrealistic expectations which most commonly result in dissatisfaction. Counselling or some form of therapy may be required to deal with intrapersonal or relationship problems before implantation can be considered. Any focus of infection must be eliminated prior to operation and it is also advisable to correct any urinary outflow obstruction. Prophylactic antibiotics are essential and these and other techniques to reduce infection will be discussed under Complications.

SURGICAL CONSIDERATIONS

The operation may be performed under general, regional or local anaesthesia and the choice depends on the preferences of the patient, surgeon and anaesthetist. Surgeons wishing to implant on a daycase basis would benefit from reading the articles on technique by Scott (1987) and Small (1987).

The original perineal incision has been abandoned and a penoscrotal incision (Barry & Siefert 1979) is the most practical. A small dorsal subcoronal incision (Jonas & Jacobi 1980) is convenient for a simple malleable prosthesis but should be avoided in the uncircumcised. The transverse infrapubic incision popularized by Kelâmi (1980) is useful but not recommended in the obese, as corporal dilatation may be difficult. It is a safe incision for the beginner to use when implanting an inflatable prosthesis with an intra-abdominal reservoir. Once the surgeon has acquired more experience, he may elect to implant the prosthesis through the inguinal canal and this may be facilitated by a transverse penoscrotal incision (Scarzella 1989).

Surgery is best learnt in the operating room but operative details may be found in textbooks of operative surgery (Hinman 1989; Montague 1986). There are also videos of operative technique and these may be obtained from the implant manufacturers.

At the conclusion of the operation, the penis is left lying on the anterior abdominal wall and inflatable prostheses are left deflated. The use of bupivacaine reduces the need for postoperative analgesics and oral medication is often all that is required. Some discomfort may persist for up to 4 weeks. Patients may be discharged as soon as

comfortable and usually on the second postoperative day. Showering is permitted after 48 hours and bathing after five days. Coitus is prohibited until the patient is pain free and the wounds have healed (usually four to six weeks). No attempt is made to inflate the hydraulic prosthesis until three to four weeks after surgery in order to allow healing and the pain free operation of the prosthesis. This may be initiated at the postoperative visit and the patient given further instruction as to its operation. A water soluble lubricant facilitates intercourse and both partners should be warned that there is a learning period in order to adjust to the new prosthesis. A further appointment is made for three months after the operation to check that all is well and the couple advised to seek further help should they have difficulties either with the mechanics of the prosthesis or with intercourse.

Complications

The overall incidence of complications varies widely and depends upon the cause of the impotence, the type of prosthesis used and the experience of the surgeon. The true incidence of complications is unknown but may be as high as 36% in some series reviewed by Kabalin & Kessler (1989a). Most of the complications were minor and 265 of the 290 patients (91%) were left with a functioning penile prosthesis, although reoperation was necessary on 152 occasions in 96 patients. Many patients are able to have intercourse satisfactorily following the loss of a single prosthesis and Krauss (1985) obtained satisfactory results when he chose to implant a single prosthesis in selected patients.

Perforation of the tunica albuginea during the operation may occur during dilatation — usually if there is an element of fibrosis. This is not important unless the perforation is through the glans or into the urethra and under these circumstances a prosthesis should not be inserted into that corpus. The safest course of events with a urethral perforation is to insert a suprapubic catheter for seven days. Should the perforation of the tunica not be at the end of the corpus, be it proximal or distal, and not into the urethra, then it is safe to implant the prosthesis provided that the two ends of the prosthesis are safely seated. Failure to recognize a proximal perforation may result in the migration of the prosthesis into the perineum. This situation may be rectified by a perineal approach to repair the tunica (Fishman 1989).

Technical failures may occur through failure of operative technique. The implantation of a prosthesis that is too short leads to the ST or Concord deformity (Fig. 14.9), whereas too long a prosthesis may produce postoperative pain and subsequent erosion with extrusion of the prosthesis (Fig. 14.10). When a prosthesis protrudes through the glans or urethral meatus, it may be easily removed and the capsule around the prosthesis prevents any bleeding. Urethral catheterization is unnecessary. It is a simple matter to exchange a short prosthesis for a larger one and it may be necessary to strengthen the distal part of the tunica albuginea with a Goretex or Dacron patch (Fishman 1989). Needle stick injuries of an inflatable prosthesis should be recognized at the time of surgery, but partial injury may cause a weak area which will subsequently cause a leakage.

Postoperative urinary retention may occur. Catheterization is avoided whenever possible and any outflow obstruction should have been corrected beforehand. Urethral catheterization may be kind if the operation is performed in the late afternoon, and the catheter is removed the next morning.

Some bruising of the penis is common, and although it may worry the patient considerably, it is rarely severe enough to warrant treatment. Penile oedema is not uncommon following the insertion of the self-contained inflatable prostheses and is more likely if there have been repeated attempts at inflation and deflation of the prosthesis. Care should be taken to avoid a constricting dressing around the penis as this may lead to gangrene. This is particularly likely to occur if the dressing has become soaked in blood and hardened and the tissues are compressed between the dressing and the prosthesis. The presence of a urethral catheter is an additional hazard as it permits the passage of urine without inspection of the penis. The glans penis should always be visible and the use of constricting tape avoided.

Infection is the major complication and results in the loss of up to 10% of prostheses. The overall incidence of infection is difficult to assess and is very low in some series. Blum (1989) and Carson (1989) have reviewed the incidence and the results are summarized in Table 14.4. Scott et al (1983) reported an incidence of 2.4% in 1300 operations to implant an inflatable prosthesis, whereas, in a personal series of 115 operations, the overall incidence of infection was 10% and the removal or extrusion of the prosthesis occurred in 18% of patients. Thanalla & Thompson (1987) found a similar incidence. The infecting organism is usually a staphylococcus epidermidis (albus) (Thanalla & Thompson 1987; Montague 1987; Carson 1989) although other organisms may be responsible.

The importance of preventing infection is shown by the number of prophylactic measures that are taken (Table 14.5).

Superficial wound infection may occur without the loss of the prosthesis but postoperative infec-

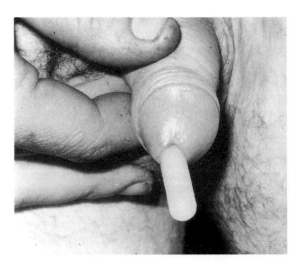

Fig. 14.10 Erosion of prosthesis that was too long.

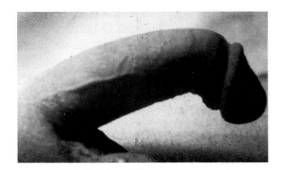

Fig. 14.9 ST or Concord deformity that occurs when the prosthesis is too short.

Table 14.4 Incidence of penile prosthesis infection (after Carson 1989).

Type of prosthesis	Number of centres	Number of patients	Number (%) of infections
Malleable rod	9	2806	50 (1.8)
Inflatable rod	2	66	4 (6)
Inflatable	9	2278	60 (2.6)

tion of the periprosthetic tissues is accompanied by pain, fever, local tenderness and swelling. Most infections are apparent within the first month but some infections do not appear for weeks or months (Montague 1987). The prosthesis usually has to be removed when infection occurs but there have been reports of successfully irrigating the cavity with antibiotic solution and reimplanting a new prosthesis (Maatman & Montague 1987; Blum 1989). A safer alternative is to wait for the tissues to heal and to implant a new prosthesis after an interval of three months, although it should be remembered that many patients are able to have satisfactory intercourse with a single prosthesis. Infection of one prosthesis does not inevitably lead to the loss of both prostheses.

Tissue necrosis and gangrene may occur rarely and usually in diabetics (Bour & Steinhardt 1984; McClellan & Masih 1985). Underlying ischaemia is an additional factor and this may be related to the original impotence or be due to a constricting dressing around the penis. The latter is more likely to occur if there is an indwelling catheter in addition to the prosthesis. Necrosis of the cavernous tissue may occur and it may be necessary to not only remove the prosthesis, but also to remove the necrotic tissue by curettage.

Some postoperative pain is to be expected following the operation and this may be mini-

Table 14.5 Prophylactic measures to reduce infection at the time of surgery to implant a penile prosthesis.

Eliminate all foci of infection
Relieve urinary outflow obstruction
Avoid catheterization
Preoperative antiseptic bath
Shave genital area in theatre
Prophylactic antibiotics
Minimize number of personnel in theatre
Minimize theatre traffic
Local antibiotics during surgery
Meticulous haemostasis

mized by avoiding excessive handling of the tissues and the intraoperative use of bupivacaine and postoperative analgesia. The worst of the pain is usually over within one week and most patients are pain free in four to six weeks, by which time the wound is healed and the polydioxanone sutures have fallen out.

Persistent pain is usually due to infection and antibiotics may dampen down the infection for many weeks. If the prosthesis is too long this may be a source of pain and the prosthesis may erode through the tunica albuginea and become subcutaneous in the penis or ulcerate through the skin. This may account for the loss of a prosthesis after many years but in some instances this will be due to a haematogenous infection.

In some patients, the pain may persist for many months and sometimes for as long as a year and then cease without apparent reason. Some patients with persistent pain are diabetics and it may be that there is a neuropathic element to the pain. On rare occasions it is necessary to explant the prosthesis on the basis of pain alone and the earliest that this was necessary was after 8 days. Before proceeding to remove the prosthesis for persistent pain, Krauss (1986) suggested injecting local anaesthesia into the corpora.

In a study of 130 prostheses implanted between 1983 and 1987 it was found that a prosthesis was removed (usually for infection) or was extruded in 30% of 30 diabetics, 3 (17%) of 17 patients with vasculogenic impotence and 2 (5%) of 39 patients with neurogenic impotence (Cumming & Pryor 1991). It was also found that only 4 (7%) of 52 Small–Carrion prostheses were removed or extruded whereas 7 of 15 AMS 600 prostheses extruded. This high incidence was probably due to the prosthesis being much more rigid and in 1987 the design was modified. In the subsequent 3 years only 3 of 30 AMS 600 prostheses were lost or extruded.

Outcome

The results of a penile prosthesis are usually satisfactory and most dissatisfaction arises when there are complications, even though these may be rectified by a further operation. Preoperative counselling of the patient, which includes information about the complications, is most important in order to obtain satisfactory results. It is most important for the patient to realize that the penis will not increase in length during intercourse.

Patients rarely complain of difficulties concealing the prosthesis and when they do it is important to check that the prosthesis is functioning satisfactorily. Some patients prefer to keep the penis against the abdominal wall whilst others prefer to keep the penis against the thigh. These measures are not necessary with the inflatable prostheses but occasionally patients complain of self-inflation of a multipart inflatable prosthesis. This occurs when the intra-abdominal pressure is raised by standing or when a capsule forms around the collapsed reservoir. It is for this reason that the prosthesis is kept deflated for the first three to four weeks after operation. The pump mechanism is sufficient to transfer fluid into the penile cylinders and stretch the capsule around the prosthesis but the return mechanism is a passive one and pressure is barely sufficient to distend the reservoir.

Dissatisfaction in the presence of a normal prosthesis usually stems from psychological reasons and further counselling is required (Schovar 1989). Dissatisfaction from a nonfunctioning prosthesis requires further operation and some of the patients resort to litigation. The legal aspects in the United States were reviewed by Irwin (1989).

Accurate information concerning the long term patient and partner satisfaction with the penile implant is incomplete and, in general, psychological assessment has been lacking (Sotile 1979; Gerstenberger et al 1979; Kaufman et al 1981; Collins & Kinder 1984; Schovar 1989; Gregoire 1992).

The study by Steege et al (1986) demonstrates that although the outcome falls far short of restoring premorbid sexual functioning or satisfaction, 90% of patients would still wish to have the procedure performed in the same circumstances.

Men undergo an implant operation for many reasons and with many different personalities.

Premorbid sexual activity, quality of the relationship and unrealistic expectations have an important bearing on the subsequent satisfaction from the operation. This has been demonstrated in both retrospective (Gee et al 1974; Gerstenberger et al 1979) and prospective studies (Berg et al 1984). Few studies have examined the partners' satisfaction. Kramarsky-Binkhorst (1978) found that 42% reported total satisfaction with the implant and, when the partner was not involved in the preoperative decision making, they were more likely to be dissatisfied. In this series, only 20% of partners were interviewed before the operation.

When a man who is in a stable sexual relationship loses the ability to obtain an erection as a result of an organic cause, it is usually unnecessary for him to undergo preoperative psychological evaluation by a mental health professional before proceeding to have an operation to restore his potency. It is desirable that the partner should be involved in the decision to proceed and counselling by a sympathetic surgeon is often all that is required. The implantation of a penile prosthesis may be the best option for many men and in others it may the the last resort after unsuccessful attempts to restore potency.

SUMMARY

The implantation of a penile prosthesis enables many men to return to successful and satisfying sexual relations. A large, and continually evolving, variety of implants is available for the surgeon to choose from, each with distinct advantages and disadvantages. Careful preoperative selection of suitable patients is essential and it is important for them to have realistic expectations. The operation provides sufficient penile rigidity for intercourse but it does not restore a normal erection and should not be expected to improve lost desire in patient or partner.

Cooperation between surgeon and mental health professional is essential if patients are to obtain maximum benefit from these operative procedures.

REFERENCES

Barry J M, Seifert A 1979 Penoscrotal approach for placement of paired penile implants for impotence. Journal

of Urology 122: 321–326
Beheri G E 1966 Surgical treatment of impotence. Journal of Plastic and Reconstructive Surgery 38: 92–97
Benson R C, Barrett D M, Patterson D E 1983 The Jonas

prosthesis: technical considerations and results. Journal of Urology 130: 920–922

Berg R, Mindus P, Berg G, Gustafson H 1984 Penile implants and erectile impotence: outcome and prognostic indicators. Scandinavian Journal of Urology and Nephrology 18: 277–282

Beutler L E, Scott F B, Rogers R R, Karacan I, Baer P E, Gaines J A 1986 Inflatable and non inflatable penile prostheses: comparative follow up evaluation. Urology 27: 136–143

Blum M D 1989 Infections of genitourinary prostheses. Infectious Diseases Clinics of North America 3: 259–274

Bogarus N 1936 Über die volle plastische wiederherstellung eines zum koitus fahigen Penis (peni plastica totalis). Zentralblatt für Chirurgie 63: 1271–1276

Bour J, Steinhardt G 1984 Penile necrosis in patients with diabetes mellitus and end stage renal disease. Journal of Urology 132: 560–561

Brown J B, Fryer M P, Randall P, Lu M P 1953 Silicones in plastic surgery. Plastic and Reconstructive Surgery 12: 374–376

Carson C L 1989 Infections in genitourinary prostheses. Urology Clinics of North America 16: 139–147

Chaikin L, Carrion H, Plitano V 1981 Complications of the Small-Carrion prosthesis: long term follow up. Journal of Urology 126: 44–45

Collins G F, Kinder B N 1984 Adjustment following surgical implantation of a penile prosthesis: a critical overview. Journal of Sex and Marital Therapy 10: 255–271

Cumming J, Pryor J P 1991 Treatment of organic impotence. British Journal of Urology 67: 640–643

Diokno A C 1983 Asymmetric inflation of the penile cylinders: etiology and management. Journal of Urology 129: 1127–1130

Dorflinger T, Bruskewitz R 1986 AMS malleable prosthesis. Urology 18: 480–485

Finney R P 1977 New hinged silicone penile implant. Journal of Urology 118: 585–587

Finney R P 1984 Finney Flexirod prosthesis. Urology 23: 79–82

Finney R P 1986 Flexiflate penile prosthesis. Seminars of Urology 4: 244–246

Fishman I J 1986 Experience with the Hydroflex penile prosthesis. Seminars of Urology 4: 239–243

Fishman I J 1989 Corporal reconstruction procedure for complicated penile implants. Urology Clinics of North America 16: 73–90

Frumkin A P 1944 Reconstruction of the male genitalia. American Review of Soviet Medicine 2: 14–21

Furlow W L, Motley R C 1988 The inflatable penile prosthesis: clinical experience with a new controlled expansion device. Journal of Urology 139: 945–946

Gee W F, McRoberts J W, Raney J O, Ansell J S 1974 The impotent patient: surgical treatment with penile prosthesis and psychiatric evaluation. Journal of Urology 111: 41–43

Gerstenberger D L, Osbourne D, Furlow W L 1979 Inflatable penile prosthesis: follow–up study of patient-partner satisfaction. Urology 14: 583–587

Goodwin W E, Scott W W 1952 Phalloplasty. Journal of Urology 68: 903–908

Gregoire A 1992 New treatments for erectile impotence. British Journal of Psychiatry 160: 315–326

Hinman F 1989 Atlas of urologic surgery. W B Saunders, Philadelphia

Irwin J R 1989 Legal aspects of urologic prosthetic devices.

Urology Clinics of North America 16: 165–174

Jonas U 1983 Five years' experience with the silicone-silver penile prosthesis: improvements and new developments. World Journal of Urology 1: 251–256

Jonas U, Jacobi G H 1980 Silicone-silver penile prosthesis: description, operative approach and results. Journal of Urology 123: 865–867

Kabalin J N, Kessler R 1989a Penile prosthesis surgery: review of 10 years' experience and examination of reoperations. Urology 23: 17–19

Kaufman J J, Boxer R J, Boxer B, Quim M C 1981 Physical and psychological results of penile prosthesis: a statistical survey. Journal of Urology 126: 173–175

Kelami A 1980 Atlas of operative andrology. De Gruyter, Berlin

Kramarsky-Binkhorst S 1978 Female partner perception of Small-Carrion implant. Urology 12: 545

Krane R J 1986 OmniPhase penile prosthesis. Seminars of Urology 4: 247–251

Krane R J 1988 Penile prostheses. Urology Clinics of North America 15: 103–109

Krane R J, Freedberg P S, Siroky M B 1981 Jonas silicone-silver prosthesis: initial experience in America. Journal of Urology 126: 475–476

Krauss D J 1985 Single cylinder penile prosthesis. Urology 26: 466–467

Krauss D J 1986 Elimination of pain caused by Small-Carrion penile prosthesis. Urology 28: 22–23

Lash H 1968, Silicone implant for impotence. Journal of Urology 100: 709–710

Lash H, Zimmerman D C, Loeffler R A 1964, Silicon implantation, inlay method. Plastic and Reconstructive Surgery 34: 75–79

Loeffler R A, Iveson R E 1976 Surgical treatment of impotence in the male. Plastic and Reconstrutive Surgery 58: 292–297

Maatman T J, Montague D K 1987 Intracorporal drainage after removal of infected penile prostheses. Urology 29 (Suppl.:) 42–43

McClellan D S, Masih B K 1985. Gangrene of the penis as a complication of penile prosthesis. Journal of Urology 133: 862

Malloy T, Wein A, Carpiniello V L 1987 Reliability of AMS 700 inflatable penile prosthesis. Urology 28: 385–387

Merrill D C 1989 Mentor inflatable penile prostheses. Urology Clinics of North America 16: 51–66

Montague D K,1986 Penile prosthesis. In: McDougal W S (ed) Rob and Smiths' operative surgery: urology. Butterworths, London, p 599–610

Montague D K 1987 Periprosthetic infections. Journal of Urology 138: 68–69

Moul J W, McLoed D G 1986 Experience with the AMS 600 malleable prosthesis. Journal of Urology 135: 929–931

Mulcahy J J 1989a The OmniPhase and DuraPhase penile prostheses. Urology Clinics of North American 16: 25–31

Mulcahy J J 1989b The Hydroflex penile prosthesis. Urology Clinics of North America 16: 33–38

Mulcahy J J, Krane R J, Lloyd K, Edson M, Siroky M B 1990 DuraPhase penile prosthesis — results of clinical trials in 63 patients. Journal of Urology 143: 518–519

Nielsen K T, Bruskewitz R C 1989 Semirigid and malleable rod penile prosthesis. Urology Clinics of North America 16: 13–23

Rowe P H, Royle M S 1983 Use of Jonas silicon–silver prosthesis in erectile impotence. Journal of the Royal

Society of Medicine 76: 1019–1022

Scarzella G I 1988 Cylinder reliability of inflatable penile prosthesis. Urology 33: 486–489

Scarzella G I 1989 Improved technique for implanting AMS 700CX inflatable penile prostheses using transverse scrotal approach. Urology 34: 388–389

Schovar L R 1989. Sex therapy for the penile prosthesis recipient. Urology Clinics of North America 16: 91–98

Scott F B 1987 Outpatient implantation of penile prostheses under local anaesthesia. Urology Clinics of North America 14: 177–186

Scott F B, Bradley W E, Timm G W 1973 Management of erectile impotence; use of an implantable inflatable prosthesis. Urology 2: 80–82

Scott F B, Fishman I J, Light J K 1983. A decade of experience with the inflatable penile prosthesis. World Journal of Urology, 1: 244–250

Small M P 1987 Semirigid and malleable penile implants. Urology Clinics of North America 14: 187–201

Small M P, Carrion H 1975 A new penile prosthesis for treating impotence. Contemporary Urology 7: 29–33

Sotile W M, 1979 The penile prosthesis: a review. Journal of Sex and Marital Therapy 5: 90–102

Stanisic T H, Dean J C 1989.The FlexiFlate and FlexiFlate II penile prostheses. Urology Clinics of North America 16: 39–49

Steege J F, Stout A L, Carsen C C 1986 Patient satisfaction in Scot and Small-Carrion penile implant recipients: a study of 52 patients. Archives of Sexual Behaviour 15(5): 393–399

Subrini L 1974 Le traitement chirurgical de l'impuissance virile par intabation prosthétique intra caverneuse. Journal of Urology and Nephrology 80: 269–276

Tawil E A, Gregory J G 1986 Failure of the Jonas prosthesis. Journal of Urology 135: 702–703

Thanalla J V, Thompson S T 1987 Infectious complications of penile prosthetic implants. Journal of Urology 138: 65–67

15. The impotent man without a partner

Martin Cole   Alain Gregoire

Many men with a sexual problem, but without a partner, find themselves in a classical 'catch 22' situation. Their problem will prevent them from forming a relationship but at the same time they need a relationship before they can begin to resolve their sexual difficulties.

Whether one agrees or not with Masters & Johnson's (1970) view that the 'relationship is the patient', and that treatment should always be focused upon the relationship, the fact remains that sex therapy programmes will have a poorer outcome in the absence of a partner. This is because, however useful psychoeducational and cognitive methods can be in the treatment of the partner-less man, there is no substitute for an in vivo behavioural approach — an approach which requires a partner. The social status of the partner is not crucial: for the impotent male she can be his wife, girlfriend, mistress or a surrogate (replacement partner). It is important, however, that whoever she is, she is as far as possible an involved partner.

More and more men are presenting with erectile problems on their own. The reasons for this are many and varied. First, the high divorce and separation rate means that many more people are living on their own without a partner, whether it is out of choice or not. Secondly, in an increasingly sexually aware society, men on their own, who might have tolerated celibacy a generation ago because of their sexual difficulties, are no longer prepared to do so. Indeed, some of these men might not have realized that they had a sexual problem but just chose not to get married (just as some women who elect not to form a relationship never realize that they are suffering from vaginismus). Thirdly, many men who are bereaved (or even divorced) in their fifties and sixties, and who would not originally have bothered to form a new relationship, will now do so because of their higher expectations. Over-exaggerated press reports of the benefits of papaverine injections and, more recently, those of hormone replacement therapy for men only serve to increase these expectations.

It has to be said that there still appears to be considerable prejudice against treating a man without a partner. It is almost as if many clinicians still hold the traditional view that a man has no need for sex until he has a relationship, or that he should be able to solve his own problems. Though there are many obvious practical difficulties to be overcome in formulating a treatment programme for the impotent single man, the negative response of some clinicians — 'Go and get yourself a partner and then come back' — has to be challenged.

ASSESSMENT AND DIAGNOSIS

Considerable attention has been paid elsewhere (see Ch. 6) to the importance of thorough history taking, a careful examination and appropriate investigations in order to ensure an accurate diagnosis is obtained before treatment begins. Obviously this is equally important for the man who presents without a partner, though his history may be complicated by two additional features. First, he may never have had the opportunity to attempt intercourse and therefore neither he nor the clinician will have any information about his responses with a partner. Furthermore, it is more likely that his problem is primary, which increases the possibility of congenital physical causes, such as venous leakage or genital abnormality.

Secondly, because he is on his own, it is sometimes difficult to anticipate precisely what is preventing him from forming a sexual relationship. Perhaps his problem is not specifically sexual but stems instead from an absence of heterosocial skills? Has he homosexual needs? Is he simply going through the motions of thinking that he ought to be sexual and ought to get married just because other people do so? Does he fear ridicule because of some real or imagined genital abnormality (a small penis or undescended testes)? Is he generally socially isolated because of psychiatric illness, such as depression or schizophrenia?

TREATMENT STRATEGIES

The treatment of a man who presents with erectile problems but has no partner can be approached in a number of ways. Attention can be focused upon any deficiencies in his social and courtship skills so that one can increase the probability that he will be able to meet a partner with whom he can form a relationship and resolve his sexual problems within the new relationship.

Alternatively, he might try surrogate therapy (see p. 222) and obtain help from a temporary, replacement partner with whom he can learn new social and sexual skills. Ideally, these strategies should be attempted at the same time. If, as a result of these approaches, he is able to form a relationship of his own then the methods used to treat erectile problems described in Chapter 10 can be used.

PSYCHOLOGICAL TREATMENTS

The methods used to help those who are socially or sexually isolated are relatively new: they incorporate four main approaches — practical advice, psychoeducation, cognitive methods and behaviour therapy. Treatment can be organized in groups (Kayata & Szydlo 1988) or singly (Stravynski 1986).

Zilbergeld & Ellison (1979), to whom the reader is particularly referred, stress the importance of social skills training in helping patients without partners and draw attention to the increasing need for this approach as therapists work more and more frequently with individuals. For example, Reynolds et al (1981), making use of teaching, homework assignments and role play, were able to help 11 men who had erectile problems but who had no sexual partners. Using these methods the patients were able to dispose of many sexual myths (see p. 220) and develop new behaviours which led to the improvement of their dating skills and in turn to the formation of sexual relationships. Employing a similar approach, Lobitz & Baker (1979), helped six out of nine partnerless men who had difficulties with erection. Finally, Stravynski (1986) gives an account of the successful treatment of one patient with erectile problems but who was without a partner. Using social skills training and a series of behavioural interventions, sexual intercourse was achieved after six weeks and was maintained after six months.

It should be obvious that organizing treatment of this kind is very difficult since it makes so many demands upon available resources. However, given good motivation on the part of the patient and the professional, it works well (Altman et al 1985) and where circumstances permit, urgent attention should be given to developing facilities of this kind.

Does the client really want a partner?

The need to have a relationship and the need for a sexual partner are, for most men, one and the same thing. However, for a variety of reasons, there are some men for whom this is not so. The sexual appetite of some men is very low and one or more platonic relationships suffice — they may present for sex therapy with erectile inadequacy, but if their 'problem' is diagnosed correctly and they are able to see it in a proper perspective, often this is all the help they require. Other men find it quite impossible to settle down with one partner because they require a large number of sexual partners, which normally places a great strain on their relationships. If these men also have erectile problems it is often difficult to help them because of the trouble they have in forming long-term relationships. Most men, however, can integrate their sexual and loving needs sufficiently well to want to form a relationship of reasonable duration and naturally this group will be easier to treat.

Before help can be provided, it is crucial to

examine the reasons why a man seeks help to form a relationship and to examine his motives for what may lead to dramatic changes in his life. He may, for example, have evolved over the years a secure and comfortable lifestyle living with his mother or be so independent surviving on his own that it would be difficult to envisage how he could adapt sufficiently to allow a partner into his life. These men may seek advice as to how they might form a relationship without having examined the consequences. Social pressures and the need to conform to the cultural norms may motivate them to try to 'settle down' when in fact it is not in their nature. In other words, if they do not *need* a relationship there is little point blaming the world at large for their isolation.

Having established that there is a genuine need for change, there are a number of specific strategies which can be used to help patients overcome their sexual and emotional blocks. Relationship formation comprises two steps: meeting a partner and forming a relationship. These will be considered in turn.

Meeting a partner

A man who lives with his family or on his own and is having difficulty in meeting someone may believe that his chances of meeting an acceptable partner who will also like him are very small. He may even believe that there is no one 'out there' with whom he can form a relationship. A moment's reflection will reveal that this is most unlikely. A quick calculation should reveal that, depending upon his age and circumstances, he might expect between about 1% and 5% of the total population of women in his catchment area to be available as potential partners, a number which could be quite large if he lives in or near a sizeable town or city.

To begin the process of setting about meeting a partner, he should be encouraged to sit down with pen and paper to work out a specific strategy to operate over a time scale of about six months to a year. The following items in this checklist need to be considered seriously and, although much of what follows simply takes the form of practical advice, the importance of this should not be underestimated. Moreover, although this seems very artifical, this strategy is in fact little more than formulating the thoughts and behaviours of most people who wish to form relationships.

- He should seek work. A man who is unwishingly without a partner and who is also unemployed clearly finds himself at a disadvantage. He will have little or no money to spend; his self-esteem may be low and to be without a job may create a poor impression upon potential partners. Furthermore, the workplace is an important social setting where he is likely to meet people in similar walks of life.

- If his resources allow, he should try to get independent transport. Admittedly, there are many men who conduct their courtships without private transport and a car is not essential, particularly if his prospective partner has one. Nevertheless, to be mobile makes his task very much easier.

- If he is living at home with his parent(s) he may wish to consider finding his own accommodation. Sometimes this makes good economic sense if he can afford a mortgage. It certainly makes good psychological sense because once away from home he can start the process (if it has not already begun) of separating from his parent(s) and obtain greater privacy and independence. In addition, he is likely to be more attractive as a potential partner. The loneliness he experiences may increase his motivation to find a partner — or he may discover that he wishes to return home and postpone his search. This isolation away from home may lead to depression and naturally this should be guarded against. Conversely, it may have the reverse effect by boosting his self-esteem.

- It is a good idea to list all the ways in which he might meet someone. The following may help:

  — Parties and dances
  — Clubs and pubs
  — Other social events
  — At work or through work
  — Sporting activities, exercise clubs and classes
  — Education, e.g. university or college
  — Evening classes
  — Public transport

— Introduction through friends
— Blind dates
— Introductory agencies; advertisements
— Chance events

- Searching for a partner on one's own can be a lonely exercise so if it can be done with a friend or friends this will help a lot. Girls often go around in groups and can be a little defensive about a man on his own and if the evening is a disaster this is lessened if one has friends to share and laugh with about the experience.

- It is a good idea to re-establish contact with people with whom you may have lost touch: friends will themselves have friends and one thing can lead to another.

- Even if one is unsociable it is sensible to entertain occasionally: the result, often, is that you get a return invitation and meet new people.

- Most local authorities publish a 'What's On' magazine which lists local clubs, societies and social and sports activities. Evening classes are also advertised and these often provide a way of meeting people. Language or art/craft classes often provide a good mix of sexes, whereas computer programming and car maintenance may be largely attended by men. It is therefore important to make an intelligent choice of subject area.

- Although opportunities to meet others with the possibility of forming a relationship often exist, these may become missed opportunities through procrastination and indecision born of anxiety. If and when opportunities do arise, however difficult it may seem at the time, he should be pressed to accept invitations and to think positively. Even if nothing comes of it, by confronting his fears he will have made his next attempt easier and gained some experience which may help him to avoid making any obvious mistakes in future.

- Whatever his circumstances, he should try to rid himself of the idea that he is too old, too ugly, too poor, too anxious or too ineffectual to get a partner. Self-judgement is rarely objective and the professional's role is to help the patient see himself objectively but in a positive context.

- He should seek the advice of others about his dress and general appearance. Many people tend to get set in the way they dress and their habits are often difficult to change. Suggestions for a dramatic revision of clothing styles will fall on deaf ears and may even be hurtful: gentle hints are much more likely to work. Cleanliness is crucial (clothes and body) and an approximation to current fashion helpful. Clothes that fit are also a good idea. Sometimes contact lenses instead of spectacles reveal attractive eyes and even a visit to the dentist or hygienist can work wonders.

- He needs to be reminded that relationships between the sexes are of many types and levels of intensity where there may or may not be a strong sexual element present. Indeed, it is often useful to be able to begin to rehearse social skills in a so-called platonic relationship. Prospective relationships should not be automatically excluded simply because there is no immediate erotic attraction present. Furthermore, it is likely to be advantageous if he can form a close, trusting relationship in which sexual failure would not be so disastrous.

- Difficult as it may be, he should try to dispose of any rigid views he has of his own needs and his expectations of others. Most people improve on acquaintance and there is much to be said for the view that propinquity is a powerful element in the bonding process. People who are thrown together often discover that a bond develops between them which would not have otherwise been forged. Relationships usually need time to mature — love at first sight is rare and often short-lived.

- In particular, he should be warned against over-investing in new relationships. This advice is often ignored but it needs to be repeated and heeded. It is very tempting, almost irresistible, for a man who is lonely, insecure, underconfident and who fears rejection to go over the top in his need to impress his partner and express his need for love and commitment. Such an approach will not only increase the risk of scaring her off, but will also add to his feelings of loss and rejection should the relationship founder.

Forming a relationship

Men who have problems with sex will often find it difficult to form and maintain relationships. There are, of course, many relationships where, for a variety of reasons, sex may play only a small part in the transaction between the couple and the relationship can be truly described as companionate. However, it has to be accepted that these relationships, particularly amongst young people, are rare and that sex does remain an important element in the process of pair-bonding.

Increasing social and sexual freedom for women has allowed them to play a much more important part in courtship, but even nowadays the male still has, generally speaking, a greater share of responsibility in initiating a relationship. Moreover, courtship rituals apart, he still needs to get an erection and to be able to hold it at the very least for a minute or so in order to, as he sees it, 'have sex' and 'please her'. If, for whatever reason, he is sexually or emotionally precarious, his penis may fail to respond and if he then begins to harbour doubts about his sexual performance and incubate these fears his performance anxieties will lead to a self-fulfilling fear of failure compounding his existing fear of underconfidence and inadequacy. Therapeutic intervention can often help those who have become victims of their own anxieties in this way and these therapies may include one or more of the following strategies: practical advice, psychoeducation, cognitive therapy or behaviour therapy.

Practical advice

The impact of the client-centred therapies has often made many professionals cautious about giving practical advice. Perhaps they believe, mistakenly, that practical advice is unsophisticated. The therapeutic value of this kind of approach is to provide the patient with new ideas and options, and to give him permission to act on thoughts, which he may well have had, but has been afraid to act on. He can then screen out those options which are inappropriate for him and retain those which seem to make sense. This directive approach can be refreshingly positive. The suggestions and ideas proposed in the earlier part of this chapter (see p. 217) should therefore be con-

sidered in this light and the patient will find that he will only try them out if they feel right.

For example, here are two suggestions which a patient may (or may not) find appropriate, remembering that advice, if given properly, is about floating new ideas, not directing people to follow a particular course of action.

- If an underconfident and sexually precarious patient is a little uncertain about whether he will achieve an erection in a first sexual encounter with a new partner, it is often a good idea for him to share his worries with his partner *before* they attempt intercourse. Doing this will help to reduce his performance anxieties to a level which may then allow him to obtain a good erection. It will also give his partner an opportunity to modify her behaviour so as to help him.
- In a new relationship, the point of readiness for intercourse is usually arrived at intuitively. However, if there are problems and the man feels the decision is up to him and he is uncertain what to do, he should realize that there is little point putting off the time of intercourse, if only for the reason that the longer he waits and his uncertainty persists, the more powerful his performance anxieties will become.

The psychoeducational mode

Allied to the provision of practical advice is that of psychoeducation or the provision of information. Clinicians should have available a short list of publications that they can recommend (see Appendix 10.1). Patients should be instructed to read and digest a few selected books. Considerable benefits can be derived from this approach, so much so that it has earned the name bibliotherapy (Trudel & Laurin 1988).

Ellis refers to this approach when he says 'therapy, however it is done, consists of largely teaching people how to look after themselves, how to undefensively see the way in which they are sabotaging their own goals and interests' (Ellis 1983, p. 37). Psychoeducation therefore aims to educate the patient by providing accurate information which will help him to see his problem more objectively. Such information would help him, for example, to begin to challenge the many sexual myths which may have contributed to his sexual difficulties in the past (Zilbergeld 1980). Thus it is useful to know, understand and remember that:

- Men normally remain sexually responsive throughout their lives and though naturally as they get older their sex drive and the speed with which they can get an erection diminishes, there is no particular cut-off point beyond which this capacity to enjoy intercourse disappears. One of the main difficulties is that men do not often communicate personally to each other about their sex lives, particularly as they get older, or if they do some of what they say may not be particularly reliable.

- As men age they require more prolonged tactile stimulation of the penis and spontaneous erections are less likely or less frequent. If necessary it is sensible to try to communicate this need to one's partner — she may be shy and feel embarrassed about taking this initiative herself. However, simply placing her hand on his penis is a very effective way of showing her that extra penile stimulation is required.

- Men are not sex machines — they do not always want sex. Many women know this but unfortunately many men believe that women expect them to be able to seduce them at fifty yards and perform instantly.

- It is important for men to realize that physical contact need not always lead to sex or that sex does not always mean intercourse. There can be a gentle progression from hand holding and kissing through to penetrative sex or one can stop and change direction at any point. Unromantic as it may appear, a few chosen words can help to make one's feelings and intent known to one's partner.

- Some men believe that by not masturbating and saving themselves they can ensure a stronger erection when the opportunity for intercourse presents itself. This is not true; indeed, if anything, the reverse is the case since a long interval between ejaculations may lead to a down regulation of the neurohormonal mechanisms responsible for sexual arousal — 'If you don't use it you will lose it' (see Ch. 4). On the other hand, occasionally one meets men who masturbate perhaps two or three times a day and are then surprised that they don't achieve a good erection in intercourse — they clearly need to reduce their number of ejaculations.

- Many men tend to project their own preoccupations with penetrative sex on to their partners. In other words, because he is preoccupied with penetration he assumes that she is too. This is particularly evident when he becomes over-concerned with giving his partner an orgasm and loses his erection in the process. Her climax may or may not be possible in intercourse but her orgasm may be less important for her than it is for him. Moreover, her capacity for a climax is her responsibility and there is only a limited number of ways in which he can help her. Since up to about one half (or more) of all women are unable to achieve an unassisted orgasm in intercourse, i.e. without some manual assistance (Sanders 1985; Kaplan 1989), clearly there are many other rewards for a woman that a man should be aware of. Closeness, intimacy, the sensuality of physical contact and the various levels of sexual arousal which may or may not end in an orgasm can all be very important to her. He should also try to discover that sexual pleasure can be a whole-body experience for him as well and that by experimenting with sensate focus on his own, for example, (see p. 151) he can discover that the rewards of non-genital arousal need not be exclusively female.

The cognitive mode

An individual's thoughts, beliefs and expectations of himself, his partner and the outside world will clearly influence and shape his sexual behaviour (Wolfe & Walen 1982) (and see Ch. 10). Cognitive therapy aims to alter a patient's perception and evaluation of himself so that he can see himself in a more positive light and hence increase the chances of experiencing pleasurable sexual encounters. For example, he should know, understand and continually remind himself (or argue with himself), if necessary, that:

- Many men are deterred from forming sexual relationships because of the fear and pain of rejection. Sometimes they may not be aware of this and it is helpful to draw their attention to this fear if it is present. Having done so, this anxiety of loss and rejection can be challenged cognitively. Patients should be encouraged to ask themselves, 'What is the worst thing that can happen if I am rejected'? They should then look closely at how they might be exaggerating and magnifying the consequences of rejection, and remember that most people have the resources to deal with these bad feelings. (For an excellent discussion of the problems of rejection and jealousy see Hauck (1981)).

- The patient's attention should be drawn to the fundamental behavioural principle that every time he runs away or backs off from a feared experience (approaching a girl for a date) the consequence will be reinforcement of this avoidance behaviour, making it much more difficult to approach her (or another) next time.

- His potential sexual partner is just as likely to be as anxious about the prospect of intimacy as he is.

- He should remember that if he can get a good erection in self-masturbation then clearly there is nothing seriously wrong with him.

- If he is unable to get an erection with a particular partner it may be that, because the penis is a sensitive barometer of his feelings, it could be telling him that this partner may not be the right one for him.

- He needs to remind himself that if he does happen to lose his erection in sex play, or even after penetration, this is not 'awful', 'terrible', or 'horrible'. Indeed, it is quite normal for this to happen, particularly in a new relationship; from previous experience he also knows that his erection will return.

The behavioural mode

As a means of modifying human behaviour there is little doubt that behavioural methods are the most effective and it is these methods which form the basis of sex therapy for couples (Masters & Johnson 1970; Kaplan 1974). However, when a patient presents with erectile inadequacy without a partner, the in vivo behavioural intervention normally used for couples is obviously not available, unless surrogate therapy (see p. 222) can be arranged. There are, however, some behavioural strategies that can be usefully employed in the treatment of the partnerless man with erectile problems.

Role play. Role play provides a very effective means of helping men without partners to deal with their anxieties about courtship, sex play and coitus, providing an opportunity for the patient to rehearse behaviours in a simulated situation which approximates to a real life experience (Stravynski 1986; Kayata & Szydlo 1988). For example, he will have an opportunity to learn to practise his social skills and, in particular, his conversational skills with a woman — who can act out either a cooperative or a 'resistant' role — to test his responses. Thus there is an informational, psycho-educational and behavioural (desensitization) component to role play if properly organized. The detached yet interpersonal element of role play allows the patient an opportunity to practise asking difficult questions of his partner, e.g. 'Will you hold my penis?', 'How does a woman masturbate herself?', or 'Sometimes I don't get a very good erection. Will you help me?'

However, it is not easy to set up either couples or groups for role play. The difficulties are obvious and often insurmountable with the result that health services provide little or no help of this kind.

David is 49 and had been happily married with no sexual problems for 25 years. He has three children who have now left home. Four years ago his wife was diagnosed as having breast cancer and she died two years later. David was devastated and found it very difficult to cope on his own. After a year grieving the loss, he felt he was ready to start a new relationship and advertised in the local papers, joined Dateline and began to try to socialize a little by going to one or two singles clubs. He met one or two women and on the third occasion, after a few drinks, he ended up going to bed with one. David had never had any sexual experience outside his marriage. It was therefore not surprising that a combination of performance anxiety, lack of experience, unresolved grief and a period of enforced abstinence during the previous three years resulted in a complete lack of sexual response on his part. David was naturally humiliated and dejected about his failure and when this happened on two further occasions he began to think there was something very seriously wrong. A few weeks later he met someone else whom he believed he really cared for and he felt that the feelings were mutual. It was at this point that he came for help.

Investigations did not reveal any organic basis to his problem and the fact that David was getting good erections in the morning, as he did when he masturbated, made it possible to stress that there was absolutely nothing wrong with him physically, that he was a physiologically intact, healthy male and that nothing could stop him achieving intercourse with his new partner when he was ready. It was also pointed out to him that it would have been more surprising if he had not failed, bearing in mind the circumstances.

He was told to try to share his feelings of insecurity and vulnerability with his new partner, to explain the reasons for his long period of abstinence, that he was not a 'macho' male and that he would prefer to begin their sex life without any preconditions or goals. Such an approach enabled him to keep command of the situation, but at the same time share his anxieties. His partner proved to be sympathetic and supportive and after one or two false starts they began a full and satisfying sex life.

Very little formal cognitive or behavioural intervention was required with David. It was, however, necessary to explain to him why he had failed before but that given a loving, supportive relationship, with a partner whom he found sexually attractive, he would be unlikely to fail again.

Masturbation and fantasy training

The idea behind masturbation and fantasy training is to help the patient initiate new fantasies or modify existing ones so that they approximate more closely to a target behaviour. In this way it is hoped that the changed fantasies will facilitate a change in behaviour. For example, some heterophobic men do not include intercourse in their masturbatory fantasies, but instead limit them to sex play. Similarly, men with erectile disorders may devise fantasies where instead of taking part themselves they play out the role of observing another couple having intercourse. In both these instances it is desirable that the patient is encouraged to include penetration and coitus in his fantasies and to play an active role himself. He should also try to synchronize his orgasm with the orgasm in his fantasy. Sometimes this change takes time and it can only be achieved by a graded series of

fantasies which increasingly approximate to the desired goal.

More specifically, masturbation training with or without fantasy can be used to help men with erectile problems. They are told to stimulate their penis to erection, then deliberately lose it and then regain it with further stimulation: this should demonstrate to their own satisfaction that lost erections can be regained and are not, as some men fear, once lost difficult to restore.

Surrogate therapy

Although there are many legal, ethical and practical difficulties involved in providing a substitute sexual partner for patients who present on their own, such an approach can prove very effective and is sometimes the only way of helping these men (Cole 1988).

The use of these so-called surrogate partners provides the opportunity to apply the normal methods of couple therapy to the treatment of erectile disorders in those men without a partner. Surrogate therapy may even have certain advantages over using the patient's own partner. This in vivo approach has one particular advantage over those psychotherapeutic methods described earlier in this chapter in that it provides an opportunity for the patient to acquire his sexual skills and achieve anxiety reduction in a real life situation. In practice, therefore, surrogate therapy simply takes heterosocial skills training one stage further to include training in sexual skills, providing an opportunity for a man to bridge the gap between being socially and sexually isolated and having a relationship of his own.

Masters & Johnson were probably the first to use substitute sexual partners. They treated 54 single men and 3 single women and achieved a 'success' rate of 78%. They described the surrogates as 'someone to hold on to, talk to, work with, learn from, be a part of and above all else give to and get from' (Masters & Johnson 1970, p. 147).

The role of the surrogate is complex, but above all she must be able to take responsibility for the patient and in so doing provide support, understanding, a listening ear, sound advice, warmth, empathy and, of course, the opportunity for tactile stimulation and sexual arousal. Of course, surrogate therapy does not always achieve all these goals but with a good surrogate, a motivated patient and a compatible mix most of these objectives can be achieved. In particular, she will be instrumental in providing the opportunity for behaviour therapy which, for these men with erectile problems, may include sensate focus together with those other features of treatment described in Chapter 10.

A major criticism that is often levelled against the use of surrogates is that because there is no 'involved' relationship between the surrogate and the patient, this form of treatment can never be successful. However, paradoxically, surrogate therapy often works well because there *is* no heavy relationship. For example, performance anxiety is reduced in surrogate therapy because the patient is not investing so much in the relationship. Indeed the element of ritual, a set appointment, payment and the constraints of time in surrogate therapy provide one way in which anxiety can be controlled. Moreover, if on occasion things do not go well, such failures will not result in a dramatic loss of self-esteem — a loss likely to be present in a more serious relationship — as there is a clear and open understanding that the patient has a problem. Finally, communication between the patient and the surrogate is normally much easier than that in a real life relationship.

In so far that information, advice and changes of attitude on the part of the patient are required in therapy of this kind, the surrogate can play a role that no girlfriend could ever achieve. Many men, for example, know little or nothing about the clitoris and to be able to ask questions, be shown where it is and to touch it as part of a learning process, instead of as part of love making, can be of great value.

Tim works as a manager in light industry. He is very achieving, ambitious and assertive and, at 31, further promotion is very likely. He is good-looking, has his own house and car but he has no girlfriends and no sex life.

He first attempted intercourse when he was 17 but was unable to get an erection even though he had been going out with his partner for the previous six months. She was less than sympathetic and he was so upset that although he subsequently took one or two girls out, he made no further sexual approaches until he was 25.

When he tried intercourse then he again failed to get an erection.

He now feels that unless he can get help he will remain single, even though he wants to get married and have a family. Thorough investigations failed to reveal any physical basis to his problem, though psychometry (EPQ) showed him to be a very anxious extrovert. Temperamentally, he was also highly obsessional and very demanding of himself and others. His social skills were more than adequate and he had no difficulty dating girls, though he was somewhat brusque and unfeeling in his approach.

Three simultaneous treatment strategies were proposed. He was made to understand and continually remind himself that it was very unlikely that there was a physical basis to his problem and that his failure to get an erection resulted from the traumatic effects of that first experience. It was explained to him that he was temperamentally vulnerable to this kind of setback, but that the effects were far from permanent. However, he had to confront these fears if he was to make any progress. He was therefore encouraged to assume that the problem would not return and to start dating again. Finally, it was arranged that he should begin a short programme of surrogate therapy.

Tim saw the surrogate on six occasions: during the first session they spent most of the time talking and the session ended with them kissing, but fully clothed. Much of the surrogate work during the early sessions was psychoeducational: she provided him with elementary information about love-making and attempted to dispose of many of the sexual myths with which the sexually inexperienced often burden themselves. In the second and subsequent sessions, they progressively became more intimate, with an initial ban on intercourse, until Tim was able to erect without any difficulty. Full and satisfactory intercourse was achieved during the fifth and sixth sessions.

Shortly after the completion of treatment Tim met a girl and, although the relationship was not a committed one, he was able to obtain a good erection and achieve intercourse on several occasions. This therapeutic approach involved psychoeducational, cognitive and behavioural therapies.

Outcome of surrogate therapy

The accurate measurement of the outcome of surrogate therapy is no easier than that of couple therapy (see Ch. 10) and follow-ups are even more difficult. A full analysis of the results of treatment of 425 patients using surrogate therapy is presented in Cole (1988). Of these, 96 presented with erectile problems. Diagnostic methods used indicated that only 10 patients out of that total had secondary erectile problems that could be attributed to psychogenicity with certainty: these patients demonstrated a mean 'therapeutic gain', using a five point scale, of 54%. The mean improvement of all the patients presenting with erectile problems, regardless of aetiology, was 28%.

PHYSICAL TREATMENT STRATEGIES

The use of physical treatments for erectile failure in men without partners poses considerable difficulties. It is, of course, possible to take a simplistic approach, isolating the malfunction of the man's penis from the man himself and his relationships (or lack of them). This approach may produce stiffness of his penis but there often remain important barriers for the man to overcome before he can have a satisfactory sexual relationship. The main reason for this is that it is virtually impossible in practice for a man to use the currently available physical treatments without the knowledge of his partner, and thus admitting to the partner that he has difficulties with his erections. This is obviously difficult unless the man is able to develop a close and trusting relationship. The only exceptions to this are the few cases who benefit from venous or arterial surgery.

GS, a 26-year-old single man, presented with intermittent inability to achieve erection adequate for intercourse. He had been involved in several brief relationships and one relationship lasting nearly a year. In each of these relationships he had been unable to obtain erections in the first few sexual encounters with his partner. In some cases this had led to the relationship ending, either because of his feelings of inadequacy, or because of his partner losing interest in him. However, with two of his partners, he had reached a stage were he was able to obtain erections on most attempts and sustained these throughout intercourse. During his longest relationship he was having reasonably satisfactory intercourse once or twice a week, with only very occasional difficulties with his erections. This relationship ended for what appeared to have been largely nonsexual reasons. In the year since that time he had three brief relationships but had not been able to achieve intercourse in any of these.

He was becoming despondent and had started avoiding contact with the opposite sex. After seeing an advertisement in the newspaper for a 'new treatment for impotence' he attended a private clinic where a brief medical history was taken and he was prescribed papaverine for self-injection. He received no form of counselling either in general terms or even with regard to the potential side effects of the treatment. He used the injections on two occasions on his own at home and obtained good erections. Several weeks later, he had sexual intercourse with a new girlfriend, having secretly injected himself in the bathroom before going to bed with her. He was able to disguise the fact that his erection did not subside following ejaculation and she apparently did not notice that anything was untoward. He made excuses to avoid her advances for further intercourse the following morning and arranged to meet her two or three days later. Unfortunately, on that occasion she interrupted him while he was in the process of preparing the injection and saw what he was doing. He then had to explain the deception. Her reaction to this and to his need for drug injections in order to achieve erections was a mixture of anger, disgust and disappointment and resulted in her ending the relationship.

This experience left him considerably worse off than he had been when he first sought treatment: his psychogenic erectile failure remained, and his reluctance to enter into relationships with women became phobic in its intensity. After several months he confided in his general practitioner who referred him to my clinic. He required regular counselling sessions over several months, which centred on controlling his by now irrational fears of rejection; anxiety management and, in the later stages, sensate focus techniques and masturbation excercises were also incorporated into the treatment.

Towards the end of the treatment he had become involved in a relationship again and had managed to confide in his new girlfriend that he had occasional sexual difficulties. Although he failed to achieve penetration on their first attempt, he was surprised to find that this was met by encouragement rather than rejection and on their second attempt, intercourse was successful and satisfying.

This case illustrates how disastrous the inappropriate use of physical treatments can be. This man, who had a psychogenic problem which later reponded well to psychological treatment, was actually considerably worse after using the treatment than he had been when he first presented.

Before launching into a discussion of the appropriate use of physical treatments in single men, the importance of adequate assessment should again be stressed. It is only through an understanding of the reasons for both the man's erectile problems *and* his singleness that a judgement can be made about the appropriate use and timing of physical treatments.

The principle that physical treatments should be accompanied by psychological approaches applies almost without exception to men without partners. It is perfectly possible and indeed quite common for men who have erectile failure to find partners who are prepared to accept their difficulty and help them overcome it. Men who feel unable to seek such relationships need the reassurance, support and advice of professionals to overcome their anxieties and feelings of inadequacy. Only then will they be in a position to benefit from physical interventions.

The decisions about if and when to employ physical treatments in single men are influenced by a number of factors. It is impossible to list these factors in a sensible hierarchy as in any individual any one factor could outweigh all others.

The cause of the erectile failure

In general, men with largely psychogenic dysfunction should be treated in the first instance with one of the psychological approaches described in the previous section. Cases of mainly organic dysfunction will at some stage require physical treatment to restore erections. In most of these cases adjunctive psychological intervention is important. These two situations are relatively clear cut. However, the use of physical treatments in the men with psychogenic impotence is controversial. There is some evidence that benefit can be derived by inducing artificial erections over a limited period of time (using intracavernosal injections of vasoactive drugs or vacuum devices). This evidence is derived from work with men in relationships who had the opportunity to use the erections obtained for sexual intercourse (see Ch. 10). Such use in single men has not been documented. Although the mechanism involved in such improvement is not established, it is likely to involve an increase in self-confidence and a decrease in performance anxiety. This increase in confidence probably stems from the experience of being able to have satisfactory sexual intercourse during which the man need not fear that his erection will disappear. In single men, this experience may not be possible and thus one would be relying on the experience of simply having an erection to boost his confidence. As men with psychogenic dysfunction are usually able to have erections at some time anyway, this experience may be of little

benefit to them. Thus we return to the need for the man to form some sort of relationship to increase his chance of benefiting from this approach.

Attitudes to sex and relationships

Men's expectation of their own sexual performance, and their beliefs about women's expectations of male sexual performance, vary greatly. Differences in such beliefs and expectations between individuals depend on factors such as social class, culture, and education. Change also occurs within individuals because of age, sexual experience and changes in their social or working environment.

These beliefs and expectations are important when considering the appropriateness and outcome of physical treatments; for example a man in his 60s who believes that a partner of his own age would automatically reject him if he needed to use IIVD is less likely to benefit from this treatment than one who knows that women in later life do not expect same age partners to be 'superstuds'. Young men who believe that relationships are based primarily on good sexual performance and an ability to obtain and maintain 'natural' erections are also likely to derive less benefit from physical treatments.

Reasons for the lack of a partner

Reasons for not having a partner are always complex. As has already been mentioned, putting it down to the erectile problem alone is denying the fact that it is also the man's response to his problem that restricts his ability to form or sustain relationships. However, in a few cases, this barrier is removed simply by the reassurance that the problem is a potentially treatable one: many men believe that impotence is untreatable and thus do not entertain the possibility of forming close relationships. In such cases, reassurance, an offer of physical treatment and a suitable time interval before starting may be all that is required to restore erections and relationships.

In many cases, however, more deep rooted problems will exist, such as low self-esteem, loss of socializing skills and lifestyle changes (burying themselves in work, social withdrawal, independent lifestyles with little room for another person). These problems are potentially treatable using psychological approaches, although this may be difficult or impossible if they reflect long-standing personality characteristics rather than a response to the current situation.

Premorbid sexual functioning

The literature on outcome following psychological or physical treatments points consistently to the importance of the quality of sexual relations before the onset of the problem (e.g. Hawton & Catalan 1986; Berg et al 1984). Such research has concentrated on men and women in relationships, but there is no reason to suppose that it does not apply equally to single men.

Thus, men who have had little difficulty in forming or sustaining sexually active relationships before the onset of erectile problems may benefit from physical treatments with only minimal psychological intervention.

Motivation

Response to psychological interventions is very much dependent on the motivation of the client (Hawton & Catalan 1986). When one is considering the outcome of physical treatments in terms of sexual satisfaction, the patient's own choice, and therefore motivation, for a particular treatment is likely to be important. Furthermore, no benefit will be derived from pressurizing patients into accepting a line of treatment which they

will simply drop out of. Thus it is entirely appropriate for the clinician to be guided to a large extent by clearly stated preferences from the patient. Of course the clinician can very effectively use the patient's chosen treatment in the first instance to gain his confidence, thus allowing the introduction of methods to which he was initially resistant. This is one of the ways in which IIVD can be usefully employed at an early stage to permit later airing of psychological issues.

SUMMARY

It is often tempting for patients and practitioners to concentrate on the single man's erectile problem and neglect the often greater problem of his lack of relationships. This attitude is often justified by taking the view that the sexual problem has caused the singleness, and that treating the former will resolve the latter. This is only rarely the case. In general, whatever the cause for the erectile dysfunction, any blocks to forming relationships should first be tackled. This may involve techniques such as simple reassurance and encouragement, social skills training, psychoeducation and cognitive behavioural therapy.

The use of physical treatment methods alone is generally inappropriate. They may, however, be an important part of a treatment package which includes some of the above psychological interventions. They are usually best introduced in the later stages of such a package. Sometimes the use of physical treatments early on may help to engage patients who are resistant to a psychological approach into a productive therapeutic relationship.

REFERENCES

Altman I, Gahan P, Jehu D 1985 Psychoeducational treatment of impotence. British Journal of Sexual Medicine 12: 55–57

Berg R, Mindus P, Berg G, Gustafson H 1984 Penile implants and erectile impotence: outcome and prognostic indicators. Scandinavian Journal of Urology and Nephrology 18: 227–282

Cole M J 1988 Sex therapy for individuals. In: Cole M, Dryden W (eds) Sex therapy in Britain. Open University Press, Milton Keynes

Ellis A 1983 Does sex therapy really have a future? Rational Living 18: 3–6

Hauck P 1989 Jealousy. Sheldon Press, London

Hawton K, Catalan J 1986 Prognostic factors in sex therapy.

Behaviour Research and Therapy 24: 377–385

Kaplan H S 1974 The new sex therapy. Brunner/Mazel, New York

Kaplan H S 1989 PE. How to overcome premature ejaculation. Brunner/Mazel, New York

Kayata L, Szydlo D 1988 Sex therapy in groups. In: Cole M, Dryden W (eds) Sex therapy in Britain. Open University Press, Milton Keynes

Lobitz W C, Baker E L 1979 Group treatment of single males with erectile dysfunction. Archives of Sexual Behavior 8: 127–138

Masters W H, Johnson V 1970 Human sexual inadequacy. Churchill, London

Reynolds B S, Cohen B D, Schochet B V, Price S C, Anderson A J 1981 Dating skills training in the group treatment of erectile dysfunction for men without partners.

Journal of Sex and Marital Therapy 7: 184–194

Sanders D 1985 The Woman book of love and sex. Sphere, London

Stravynski A 1986 Indirect behavioral treatment of erectile failure and premature ejaculation without a partner. Archives of Sexual Behavior 15: 355–361

Trudel G, Laurin F 1988 The effects of bibliotherapy on orgasmic dysfunction and couple interactions: an experimental study. Sexual and Marital Therapy 3: 223–228

Wolfe J, Walen S 1982 Cognitive factors in sexual behavior. In: Grieger R, Grieger I (eds) Cognition and emotional disturbance. Human Sciences Press, New York

Zilbergeld B 1980 Men and sex. Fontana/Collins, Glasgow

Zilbergeld B, Ellison C R 1979 Social skills training as an adjunct in sex therapy. Journal of Sex and Marital Therapy 5: 340–350

Index